From passionate self-taught cook and nutritionist Radhi Devlukia-Shetty, *JoyFull* is abundant with more than 125 plant-based recipes. Wide-ranging and designed to honor the deep flavors and satisfying, healthful meals Radhi is known for, this inviting collection is for anyone who wants to feel good and eat well.

Radhi offers fuss-free recipes attuned to the rhythms of the day, such as Chai Oatmeal and Veggie Frittata Muffins for morning energy, and a beautiful balance of lighter and heartier dishes for later, such as the crowd-pleasing Mexican Lasagna, the Ultimate Veggie Lentil Soup, and easy Chilled Soba Noodle Salad. For comfort-food cravings, there are Cheesy Bread Two Ways and Spicy Bean Burgers, among dozens of other irresistible dishes—and, of course, there are sweet treats, too, ranging from simple Oatmeal Raisin Cookies to Chocolate Mud Pie.

And because food alone cannot sustain us completely, Radhi shares daily wellness practices: her revitalizing morning skincare routine, meditations for staying present, and breathwork that will carry you from dawn until night. A stunning go-to resource, *JoyFull* will show you how to connect to your best health inside and out.

JOYFULL

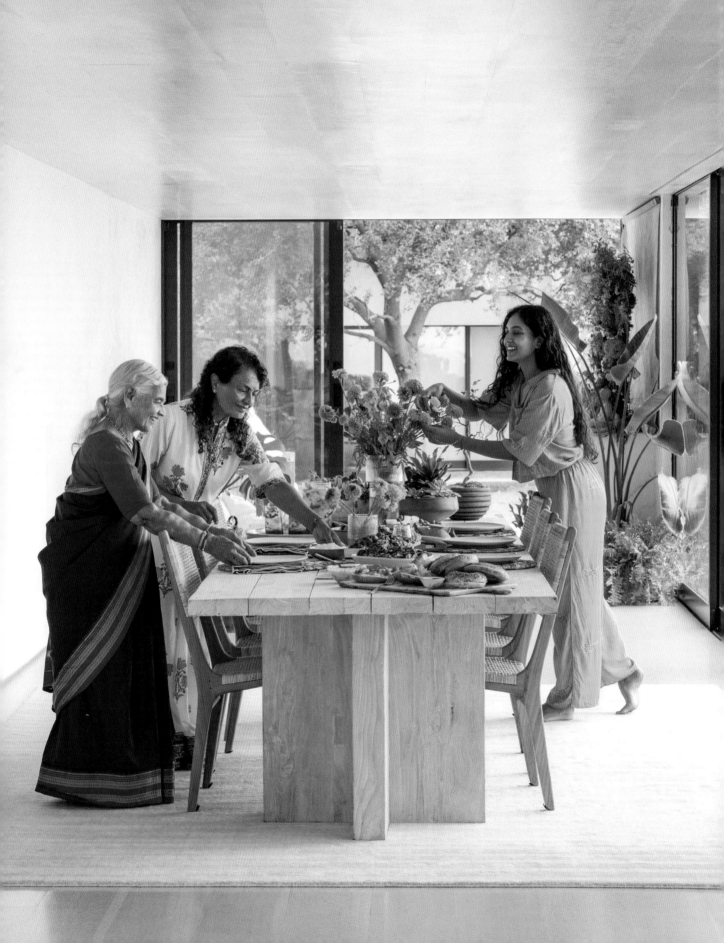

JOYFULL

COOK EFFORTLESSLY, EAT FREELY, LIVE RADIANTLY

RADHI DEVLUKIA-SHETTY

With Rachel Holtzman

PHOTOGRAPHY BY ALANNA HALE

SIMON ELEMENT

New York London Toronto Sydney New Delhi

SIMON ELEMENT

For information about special discounts for bulk purchases, please contact Simon & Schuster Special Sales at 1-866-506-1949 or business@simonandschuster.com.

The Simon & Schuster Speakers Bureau can bring authors to your live event. For more information or to book an event, contact the Simon & Schuster Speakers Bureau at 1-866-248-3049 or visit our website at www.simonspeakers.com.

Interior design by Laura Palese

Manufactured in China

1 3 5 7 9 10 8 6 4 2

Library of Congress Cataloging-in-Publication Data has been applied for.

ISBN 978-1-9821-9972-2

ISBN 978-1-9821-9973-9 (ebook)

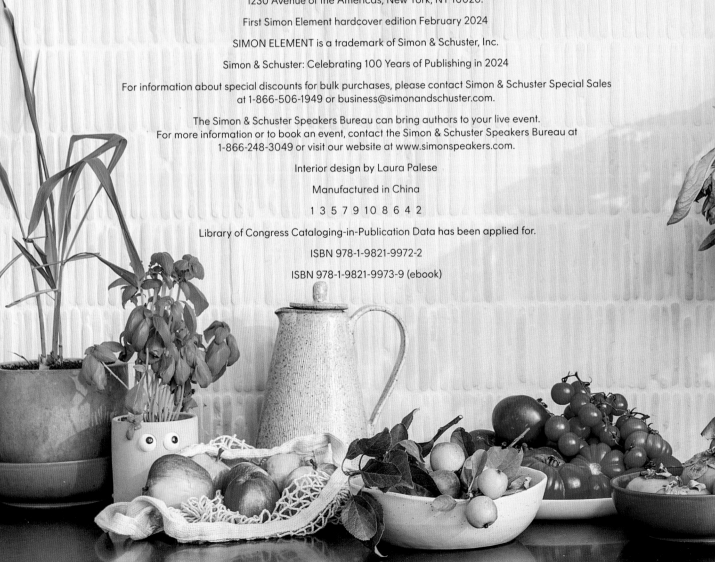

I DEDICATE THIS BOOK TO

My baa, whose unlimited love and prayers got me to where I am today

My mum, my first and best teacher in the kitchen, who showed
me daily what it truly means to cook with love

My dad, the best sous chef to ever exist and my constant cheerleader

My sister, who paved the way for us all toward conscious eating
and helped me to find my voice through writing

My husband, who through example has always been a beautiful reminder
to do everything with deeper meaning and purpose

My family and friends, who contributed to this book
through recipes, inspiration, and taste testing

And, most important,
My spiritual teacher, His Holiness Radhanath Swami,
for whom I first began creating recipes

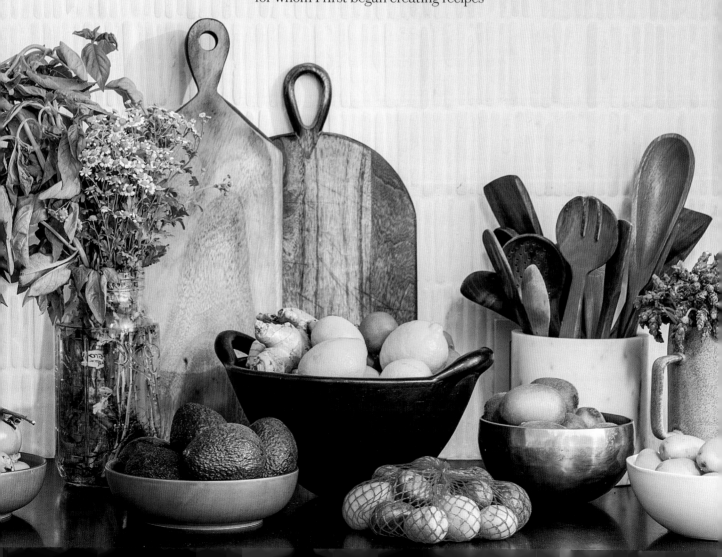

ACKNOWLEDGMENTS

Just as creating a beautiful, balanced, delicious dish requires all the right ingredients, equipment, and skills, this book would not have been as spectacular without its beautiful *JoyFull* community. This book was marked not only by these individuals' physical contributions but also by their spirit, which truly helped *JoyFull* live up to its name. A special thank-you to:

My writing collaborator, Rachel Holtzman, who has patiently spent days with me and fielded innumerable phone calls, emails, and edits to curate and share so eloquently what you have read in this book.

My wonderful, loving editor, Doris Cooper, who from day one had unwavering faith in my vision and dream and made all my outrageous requests a reality!

My publisher, Richard Rhorer, who brought calm amid any storms that came our way.

My photographer, Alanna Hale, who captured not just the food (in the juiciest way possible) but also the most magical memories and moments with my family that I will forever hold close to my heart.

Carrie Purcell, Nidia Cueva, Max Rappaport, Malina Syvoravong, Audryana Cruz, Rebecca Richard, and Tomo Kostygina, who brought life and vibrance to the recipes and made the three weeks of shooting so much fun!

Lysbett Valles, who had the tiresome job of making sure I met deadlines and got this book written, and who was also my confidante and creative partner, and an assertive voice when I couldn't find my own. She is a force to be reckoned with.

Kelsey Lapolla, who helped me to design my dream book cover and didn't stop until I got it.

The Simon & Schuster team—Elizabeth Breeden, Jessica Preeg, Patrick Sullivan, Kristina Juodenas, Katie McClimon, Allison Har-zvi, Jessie McNiel, Benjamin Holmes, and Ingrid Carabulea—who are like the spices and seasoning, enhancing a recipe in nuanced and powerful ways.

My literary agent, Pilar Queen, whose constant support and enthusiasm were so appreciated.

My sweet friend Aadil Abedi, who drew and designed the Holy Basil art on the cover of the book.

My brother-in-law, Sandeep, who kindly contributed some of his special recipes.

Every single person who has supported me through love, food, ideas, space, feedback, a shoulder to cry on, enthusiasm, and laughter during these two years. I thank you deeply.

CONTENTS

THE JOYFULL KITCHEN

*Hi! I'm so happy you're here! I thought
I would begin by sharing a bit about myself
and how I came to write this book.*

To be honest, I never, ever thought I would write one. Until now, I had always seen myself as a perpetual student. Maybe that identity allowed me to satisfy my deep desire to learn. Or maybe it was just a good way for me to avoid imposter syndrome (or subconsciously avoid adult responsibilities!). Whatever the reason, I was—and still am—a serial seeker. That curiosity has led me to great places: I earned a degree in nutrition and dietetics; I trained as a yoga teacher; and I spent years studying Ayurveda, an ancient, though incredibly relevant, approach to mind-body wellness that has completely changed my life. I experienced firsthand how powerful these teachings are. I saw how inviting sattvic or healing plant-based foods to my plate, gratitude to my mind, and love to my heart could bring me a deeper sense of contentment and vitality. I knew that I wanted to one day help others feel it themselves, but when it came to actually *being* the teacher, I wasn't sure these gifts were mine to share just yet. I still saw myself as the baby of the family who followed her big sister's every move (including switching from vegetarian to vegan after she read Jonathan Safran Foer's *Eating Animals*), never making decisions for herself (down to the cutlery set I bought for my first flat), and generally feeling unsure of what I really had to offer.

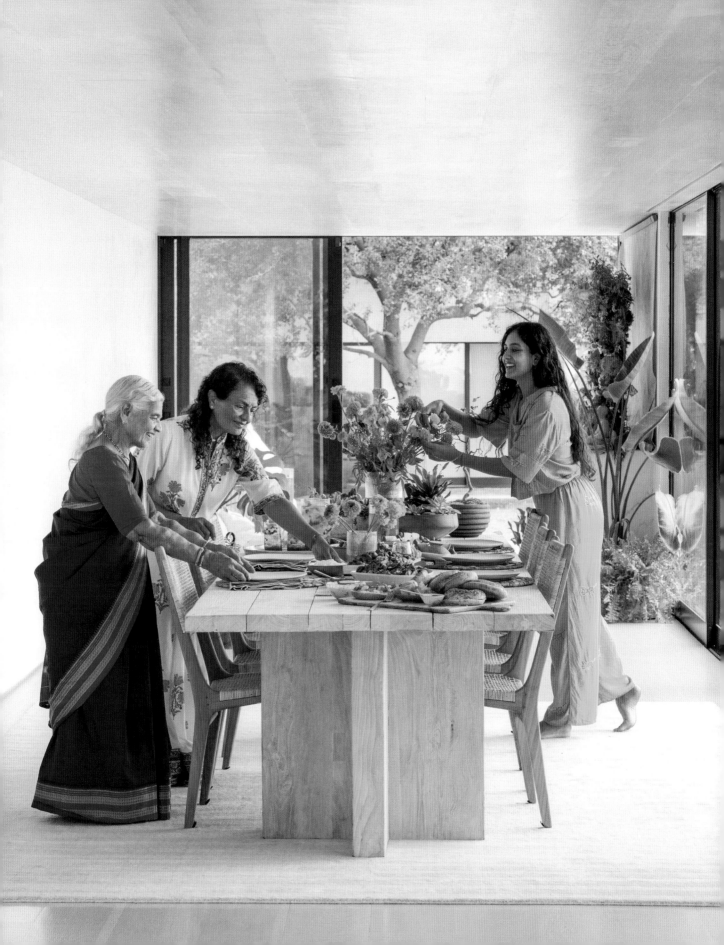

Then one day, my spiritual teacher, His Holiness Radhanath Swami, said this: "Knowledge is useless unless it is shared." It felt like he was telling me exactly what I needed to hear in that moment of my life. And when the Universe sends you that kind of message, you listen. In that instant, I knew what I needed to do: Stop searching for that next rabbit hole to immerse myself in (probably some sort of aromatherapy massage course) and instead find a way to put his advice into practice. I had finally realized that everything I had learned boiled down to this: **What you eat—along with your daily habits and the thoughts you think—has the ability to** *completely transform every aspect of your health.* And I wanted to be a vessel for that message.

Since that major aha moment six years ago, I've connected with a big, beautiful online community where I've shared plant-based recipes and Ayurveda-inspired wellness advice (plus some dance moves I was sure no one wanted to see!). Over the years, I've gotten to hear about all the ways that people have dramatically improved their sleep, naturally supercharged their energy, balanced their digestion, sharpened their focus, and felt lighter and brighter overall. I remember when I was once on a hike in LA, way up in the hills, and a woman seemingly miles below called out to me, "RADHI! I drink water the right way because of you!" (And so will you once you read this book!)

These experiences have taught me that even the smallest shift can have a big impact. Even if it's just one person I've reached, then it will have been worth it, because they, too, become a channel for that change, which then creates a beautiful chain reaction for us to elevate one another.

FROM ME TO YOU

The approach that I've taken to writing this book reflects what I'm doing every day in my own life. I combine science-based nutrition with ancient healing traditions, shake it up a bit so it doesn't take itself quite so seriously, and make room for the joy. It's a kind of mash-up that I credit for making meaningful change that much easier and sustainable. I call it "the playful and the profound."

It's an idea introduced to me by my husband, Jay, who says that our relationship works well because of our playful and profound dynamic. (I tend toward the playful while he leans toward the profound.) Of course, neither of us is serious or silly all the time, but I think it provides a lovely balance!

This same idea applies to cooking and wellness. Ultimately, my goal is to inspire you to get into the kitchen and just *play*. Every meal should feel easy and flexible. The recipes I've shared can be used as foundations, but you can also be guided and shaped by your intuition as you choose from an abundance of whole, plant-based foods and spices to suit exactly how you're feeling physically, emotionally, and spiritually in the moment. When you do, you will experience a deep satisfaction and fullness. Not in the sense of needing to change into stretchy pants, but rather full of gratitude, full of contentment, and full of what your body needs to live optimally. What could be more joyous than that?

WHY IT WORKS

There is a natural rhythm to everything—our body's cycles, the days, the seasons—and to live out of sync with them is to live in a constant state of friction and imbalance. That's a recipe for feeling run down, burned out, overwhelmed, or even sick. When you think about our fast-paced lives filled with on-demand access to just about anything, anytime, without any adjustment for day, night, spring, or summer—it's no wonder so many people suffer from poor digestion, disordered sleep, hormonal imbalance, aches and pains, and why they generally feel blah. **But if you can get back in sync, choose your meals with intention, and sprinkle in a few simple but well-timed habits throughout the day, you will begin to experience what balance feels like.**

In Ayurveda, it's believed that the combination of eating plant-based foods in harmony with the day's rhythm and enjoying them with gratitude and presence of mind creates what we call prana or "life force" in the body. And that promotes proper digestion, stronger immunity, less inflammation, vitality, hormonal stability, emotional steadiness, and complete spiritual ignition. All of this comes together to give you that special, radiant inner and outer glow, which in Ayurveda is referred to as ojas, the "essence of vitality."

Kind of makes you think about dinner a little differently, doesn't it?

BRINGING HOME THE JOY

In this book, you'll find some of my favorite recipes that I've collected and created over the years. They are just as much a reflection of my love for cooking as they are a product of my grandmothers' traditional Indian recipes, my mum's magic touch for blending different cuisines and flavors, my dad's opinions about how to make a recipe absolutely perfect (which is why he's my official taste tester), and my passion for infusing simple, seasonal ingredients with bright punches of flavor and *all* the saucy, creamy, crunchy condiments. They will satiate you at every meal and scratch the itch when cravings arise. No one said the road to enlightenment couldn't include a pit stop for breads and sweets!

And while we're nourishing your body with vibrant, plant-based dishes, we'll be working on getting you back into rhythm with nature. By embracing simple but powerful habits such as creating meals that balance all six essential tastes, eating with all your senses, practicing breathwork to help you transition through the phases of the day, and cooking and eating with gratitude and presence of mind, you'll be creating a strong foundation for health and vitality in body and spirit.

I hope this book sparks in you the same love for this conversation with nature that's brought so much of the good stuff to my life. And I hope it helps you take the next step (even if it's just a baby step!) toward nourishing yourself from the inside out. As with everything in life, the more you commit, the more benefit you will receive. It is, after all, the law of nature.

As you begin this new chapter, I'll leave you with this affirmation:

What I feed my mind, body, and soul becomes who I am, and I choose to be full of joy; I choose to be joyFULL.

With love and gratitude,

Radhi

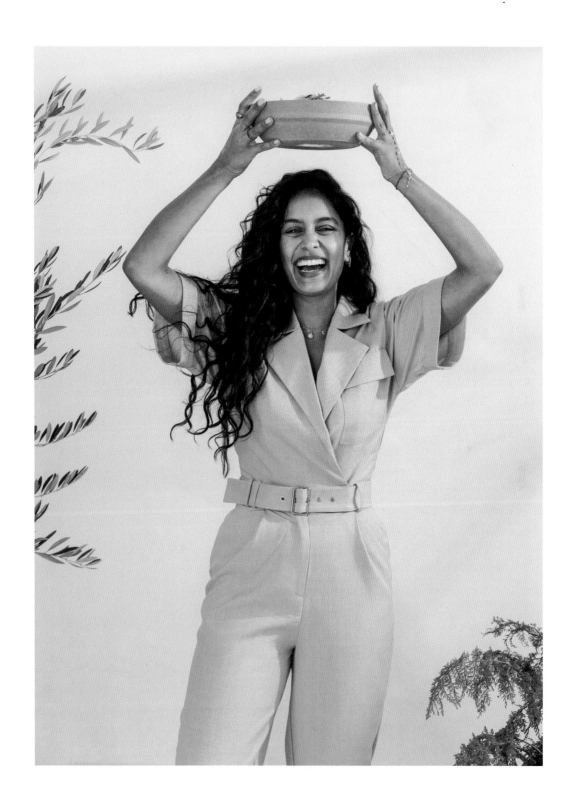

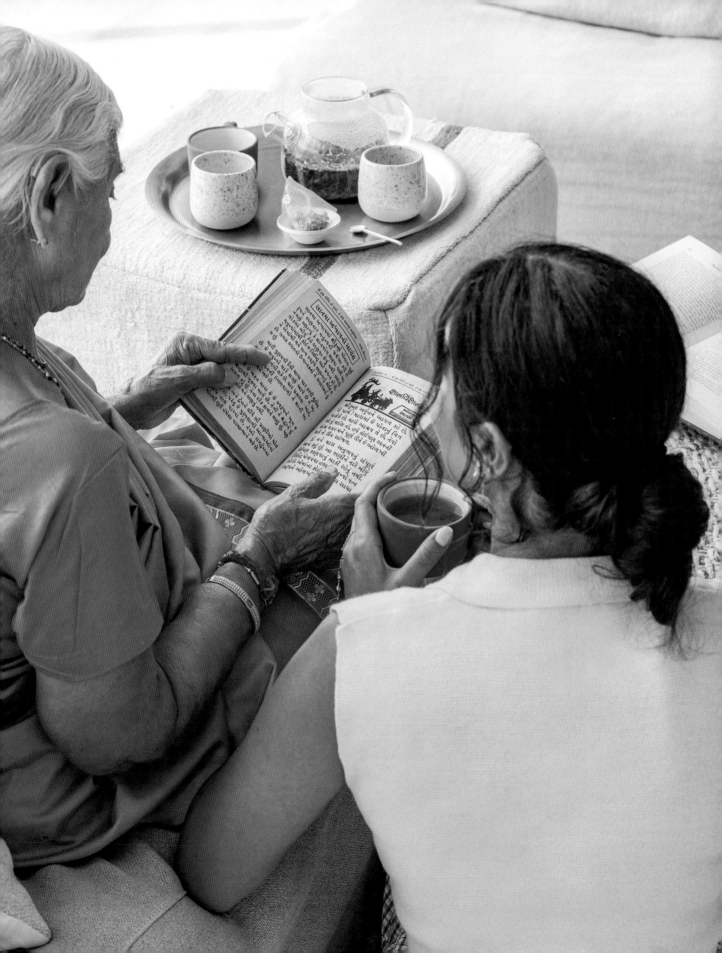

YOUR INVITATION TO

AYURVEDA

In Sanskrit, Ayurveda translates to "the science of life" (*ayur* is life, *veda* is knowledge). As a more-than-five-thousand-year-old discipline—the oldest health science to exist—we could spend years unpacking all the knowledge that Ayurveda has to offer. Instead, I want you to think of this book as a bridge providing the fundamental principles and lessons that will help you dig even deeper. What you're about to learn here is just the beautiful, and essential, beginning to your journey.

Some people refer to Ayurveda as "The Mother of Healing" because it teaches you how to create the ideal environment—internally and externally—for optimal health. Unlike most applications of Western medicine, which focuses on the cure, Ayurveda puts the emphasis on prevention—as in, how we can keep from getting ill in the first place? And by ill, I'm not necessarily talking about the biggies like heart disease, arthritis, or diabetes—though these are absolutely what we're looking to avoid—but we're also focusing on the smaller, more subtle irritations that take away from our everyday quality of life, like aches and pains, poor sleep, and sluggish digestion. Just as important, Ayurveda addresses more understated conditions that are often the initial signs of illness or imbalance in the body, such as dull skin, brittle hair, and low mood and energy. Because the outside of your body communicates what's happening on the inside of your body.

I fell in love with Ayurveda because of its key idea that we have the power not only to recognize our symptoms of imbalance before they build to something more damaging but also to treat them by creating subtle shifts in our routines, whether it's what we eat, how we move, or the habits we keep in our spiritual practices or our living space.

Ayurveda demonstrates how each of us has our own natural disposition, and because of that, your long-term recipe for health will look different from anyone else's. It's far from a one-size-fits-all prescription.

My guidelines and recipes are designed to help you tune in closely to what your body might be asking of you and what it needs to feel good and nourished. But instead of getting *too* caught up at this moment with what you "should" or "shouldn't" be eating based on your type or prakruti (as one's overall constitution is called in Ayurveda), or getting too bogged down in the many, many layers of philosophy behind these recommendations, I'd rather you first embrace more general practices, rooted in Ayurveda, that *everyone* benefits from. These are simply:

1. Eating more plants and spices
2. Living in rhythm with nature and your own body
3. Surrounding yourself with the energy, attitude, intention, and feelings with which you want to fill yourself

And that's pretty much it; easy-peasy, right? Okay, maybe not exactly a quick fix (nothing that really works is!)—but hey, when was the last time someone told you to eat delicious food in a deeply satisfying way as a prescription for feeling amazing?

Once you've started implementing the changes above, you'll be able to hear that voice saying *This is what I want* or *This is what I need*—and you'll know the difference between the two (and, yes, hopefully that voice is kind and sweet and doesn't sound like Darth Vader!). Trusting your instincts will empower you to be the authority on your own health. You will know what you need to tweak and fine-tune as you evolve.

ENJOY MORE PLANTS

When I was studying nutrition, I learned how food impacts the body, especially plants. They are the very best source of vitamins and minerals, and maintain and nourish our organs and tissues. They are rich in antioxidants, which protect our bodies from environmental stressors and cellular damage. They are full of fiber, which sweeps through our digestive system, clearing the body of toxins and promoting the internal movement on which our life force depends. Plant foods are all we need to deliver the necessary fuel—carbohydrates, fats, and proteins—that every physiological system (digestive, cardiovascular, neurological, immune, etc.) needs to work optimally.

Although I have a degree in nutrition, it is being a student of Ayurveda that has given me the most appreciation for how food affects not just your body but also your mindset, mood, and spirit. Ayurveda teaches that everything in the living world, including the food we eat, can be divided into one of three gunas, or modes:

SATTVA: the mode of goodness
RAJAS: the mode of passion
TAMAS: the mode of ignorance

At the bottom of the food chain, as it were, are tamasic foods. These are considered "low-vibration" foods and have the same vibration-lowering effect on you. Think deep-fried foods, foods that have sat for a long time in the fridge and are sapped of their original nutritional value, and food that involves suffering, such as food derived from animals. These foods require extra energy and effort to digest, and they don't lift your consciousness or your energy. As a result, they will often leave you lethargic, unmotivated, and *meh.* They are frequently at the root of many health issues.

Rajasic foods can give you energy, but often only fleetingly and with an aggressive edge. Think processed foods, sweets, and caffeine—things that stimulate you but only with

Trusting your instincts will empower you to be the leader when it comes to your own health.

a temporary burst, often followed by a crash in mood or energy. They feed the body at the expense of the mind and long-term health. Rajasic foods can also be plants that possess overstimulating, agitating qualities, such as onions, garlic, chiles, and coffee. That's why you won't find many of those ingredients in my recipes—but more on that in a moment.

And then there are sattvic foods. These are free of additives and preservatives and are typically plants in their whole, unprocessed form. Think whole grains, fresh fruit, nuts and seeds, and vegetables. They are easy to digest, elevate the happy hormones in your body (serotonin, dopamine, oxytocin, and endorphins) to lift your mood and help you feel balanced; and they raise your consciousness and your vibrations. It is believed that merely by enjoying more sattvic foods, you are nourishing your mind and making it more receptive to reflection, clarity, and wisdom. This is because sattvic foods produce what's called ojas. In Sanskrit, ojas translates to "vigor" or "essence of vitality," and is described as health, vitality, strength, longevity, immunity, and emotional well-being. It is an essential energy for the body and mind.

When we properly digest sattvic foods, we are creating a sort of ojas smoothie for the body that nourishes all seven layers of our tissues, including our plasma (rasa), blood (rakta), muscle (mamsa), fat (meda), bone marrow (majja), nerve tissue (asthi), and reproductive tissue (shukra). All that goodness squeezed from sattvic foods accumulates over time as a sort of life force, a nectar. When ojas is flowing, you feel grounded, balanced, and stable. Your digestion is robust; you don't pick up every cold and flu that comes around; you feel light and energized, and while you may sometimes feel tired, you're not exhausted or defeated. Your hair looks shiny and lush, your skin supple, and eyes white and bright. Ojas is nature's purest source of life force and energy.

That said, while eating sattvic foods is one powerful way to create more ojas in your life, if you're doing it in a way that is at odds with the flow of nature, then you're still going to feel that friction. So it's also important to live a sattvic *lifestyle*—one that honors and supports the 24-hour cycle of our bodies.

LIVE IN RHYTHM WITH THE DAY

Here's the main thing to understand when it comes to "eating and living in rhythm": Your body is just as much a product of nature as the sun and the moon. So it makes sense that our internal processes (waking, sleeping, digesting, moving, repairing) follow the same 24-hour tempo. Think about it: The sun rises and brings its light, heat, and radiant energy, which gradually builds and builds until it peaks at midday. After that, the light, the heat, and the energy begin to fade, making way for the moon to rise. As it does, the air cools and the energy shifts toward a slower, sleepier pace. Your body is built to be doing that exact same thing every single day, and our job is to follow its lead. You may have noticed that when you sleep in, you feel sluggish or tired for the rest of the day. Or that you get hungry when you've stayed up late into the night. Or that when you eat a late-night meal, you often wake up in the early hours of the morning with your mind racing. All of this makes complete sense once you understand this rhythm.

Ayurveda describes this 24-hour cycle using the three main doshas: pitta, vata, and kapha. While you may have heard these terms used in quizzes, such as "Which Dosha Are You?" (and it's true that these doshas can hold the key to better understanding your unique constitution), here we're using them to describe the different phases of the day. Understanding how each of these doshas "governs" certain times of the day-night cycle will give you insight into how you can better eat, move, and live in harmony with nature.

Think of the day as being divided into six equal pieces:

6 A.M. TO 10 A.M.: KAPHA

Kapha's elemental makeup is earth and water and is, by extension, stabilizing, solid, and strong. Waking up just before this period or in the very beginning of this window is optimal—closer to 6 a.m. than 10 a.m. Getting out of bed toward the middle or tail end of this phase can leave you with the "I just slept for 10 hours but still don't feel rested" feeling. It's often the best time to exercise because you can bring gentle stimulation to all your body's physiological systems and ease them out of the stagnation of being asleep. While your body isn't quite ready to accept its first proper meal of the day, you can prepare the digestive system with something light and easy to digest such as Spiced Stewed Apples (page 64) or a beverage such as CCF Detox Tea (page 49) or Masala Chai (page 46).

10 A.M. TO 2 P.M.: PITTA

Pitta is linked to fire; it is dynamic and action-oriented. Just as the fire of the sun is carving its way to its peak in the sky, so too is your digestive fire revving up. In Ayurveda, we really do use the term *agni* or "fire" to describe the furnace churning in your belly that converts food into the energy that fuels the body's engine. Just as this time of day is ideal for using that fire to metabolize bigger meals, it's also perfect for metabolizing your biggest thoughts and tackling your biggest tasks.

2 P.M. TO 6 P.M.: VATA

Vata is ruled by air and ether and governs the nervous system. Since this is the phase when the nervous system can be heightened, think about leaning into the vata qualities of creativity, movement, and flow as a way to balance and ground yourself. Think about creating a peaceful environment, shifting from the left-brained analytical work you did in the morning to softer, more imaginative and creative right-brained tasks, and partaking in activities that calm rather than excite or stimulate. This will serve you as you transition between the events of the day and the preparation for evening.

6 P.M. TO 10 P.M.: KAPHA

The sun setting brings a return to kapha in its slowest, most grounded form. Your digestive fire dwindles, which means meals during this time should be light and easy to digest (the reason why I particularly love soups for dinner). This is also the time to help your body wind down and transition to sleep. Getting into bed by the end of this phase is ideal for falling asleep more easily and getting the deepest, most restful sleep. Many people find that if they miss this window for bedtime, they get a second burst of energy that makes sleep difficult. (Which is not such a mystery once you see what happens during the next window!)

10 P.M. TO 2 A.M.: PITTA

Even though you are at rest during this time, your body's systems are kicking back into gear for their night shift. This is when your digestive system, circulatory system, and nervous system metabolize and process the day. They take out the trash by flushing unwanted toxins from the brain and the digestive tract, as well as rebuild and repair your cells. However, if you're awake during that time, or more significantly, digesting a meal during that time, it inhibits those processes from happening. Can you think back to a night when you went in for a late-night pizza and woke up feeling groggy and sluggish? When you're asking your body to take on too much work at night, your sleep will suffer.

2 A.M. TO 6 A.M.: VATA

Another transitional moment of the day as the sun prepares to rise and the body prepares to be awake. Just as the afternoon vata window is a time of creativity, this moment is one of receptivity to information, ideas, and energy. Many practitioners of Ayurveda believe the optimal time to wake and meditate is before sunrise or before the energy shifts from moon to sun.

The goal here is to simply allow yourself to feel the qualities of these moments in the day—the lightness of vata as your body first stirs and takes in the sun's early rays, the urgency of pitta powering the afternoon's big wave of energy, the heaviness of kapha as you turn down the lights and bury yourself in the blankets with a book. If you are like most people (including me before I began my own healing journey), this will take some getting used to. We're so accustomed to living our lives against these currents that we don't often experience them. But the more you participate in these ebbs and flows and support them with the meals you eat, the practices you choose, and the thoughts you think (aka following the advice shared in this book!), the more in alignment you will become.

While every day may not look just like this, what will naturally happen over time is that you'll realize how much better you feel when it does. If you want more restful sleep, or you want more energy in the morning, or you want better concentration in the afternoon, the solution isn't to hyperfocus your efforts on that time of day. Instead, when you're supporting *all* of the shifts throughout the day, the benefits are cumulative.

THE RECIPES FOLLOW THE CYCLE OF THE DAY

To help you get and stay in rhythm, I've organized the chapters to reflect which meals you'd reach for at certain times of day. Recipes early in the book (drinks, breakfast) are perfect for lighter morning meals, while recipes in the middle of the book (pasta, lentils, breads, salads, main dishes) are better suited for midday, when your digestion is more robust. Toward the end of the book (soups), we're returning to lighter dishes that suit a body preparing for rest (although these dishes would be just as appropriate earlier in the day, too).

When choosing a recipe, ask yourself: *What does my body need right now? What is it truly hungry for? What sounds delicious to meet that need?* Honor the voice that responds.

Another part of this tuning-in process is **Living with the Sun and Moon**. Each of these bodies has its own powerful vibrations. Thinking about their qualities and the time of day when they "rule" as you consider what nourishment your body needs helps you to live in vibration with them. For example:

Sun vs. Moon

Energizing vs. Calming

Heating vs. Cooling

Activating vs. Relaxing

Strength vs. Flow

Creation vs. Preservation

Activating vs. Surrender

For both men and women: Masculine (active, doing) vs. Feminine (processing emotions, soothing, nurturing)

BRING INTENTION INTO THE MIX

Practitioners of Ayurveda believe that the energy, attitude, intention, and feelings you have while cooking are infused into the food—which is then absorbed and digested into the person receiving it. That's why one of my very favorite things to do is feed people when they come to my home. I love putting thought into what nourishing, delicious meal I can prepare for them, and then actively reflecting on and praying for their well-being as I cook. And what's amazing is that my guests often tell me that they can actually sense that.

It may sound woo-woo, but the thoughts you think and the intention you bring to the simplest acts, including preparing your food, are powerful. That means that cooking with love, devotion, gratitude, and kind energy is just as healing—for both body and mind—as the food itself. In Ayurveda, we call this Prashad. I often describe it as food cooked with devotion, sealed with a prayer, and served with love. In your everyday life, you can think of it as **conscious cooking**. Conscious cooking is just what it sounds like: cooking with your mind turned *on*. It is not throwing together ingredients as you rush to get to work or zone out to your favorite show (although there is definitely a time and place for that). It is a simple daily practice that elevates the humblest meals, and here are a few ways to do it.

- Envision the meal you are going to prepare, the people you will feed, and how it will nourish them—even if it's just yourself.

- Cook without distraction so you can focus your energy on the food and the act of preparing it.

- Imagine how this food will give your body the energy to do good in the world through whatever unique skills you have.

- Speak affirming words, listen to a meditation or uplifting songs, or even sing to your food as you prepare it! It may sound silly, but scientists have compared the effects of music and words on water molecules and found that soothing words and music create lovely, snowflake-like structures, while angry words and music create more of a chaotic, disjointed formation. If words and music have the power to do that to water, imagine what they can create in your body, which is 70 percent water!

- Offer gratitude for these ingredients and this moment of being alive on the planet, whether it's to God or the Universe. For me, this is a key part of my consciousness-raising practice.

CONSCIOUS EATING

Equally as important as cooking with intention is *eating* with intention—or **conscious eating**. And just as preparing food mindfully and joyfully translates into a more nourishing meal, so does receiving it mindfully and joyfully.

The craziest thing—and the most beautiful—is that when I started eating food more mindfully and presently, whether it was with my mum, in the temple I visited regularly, or at the tables of the teachers and practitioners of this philosophy, I could feel a shift. It wasn't only in my body but in my consciousness, too. It felt purifying, uplifting, and spiritually enhancing.

Think of it as the exchange of a gift—when someone gives you a gift and you accept it with heartfelt gratitude, it is an energetically complete experience. Similarly, when you take a moment to be quiet and present with your food, express gratitude for it, put down your utensils between bites, and savor the individual flavors as you slowly chew, that creates a more positive, healing, uplifting experience.

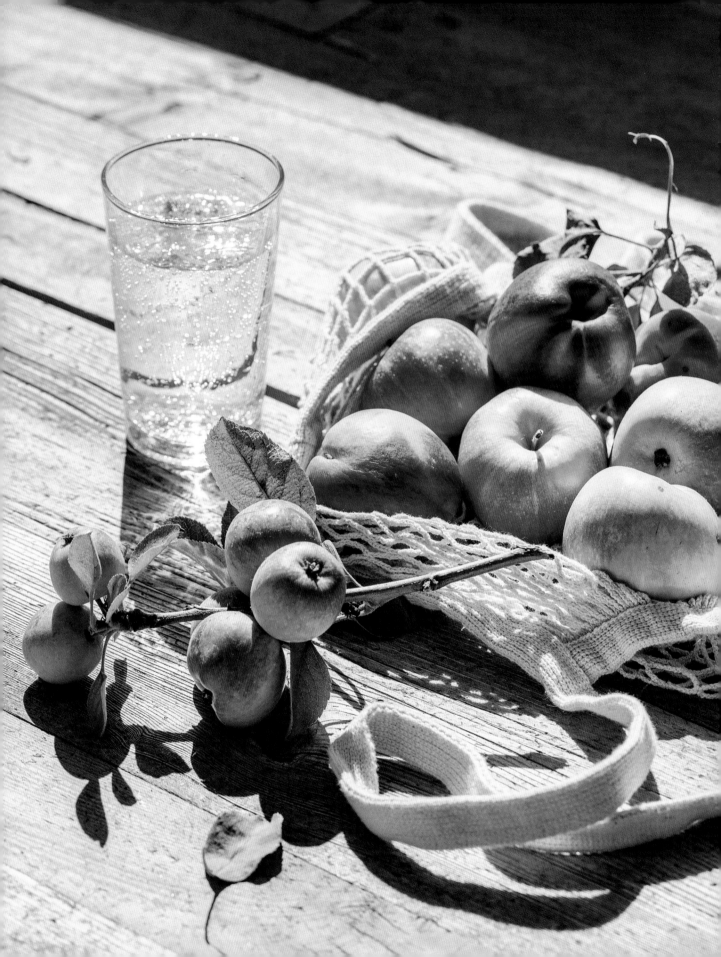

EASING IN

In this book you'll find all the tools you need to live a *Joyfull* life, from creating plant-based meals that support living in rhythm with nature, to harnessing the power of spices, to balancing the types of flavors on your plate (both for more pleasurable eating *and* more efficient digestion), to cooking with intention, to eating mindfully and with all your senses, to breathwork and rituals to transition you through the day. The foundation of the book, however, is the recipes. They are designed to maintain balance, health, and satisfaction—in addition to being very, very delicious.

> Here you'll find the information that will be most *valuable* at the start of your journey.

Instead of packing every single useful tidbit here in this chapter, I've broken things up a bit. Here you'll find the information that will be most valuable at the start of your journey. Throughout the book, I've tucked more lessons and insights so you can build and layer your practices at your own pace. Incorporate new habits as it suits—one day at a time or maybe just one meal at a time. Be curious, explore, and let go of any pressure to do more.

To help you make sense of all this new (but very old) information, here is what I'd like you to know:

YOU'RE GOING TO GET EVERYTHING YOU NEED

People who are transitioning to a plant-based diet are sometimes concerned that they're going to miss out on certain nutrients by not eating animal foods. But you can get *everything you need* from eating a variety of plants—and without the discomfort- and disease-causing qualities of tamasic and rajasic animal foods. Plant foods satisfy all your nutritional needs and provide the robust benefits shown in the following chart:

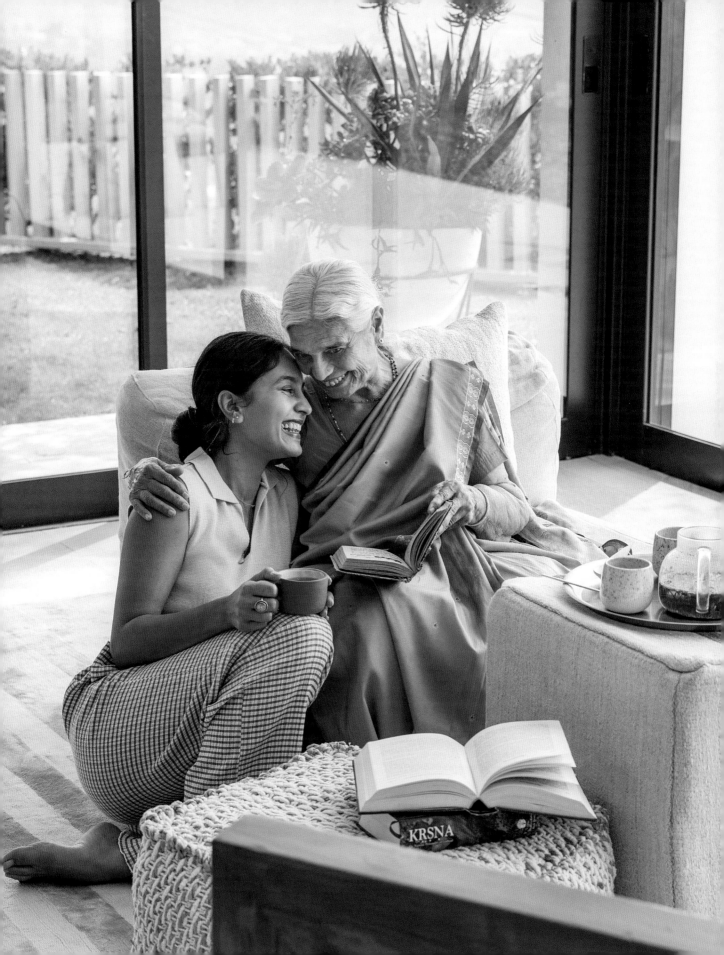

Nutrient	Benefits	Sources
MACRONUTRIENTS		
Protein	• Supports immune function, muscle contractions and movements, and the growth and maintenance of cells • Makes essential hormones and enzymes • Assists in the growth and maintenance of muscle	• Beans • Buckwheat • Edamame • Lentils • Nuts and nut butters • Quinoa • Seeds and seed butters • Tempeh • Tofu • Whole grains
Healthy Fats	• Protect your organs • Provide energy • Regulate cholesterol and blood pressure • Support cell growth • Help the body absorb vital nutrients (especially vitamins A, D, and E) • Great source of vitamin E, which is important for vision, brain health, and skin	• Avocado • Coconut • Extra-virgin olive oil • Nuts • Seeds
Carbs	• Are the body's primary source of energy • Essential for the functioning of the central nervous system, kidneys, brain, and muscles (including the heart) • Provide fiber, which is necessary for optimal intestinal health and digestion	• Beans • Fruits and vegetables • Lentils • Whole grains and whole-grain foods
MICRONUTRIENTS		
MINERALS		
Zinc	• Required for the creation of DNA, growth of cells, building proteins, healing damaged tissue, and supporting a healthy immune system • Aids wound healing and your sense of taste and smell	• Beans • Lentils • Nuts (especially walnuts and cashews) • Quinoa • Seeds (especially chia, hemp, pumpkin, and ground flaxseed) • Tofu • Whole grains and whole-grain foods
Calcium	• Necessary for healthy bones and teeth • Plays a role in blood clotting, muscle contractions, regulating a normal heart rhythm, and nerve function	• Blackberries • Broccoli • Dark leafy greens (especially bok choy, kale, mustard greens, turnip greens, and watercress) • Figs • Fortified plant milks and juices • Nuts and seeds • Oranges • Soy products (soybeans, tofu, soy milk)

Nutrient	Benefits	Sources
Iron	• Used for making hemoglobin, a protein in red blood cells that carries oxygen from the lungs to all parts of the body • Necessary ingredient for myoglobin, a protein that provides oxygen to the muscles • Used to make some hormones	• Beans • Cashews • Flaxseed • Fortified cereal • Kale • Lentils • Quinoa • Raisins • Spinach • Tofu
Selenium	• Helps make DNA and protects against cell damage and infections • Essential for the production of the thyroid hormones that regulate hair growth	• Beans • Brazil nuts • Soy products (soybeans, tofu, soy milk) • Whole grains
Magnesium	• Supports muscle and nerve function, and energy production • Regulates blood sugar levels and blood pressure • Necessary for the building of proteins, bones, and DNA	• Spinach • Whole grains and whole-grain foods • Nuts • Seeds and seed butters • Beans • Lentils • Soy products (soybeans, tofu, soy milk) • Molasses • Cocoa powder
Potassium	• Helps maintain normal levels of fluid inside the cells	• Adzuki beans • Apricots • Avocado • Broccoli • Figs • Hemp seeds • Pistachios • Potatoes • Pumpkin seeds • Seaweed • Soybeans and tofu • Spinach • Squash • Tempeh
Iodine	• Produces the thyroid hormones thyroxine and triiodothyronine, which assist with the creation of proteins and enzyme activity, as well as regulating the metabolism	• Cranberries and cranberry juice • Lima beans • Navy beans • Potatoes (skin on) • Seaweed • Strawberries

Nutrient	Benefits	Sources
VITAMINS		
Vitamin A (carotenoids)	• Carotenoids are pigments that give yellow, orange, and red fruits their color. Your body is able to convert some carotenoids into vitamin A, which supports energy production, as well as healthy hair, skin, nails, and eyes.	• Butternut squash • Carrots • Pumpkins • Spinach • Sweet potatoes
Vitamin B_1 (thiamine)	• Helps cells convert food into energy • Contributes to the metabolizing of fats and proteins	• Asparagus • Beans • Green peas • Seeds • Squash
Vitamin B_2 (riboflavin)	• Protects cells from damage and reduces inflammation of the nerves • Helps to break down fats, proteins, and carbohydrates • Encourages the absorption of iron	• Artichokes • Avocados • Currants • Molasses • Mushrooms • Nuts
Vitamin B_3 (niacin)	• Converts food into energy • Keeps the nervous system, digestive system, and skin healthy • Required for the production of stress and sex hormones • Reduces inflammation	• Beets • Buckwheat • Chili powder • Peanuts • Seitan • Yeast
Vitamin B_5 (pantothenic acid)	• Helps break down fats and carbohydrates into energy • Critical to the production of red blood cells and sex and stress-related hormones made by the adrenal glands • Aids in absorption of other vitamins • Important for maintaining a healthy digestive tract	• Broccoli • Split peas • Sunflower seeds • Sweet potatoes • Tahini • Yeast
Vitamin B_6	• Aids detoxification, cognitive function, and prevents anemia	• Soy products (soybeans, tofu, soy milk) • Bananas • Figs • Watermelon • Peanut butter
Vitamin B_7	• Assists with energy production, blood sugar regulation, and metabolism	• Almonds • Chia seeds • Oats • Peanuts • Sweet potatoes

Nutrient	Benefits	Sources
Vitamin B$_9$	• Important for brain development and red blood cell health	• Beans • Lentils • Lettuce • Spinach • Tomatoes
Vitamin B$_{12}$	• Supports nerve and blood cell health as well as DNA creation	• B$_{12}$ supplements (sometimes necessary for vegans *and* non-vegans, as it's more difficult to come by in non-fortified food sources) • Fortified cereal • Fortified vegan milk and yogurt • Nutritional yeast
Vitamin C	• Aids iron absorption • Protects against free radicals (unstable molecules made during normal cell metabolism that can cause damage to DNA and proteins)	• Broccoli • Oranges • Peppers • Strawberries • Tomatoes
Vitamin D	• Enhances calcium absorption • Contributes to healthy bones, teeth, and muscles	• Fortified cereals • Fortified plant-based milks • Mushrooms • Sunshine • Vitamin D supplements (sometimes necessary for vegans *and* non-vegans)
Vitamin E	• Protects against free radicals • Supports eye health • Strengthens the immune system	• Almonds • Hazelnuts • Peanuts • Sunflower oil • Sunflower seeds
Vitamin K	• Encourages healthy blood clotting and wound healing	• Brussels sprouts • Green beans • Kale • Spinach • Swiss chard
ADDITIONAL		
Omega-3 fatty acids	• Regulate hormones • Encourage healthy blood clotting • Support brain health and memory, menstrual health, skin and sleep	• Algae (especially spirulina and chlorella—where fish get their omega-3s from!) • Avocado • Chia and flaxseeds • Hemp seeds • Soy products (soybeans, tofu, soy milk) • Walnuts

But Will I Get Enough Protein?

This is quite possibly the most common question vegans are asked. To be honest, that was my concern, too, when I transitioned from being a vegetarian to a vegan. Luckily, there are numerous studies that offer peace of mind. In 2013, the *Journal of the Academy of Nutrition and Dietetics* published the largest study to date that compared the protein intake of 71,000 vegans, vegetarians, and nonvegetarians. On average, the vegans and vegetarians actually *exceeded* their protein needs by 70 percent. If you are eating an assortment of plants throughout the week, you will get the nutrition you need.

WHAT ABOUT "COMPLETE" PROTEINS?

I've often heard people argue that animal proteins, unlike those from plants, provide what's sometimes called a "complete" protein, meaning you're getting all nine essential amino acids (compounds essential to the body's biological processes, such as transporting nutrients and healing cells, and nourishing hair, skin, and nails) in one place. The truth is, so long as you're getting all nine essential amino acids, it doesn't matter whether they come from a single food source or multiple. I like to make the point that even if you are eating a complete protein (such as tofu), it gets broken down into amino acids anyway, so you might as well get them with a side of antioxidants, phytonutrients, and fiber (versus the inflammation, hormone disruption, calcium malabsorption, and heart disease and cancer risk you'd get from animal foods). Ultimately, if you eat animals, you're only getting as much nutrition as that animal gets through the plants they eat—so why not go immediately to the source and get your protein from plants themselves?!

WHAT IF I'M STILL CONCERNED?

First, I'll give you an example of a protein-filled meal: 1 cup cooked oatmeal has 6 grams of protein. Swirl in 1 tablespoon peanut butter (4 grams of protein) and a ½ cup soy or nut milk (4 grams of protein) and you have 14 grams just from breakfast—about 30 percent of the average person's daily requirement. In addition to looking at the total amount of protein you're eating, you can also make a point of eating "complementary" combinations of foods to get a full set of essential amino acids. Primary among these is the combination of beans and legumes plus grains, as well as nuts and seeds. It's not a coincidence that many of the recipes in this book feature these ingredients together!

Last, it's important to point out that your body's preferred source of energy is actually not protein—it's carbohydrates! They're the fuel that the body requires—especially your brain and muscles.

YOU'RE NOW LIVING THAT NONG (NO ONION, NO GARLIC) LIFE (BUT YOU WON'T MISS THEM, I *SWEAR*!)

You'll notice that none of the recipes in this book calls for onion or garlic. I know that may come as a shock, and yes, used in small quantities, these plants do have health benefits. But they have become so pervasive in our food that it adds up to a lot. All foods carry energetic properties, and for onion and garlic, those properties can be overly stimulating. In Ayurveda, onion is considered tamasic, meaning when it's eaten in large quantities, it can cause irritability and agitation. Garlic, on the other hand, is considered rajasic, meaning it can be heating, energy-draining, and sleep-disturbing. Plus, they're both members of the nightshade family and are inflammatory when eaten regularly. (See A Note About Nightshades, page 36.)

When I was starting my spiritual journey, I wanted to create the quietest, most peaceful internal environment to support my new yogic and meditative practices, so I altered my cooking accordingly. That's saying a lot, considering I used to *love* a good super-garlicky pasta! (You know—the ones that you can smell coming out of your pores for days afterward . . .) When I'm eating outside the house or ordering in I do occasionally partake, but I promise you that the meals you will create from this book are far from bland because you will become an expert in layering spices.

People can't believe it when I tell them after their meal that it was onion- and garlic-free, and I think it's because of my use of spices, including one in particular that mimics this savory flavor profile. Asafoetida (aka hing) is a pungent spice made from a variety of giant fennel, where the sap is extracted and the root is dried to make a vibrant yellow-colored resin. Once it's cooked, it comes "alive"—the aroma changes and creates a beautifully savory substitute for onion and garlic. You can find it in Indian markets as well as online; just be sure to purchase a pure form that hasn't been diluted with other ingredients such as rice flour, since that can also dilute the flavor (and will affect how these recipes turn out). Also, one gentle warning: Just as onion makes you cry with its pungent essence, asafoetida is extremely strong-smelling and can take a little getting used to. Be sure to store it in a tightly sealed container!

THERE IS NO SUCH THING AS "WINNING" AYURVEDA

Start slow and be gentle with yourself. Don't feel that you need to follow every single recommendation in this book at once! Simply following a plant-based diet and adopting some of the mindful rituals in this book is a powerful shift. Then, see if you can challenge yourself to focus on one or two new practices a day, depending on what feels significant to you at that moment. Maybe it's saying a few words of gratitude before your meals, then putting your utensils down between bites, or committing to turning off the television and phone during mealtimes. **This book is not meant to be a checklist**, and it's certainly not meant to stress you out. What's most important is *consistency*. Start slow, be gentle with yourself, and remember that what may feel slightly uncomfortable or unnatural now will eventually deliver substantial benefits. And once you experience those benefits, I assure you that many more of these practices will easily become part of your everyday life.

I'M ABOUT TO SPICE UP YOUR LIFE

Coming from an Indian family, I feel like I've known since birth how incredible spices and herbs are when it comes to creating bold, flavorful meals. But now that I understand their natural healing properties, I turn to my spice box as my medicine cabinet. Spices possess the power to lower your stress hormones, reduce inflammation, regulate blood sugar, keep you feeling more grounded, flush toxins from your body, improve digestion, and alleviate discomfort. They are your secret weapon to feeling happy and healthy. Spices are easy to use, even if they are not called for in a recipe: Sprinkle them on food, steep them in water for tea, stir them into coffee, blend them into smoothies, fold them into baked goods—there's no wrong way to enjoy them! See the appendix for a detailed chart of all the herbs and spices available to you, their benefits, and the best ways to use them.

Just remember that spices have more prana or vital life force, and therefore more medicinal potency as well as flavor, when freshly ground. You can grind them with a coffee grinder or mortar and pestle. And, as you'll see in the table below, the spices' flavors are released and medicinal properties activated when you cook them in fat before eating them.

BUILD MEALS WITH THE SIX TASTES IN MIND

In Ayurveda, we believe that there are six essential tastes, and to enjoy them in harmony not only creates more balanced meals but also recalibrates our body, mind, and spirit.

When each of the six tastes, or flavors, are combined on your plate, your meals will become even more deeply satisfying. This is in part because all your different taste buds are being stimulated. But on a much deeper level, these tastes have different effects on your physiology. Sweet is grounding, sour awakens digestion, salty aids the absorption of minerals, pungent improves circulation, bitter is detoxifying, and astringent clears the mind. The key is maintaining a balance between these tastes, which in turn preserves balance in the body. My recipes include these tastes in some combination (namely so you don't even have to think about it!), and whatever doesn't appear on your plate can easily be added through herbs and spices (see the chart on pages 280–83).

The six tastes are:

1. **SWEET:** Fruits, sweet vegetables such as pumpkin and sweet potato, grains, natural sugars, and nut milks, as well as spices such as cinnamon, cardamom, and coriander
2. **SOUR:** Sour fruits (lemons, limes, tamarind), yogurt, and other fermented ingredients
3. **SALTY:** Seaweed, celery, black olives, tamari, soy sauce, and salt in all forms
4. **ASTRINGENT:** Beans, pulses/legumes, some raw fruits (persimmon, fresh cranberries, pomegranate, green grapes, citrus zest, unripe bananas), alfalfa sprouts, okra, turmeric, and green and black tea
5. **BITTER:** Dark leafy greens, arugula, eggplant, sesame seeds, some fresh herbs (such as parsley, thyme, dill), and some spices (such as fenugreek, turmeric, and cloves)
6. **PUNGENT:** Chiles, garlic, ginger, asafoetida, mustard greens, spinach, spelt, and buckwheat, plus some spices (such as black pepper, mustard seeds, paprika, cayenne) and herbs (such as oregano, rosemary, and sage)

A Note About Nightshades

There's a group of plants called "nightshades" that, according to Ayurveda, are not recommended as part of your regular diet. These include eggplants, tomatoes, peppers, and potatoes, and the thinking is that these foods are rajasic, or overstimulating, overheating, and inflammatory—similar to garlic and onion. However, I've included recipes with these ingredients because I see the vitamin- and nutrient-filled merits of eating them—plus I love them so much that I'm not quite ready to let them go! So while it is not my personal rule to avoid these foods, I do recommend eating them in moderation and monitoring how you feel after you do so.

HYDRATE, HYDRATE, HYDRATE

Nature shows us what happens when living beings don't get enough water—just look at how plants start whimpering and wilting on a hot, dry day. That same thing happens to people who don't drink enough water. Water delivers nutrients throughout the body and promotes growth and lubrication. That translates to much-needed support for your brain, kidney, liver, and other organs, your digestion, your joints—all the essentials—not to mention glowing skin and bouncy hair. So, to keep things nice and supple, you have to hydrate. The recipes in Liquid Love (page 45) are meant to make this a little bit more exciting.

One thing to note: Be sure to drink the majority of your fluids between meals, not with your meals. Drinking water with meals dilutes the acid that is breaking down your food, and so it takes longer to digest it.

PLAY WITH YOUR FOOD

While these recipes will satisfy every single time if you make them as written, know that they are flexible and can be tailored to your preferences and the contents of your fridge or pantry. After all, following your intuition is the foundation of conscious cooking. I also never want you to feel like you won't reap the benefits of these dishes or that they won't be maximally delicious if you want or need to improvise—that's life! Mix and match the veggies, layer in or remove a spice, swap in (or add!) a different sauce or condiment. To help you loosen up a bit in the kitchen, here are some universal substitutions that will work in every recipe here. I also highly recommend getting inspired by Crunchy Bits (page 111) and Drizzles and Dollops (page 111).

These are all interchangeable:

- Cashews and sunflower seeds
- All unsweetened vegan milks
- All nut and seed butters (the flavor may change slightly)
- Garlic and asafoetida
- Dried and fresh herbs
- Dried and fresh curry leaves
- Ground cumin and cumin seeds

- Ground CCF Masala (page 49) and garam masala
- Coconut sugar and jaggery
- Maple syrup and agave
- Liquid aminos and soy sauce or tamari
- Cornstarch and tapioca starch
- Plain bread crumbs and almond flour
- Coconut milk and vegan cream

LOVE YOUR LEFTOVERS

In the same spirit of being playful and flexible in the kitchen, give yourself permission to reinvent your leftovers as brand-new meals. Think outside the bowl!

- Toss them with grains
- Heap them over greens
- Stuff them into a sandwich
- Scoop them onto naan, tortilla, or flatbread
- Puree them into a soup (you'd be amazed how well this works with the dishes in the Hero Veg chapter!)
- Reheat and enjoy with a simple salad on the side

The same goes for leftover ingredients. Sometimes you may find yourself with a stray cup or two of cooked noodles, grains, beans, lentils, canned tomatoes, a handful of chopped vegetables, and so on. You've pretty much just gifted yourself your next meal or two! These foundational ingredients will keep in your fridge for about 3 days and can be used in all sorts of delicious ways that are not difficult to prepare (even if you're a cooking newbie, I promise!). Here are some of my favorite go-tos, which you can dress up with your favorite spices (see Appendix: Spice Up Your Life), Crunchy Bits (page 111), and Condiments (page 231).

- Mix them into a stir-fry.
- Simmer veggies and canned tomatoes into a soup. Make it extra hearty by stirring in grains, beans, lentils, or pasta.
- Toss them in a blender with some olive oil and spices for a dip.
- Fold them into a tofu scramble.
- Sprinkle them over greens for a salad.
- Add a scoop of dip or vegan mayo to lentils or beans for a sandwich-stuffer.

HERE ARE A FEW OF MY FAVORITE THINGS

If you're new to buying plant-based products or would like some guidance on which pantry and fridge staples to choose, here's a list of some of my favorite items. You will most likely be able to find them at your grocery store or a natural foods store.

- **BUTTER:** Miyoko's Creamery
- **YOGURT:** Kite Hill (in the UK: Nush or Alpro plain)
- **SOUR CREAM:** Kite Hill
- **MILK:** Oatly or Minor Figures for thick, creamy oat milk; Califia Farms for almond
- **COCONUT MILK:** Thai Kitchen or Native Forest (in the UK: Biona or Natco)
- **MAYO:** Follow Your Heart Vegenaise (in the UK: Hellmann's Vegan Mayo)
- **MOZZARELLA (THAT MELTS!):** Miyoko's Creamery (in the UK: Julienne Bruno, MozzaRisella, and Sheese)
- **SHREDDED CHEESE:** Violife or Follow Your Heart (in the UK: Cathedral City)
- **CREAM CHEESE AND RICOTTA:** Kite Hill (in the UK: Julienne Bruno and Crematta)
- **GARLIC- AND ONION-FREE TACO SEASONING:** Fody

AND SPEAKING OF KITCHEN NECESSITIES . . .

I've made a point of not requiring fancy gadgets or tools to make these recipes—mostly because I don't use them myself! But if there is one item to invest in, it's a high-powered blender. It is the secret to creamy sauces, soups, purees, and dressings and will save you the heartache of throwing all your lovingly chopped ingredients into a standard blender only to realize that it's not up to the task. Plus, it will last you half a lifetime.

Close second and third appliances would be a food processor and an electric pressure cooker for making quicker and easier work of your prep and cooking, but they are by no means required to make the recipes in this book. Other kitchen staples for me include:

- Chef's knife
- Mandoline
- Cutting board
- Measuring cups and spoons
- Mixing bowls (large, medium, small)

- Silicone or rubber spatula
- Cast-iron skillet
- Rolling pin (whichever type you like)
- Fine-mesh sieve
- Colander

PRACTICE KITCHEN SELF-CARE

While many of these recipes can be made in under 30 minutes, there are many shortcuts you can take that will save you time while also allowing you to focus on eating delicious food rather than on the effort it took to make it. Give your future self the gift of cooked grains and legumes, a couple sauces or dressings stored in the fridge, and, if you have a little extra time in the evening or on the weekend, various components of dishes that can be prepped ahead. At the very least, give all your produce a rinse and a pat dry before putting it away so you don't need to do it come mealtime.

LAST BUT NOT LEAST: CHOOSING A PLANT-BASED LIFESTYLE IS A PERSONAL CHOICE, AND THERE IS NO RIGHT OR WRONG REASON TO DO SO

My own journey from vegetarian to vegan started after I read Jonathan Safran Foer's *Eating Animals*, and I could never unlearn what he described. I realized I could no longer justify eating another sentient being or causing suffering just to satisfy my taste buds or fashion sense. But that was my journey and my truth. This is not a space for judgment or guilt; my goal is simply to share information and my perspective. If you're going down this path because you want your skin to look better and you're tired of getting blemishes when you eat dairy, that's great! You don't necessarily need to be doing it (for now) because you care too much about the animals, and it doesn't have to be an all-out mission to save the world. But what I think you'll find is that as you raise your consciousness, and as you remove suffering from your personal food sources, the more connected to the world you'll become.

9 Tips for Living Joyfully

1. COOK AND EAT WITH LOVE

Remember to infuse your meals with the energy that you want your body to receive. Think positive thoughts, talk or sing to your food (I said it once and I'll say it again—it's silly, but it works!), picture each element of a dish and what it's doing to benefit your body. Then, before you tuck in, take a moment to say thank you for this beautiful meal—even if it's just toast. Give gratitude to the hardworking people who grew these plants, to the plants themselves for what they're about to give your body, to God or the Universe or Mother Nature for providing all we need to live another day with good health and abundance, to the person who created the meal, and to yourself. If you'd like to say a little blessing or prayer, I've included some of my favorites on page 112.

2. EAT UNTIL SATISFIED, NOT STUFFED

Ayurveda recommends that we eat until we are three-quarters satisfied versus 100 percent full. Overeating increases the production of free radicals, or unstable molecules that build up in the cells and can cause damage to other molecules, such as your genetic material (DNA) and proteins (the building blocks of just about everything in your body). This overwhelms and weakens the digestive fire, which can inhibit your ability to break down foods and in turn lead to chronic health issues. When you really give yourself a chance to tune into how your body feels as you eat (such as by limiting distractions, see #5), you're much less likely to overeat while still providing your body with the nourishment it needs.

3. CHEW YOUR FOOD

Chewing breaks down your food, which makes it easier for your body to absorb and utilize the nutrients in the food. You're also stimulating the production of digestive enzymes. But what's also truly powerful about chewing is that it allows you to experience your food—notice the textures, the sour, the sweet, the heat. It turns eating into a sensory experience, which (as you will learn more about in Eating with Your Senses, page 212) is yet another way to aid digestion while also leaning into the pure bliss of your food. The act of chewing seems really obvious, but

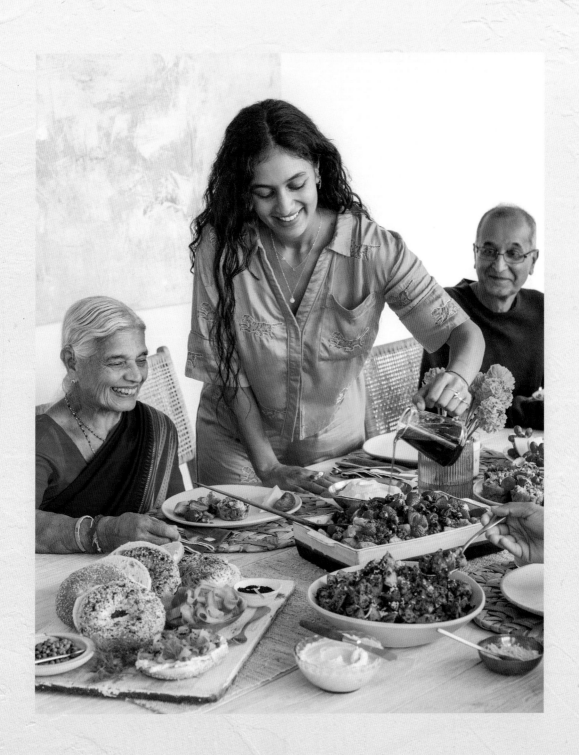

you'd be surprised how few of us actually chew (myself included!). The recommended amount to chew is *thirty* times. Per bite. That's right. But I say start with fifteen, since chewing a mouthful of rice thirty times can seem a little tedious at first! As you practice chewing more completely, you'll see what it feels like for your food to be ready to move on to the next phase of digestion.

4. EAT (AND COOK) WITH YOUR HANDS

One of the easiest ways to connect your senses with your meal is to physically touch your food. I realize not every dish lends itself to eating with your hands, but many do—especially when you add a side of Proper Good Naan (page 156) for scooping. And no one said you can't pick at a salad with your fingers! This also extends to preparing meals—tossing salads, arranging elements on a plate, and sprinkling fresh herbs over a dish are all lovely ways to *feel* your food and impart that much more of yourself when you cook because touching the food directly connects it to you and your love.

5. EAT WITHOUT DISTRACTIONS

If you are eating while watching TV/working/chatting, it increases the chances of overeating and not chewing your food adequately. Not only are you missing out on the nourishing experience of eating but you're also making it more difficult for your body to digest your food. Remember that food is the main source of nourishment for your body—it's a sign of respect to honor it with your full attention! Or at the very least be mindful of what else you're exposing your senses to. If you do want to have a conversation over a meal or listen to music, make sure it's relaxing and calm. (This should make you think twice about who you invite over for dinner!)

6. AVOID COLD DRINKS AND ICED BEVERAGES

If your digestion is like a fire, then imagine what introducing a cold drink can do to that flame. Anything that dampens that fire will make digestion more difficult. In scientific terms, cold beverages cause your blood vessels to constrict, which can hinder digestion and the process of absorbing nutrients. Every once in a while is fine—like a little Iced Matcha Tahini Latte (page 50) on a summer's day—but overall, most of the beverages I recommend are enjoyed warm or at room temperature. Similarly, drinking large amounts of liquid during your meals can slow down your digestion because the added fluid dilutes the stomach acids that break down your food. Try to stick to ½ cup hot water, warm water, or room-temperature water at mealtime.

7. AVOID SNACKING

Your body needs at least 3 hours to digest a meal, so eating between meals can disrupt the digestive process and lead to incomplete digestion. Over time, this can result in the accumulation of ama or toxins, which can present as any number of mild to moderate symptoms, such as bloating, gas, grogginess, diarrhea, lack of appetite, fatigue, bad breath, residue on the tongue, and strong-smelling sweat.

8. EAT YOUR DESSERT BEFORE DINNER

If you're following Ayurvedic practices to the letter, then ideally you would enjoy sweeter indulgences before a meal, not after. That's because sweets are always digested first, so if any other food is in your system, your body will stop digesting it in favor of the sweet, leading the undigested food to ferment and toxins to accumulate in your digestive system. However, sometimes having a little sweet something after dinner is just what needs to happen. When it does, reach for one of my recipes in Sweet Treats (page 259), which are meant to be decadent and delicious but gentle on the body.

9. GO FOR A WALK

While sitting or lying down after a meal may be tempting, try to resist. Sitting essentially squashes the digestive tract and slows digestion. It can even lead to indigestion. Instead, go for a little stroll, a lil' dawdle—nothing crazy, just 10 to 15 minutes—then come home and get cozy on that sofa.

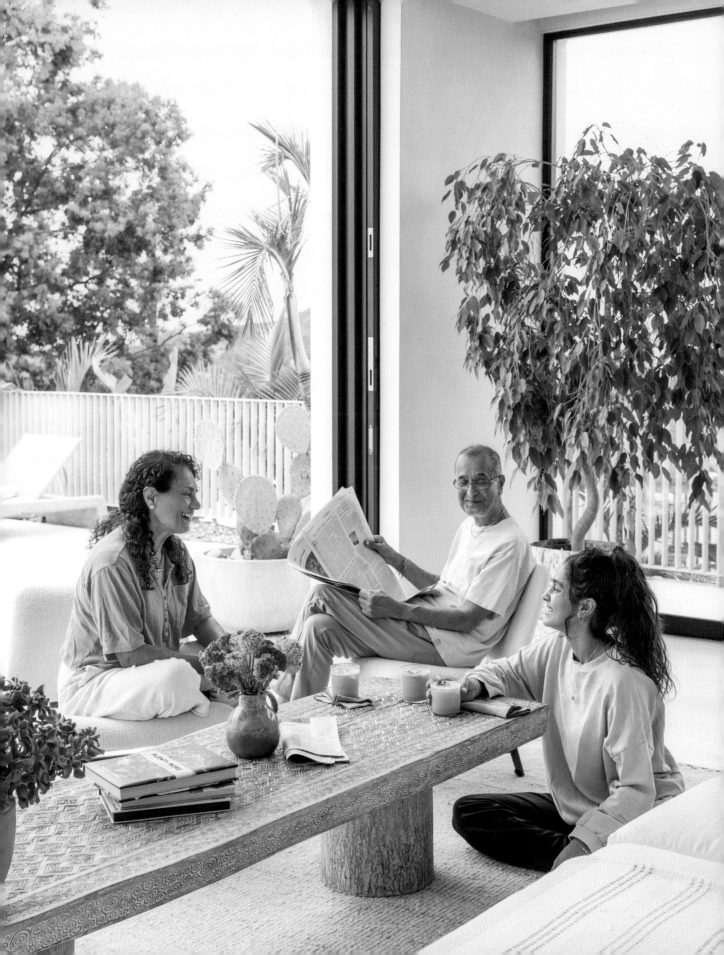

DRINKS

Whether you need a gentle energy bump in the morning, something warm and soothing to help you drift into sleep in the evening, re-energizing postworkout sustenance, or a little celebratory sip to share with guests, these recipes are your quick hits for mindfully dropping into the moment. Making them can be a ritual unto itself—practicing patience and stillness as you wait for the elements to come together—the liquid to boil, the tea to steep, the spices to bloom.

Inhale, exhale.

MASALA CHAI

Masala chai is a staple for my parents, and I grew up smelling the beautiful blend of spices that would waft through our house when they prepared it as a midday pick-me-up. I now often prepare this fragrant milk tonic in the morning as a gentle way to wake up, but I also love to snuggle up with it on a cold afternoon. You can enjoy it on its own or with a black tea bag (or two) for a little extra boost. You'll notice that in this recipe you bring the liquid mixture to a boil multiple times. This is to ensure that you end up with a rich, creamy chai.

SERVES *2*
TOTAL TIME: *10 minutes*

- 1 to 2 black tea bags (optional), to taste
- 1 teaspoon Homemade Chai Masala (recipe follows), or store-bought
- 1 sprig fresh mint
- ¼ teaspoon minced or grated fresh ginger (optional)
- 1 cup unsweetened vegan milk
- 1 teaspoon coconut sugar, plus more to taste

In a medium saucepan, bring 1 cup water to a boil over high heat. Add the tea bags (if using), the masala, mint, and ginger (if using) and return to a boil. Reduce the heat to a simmer, then immediately return the mixture to a boil. Repeat this once more and then bring the mixture back down to a simmer. Stir in the milk and sugar and return to a boil once more, breathing in the lovely aromas that will now be rising from the pan. Remove the pan from the heat, strain half the mixture over a mug, and do the same over a second mug with the remainder of the mixture and serve.

Homemade Chai Masala

Masala simply means "spice blend," and here I've combined a particularly warming medley that's powerful for digestion. This aromatic mixture will last in a sealed container for up to 2 weeks, and you can use it in multiple ways—stirred into chai, soups, stews, and curries; sprinkled over vegetables before they roast; or shaken into dressings. Just remember, when making this masala, as with any spice blend, it's ideal to start with whole spices and grind them fresh.

MAKES *about 2 cups*
TOTAL TIME: *10 minutes*

- ¾ cup ground ginger
- ½ cup ground cardamom
- ¼ cup freshly ground black pepper
- ¼ cup ground cinnamon
- ¼ cup ground cloves
- 2 tablespoons ground nutmeg

Use a mortar and pestle or spice grinder to grind the spices together into a fine powder. Transfer the mixture to a tightly sealed jar and store in a cool, dark place for up to 2 weeks.

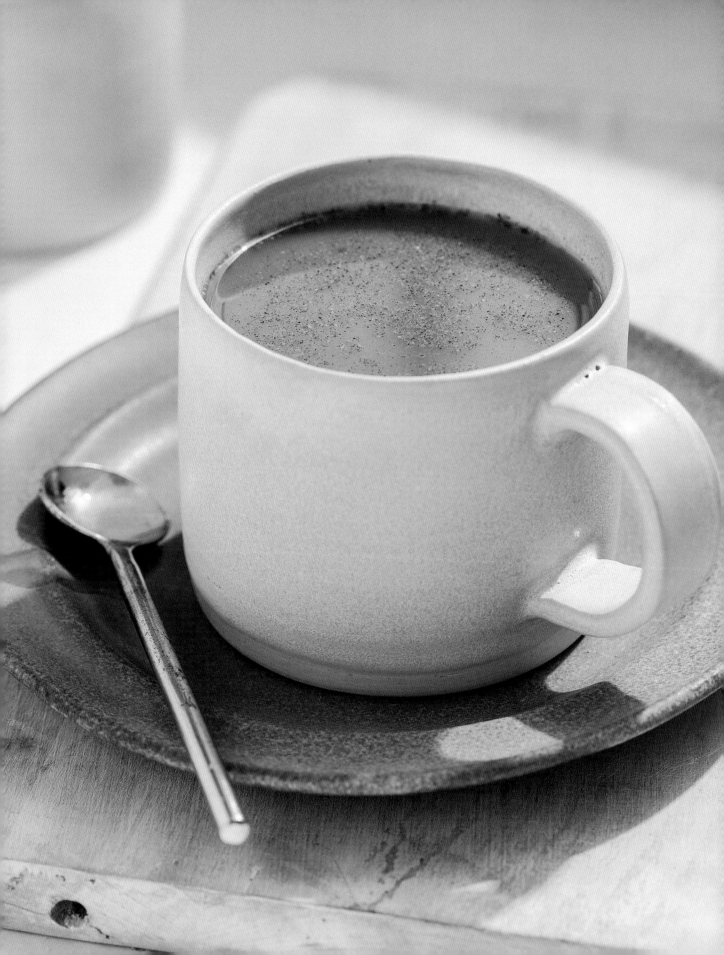

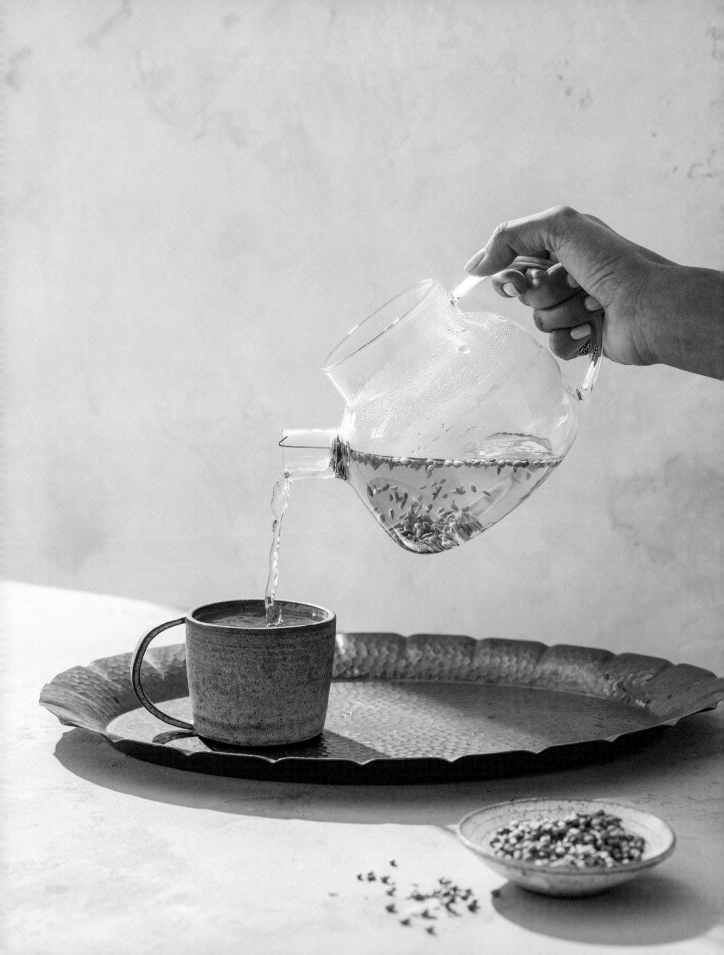

CCF DETOX TEA

"CCF" stands for coriander, cumin, and fennel, which in Ayurveda is a digestive partnership. It increases the absorption of nutrients and supports the body's natural detoxification process—which is a pretty impressive gift from just a small palmful of seeds! Not to mention the fact that this blend is also earthy and delicious. A mug of CCF tea is often the first thing I invite into my body in the morning. I'll also grind the spices into powder and sprinkle them into my meals, or use them as seasoning in my cooking—which you'll see called for in these recipes, especially the Indian-inspired dishes.

SERVES *1*

TOTAL TIME: *10 minutes*

- 1 teaspoon coriander seeds
- 1 teaspoon cumin seeds
- 1 teaspoon fennel seeds

In a small pot, combine the coriander, cumin, fennel seeds, and 2 cups water. Bring to a boil over high heat and boil for 5 minutes, taking a deep inhale of the spices' fragrance as they bloom.

Strain into a mug and drink hot or at room temperature.

NOTE   You can make a bigger batch of this tea by combining 1 cup of each spice in an airtight container. Use 1 tablespoon of the blend and steep as directed.

VARIATION   *Big Batch Blend:* Combine 1 cup of each spice in an airtight container. Add 1 tablespoon of the mixture to your water every morning. *Ground CCF Masala:* Grind equal measures of coriander seeds, cumin seeds, and fennel seeds to a fine powder. Store in an airtight container at room temperature for up to 1 month.

ICED MATCHA TAHINI LATTE

I like reaching for this rich, creamy coffee alternative mid-morning or afternoon, or whenever I want a gentle boost. (Although not first thing in the morning—I like to give my natural energy the opportunity to kick in first.) Matcha is a lovely tool for energy because while it delivers caffeine, it doesn't give me the jitters the way coffee does. So this latte supports a serene, focused mind. It's sweet from the maple syrup, which is complemented by the nutty tahini—a toasted sesame seed paste that is rich in healthy, brain-boosting fats.

MAKES *1 latte*
TOTAL TIME: *5 minutes*

2 tablespoons boiling water

2 teaspoons matcha powder

2 cups plain unsweetened oat milk

2 tablespoons tahini

1 tablespoon maple syrup, plus more as needed

¼ teaspoon ground cinnamon

¼ teaspoon vanilla extract

Ice, for serving (optional)

In a small bowl, whisk together the hot water and matcha powder until smooth.

In a high-powered blender, combine the matcha mixture, oat milk, tahini, maple syrup, cinnamon, and vanilla and blend until smooth. Add more maple syrup to taste, if you like. Serve over ice, if desired.

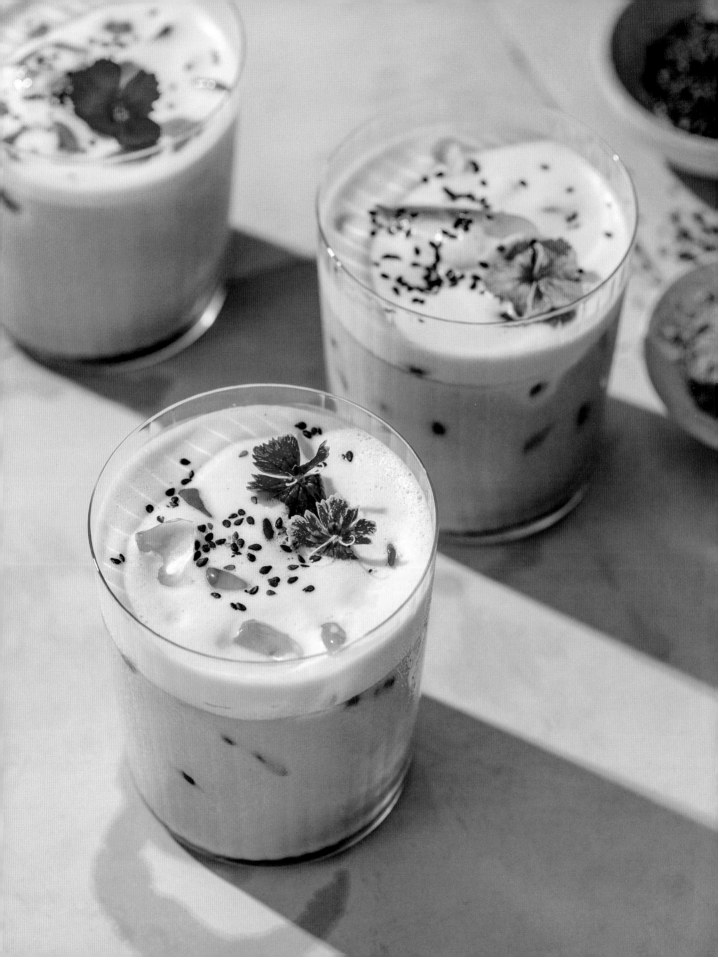

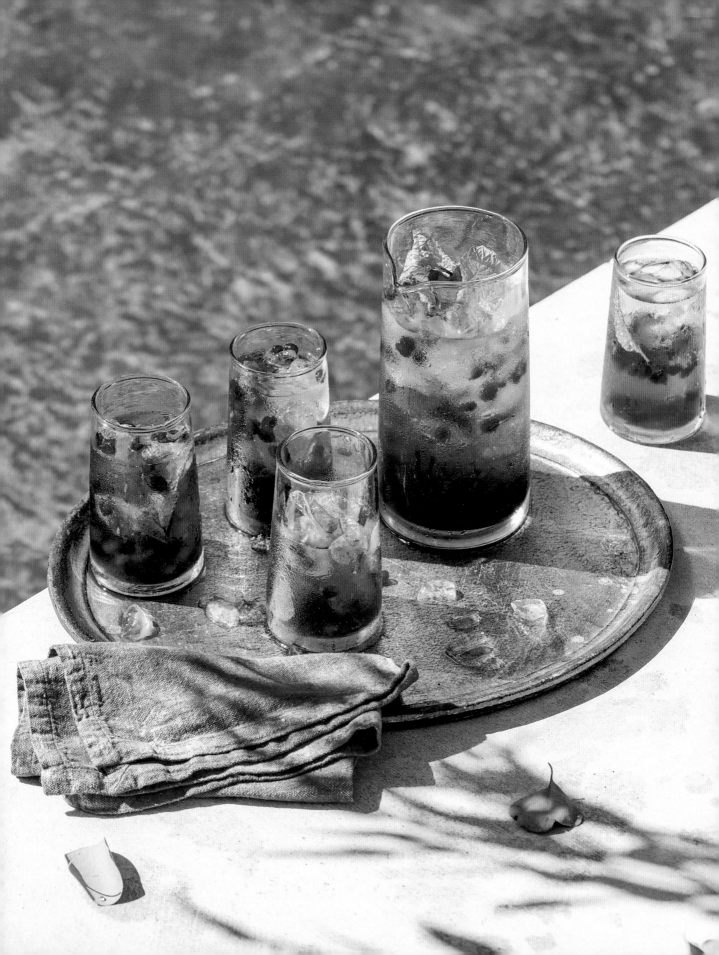

POMEGRANATE SPRITZER

I don't serve alcohol in my home, but I do like to give my guests a little something special and fancy with their meals so that they feel like they're partaking in the drink-with-dinner ritual. I came up with this gem-colored spritzer, which looks enticingly fizzy and festive, especially when served in a wineglass. You could also enjoy it as an afternoon treat, perhaps in place of soda, if that is a habit you're looking to change.

MAKES *2 spritzers*
TOTAL TIME: *5 minutes*

- 1 cup pomegranate juice, chilled
- ½ cup sparkling water, chilled
- ¼ cup pomegranate seeds
- 2 to 3 sprigs fresh mint

In a small pitcher, stir together the pomegranate juice and sparkling water. Divide the mixture between two glasses and garnish with the pomegranate seeds and mint sprigs. Cheers to a small moment worth celebrating!

STRAWBERRY MINT LEMONADE

Sometimes a drink isn't so much about what's in it as the moment it can create when it's enjoyed. Many of my most vivid memories are rooted in experiences having to do with eating and drinking. I may not be able to recall all the details, but I distinctly remember the *feelings*, like the pure delight that came with sipping cold lemonade on a hot summer day. So while this recipe might seem like a simple refreshment you've had before, I like to think of it as an opportunity to take a beautiful snapshot in time.

SERVES *4*
TOTAL TIME: *5 minutes*

- 2 cups strawberries, hulled, plus a few halved strawberries for garnish
- ½ cup agave nectar
- ½ cup fresh Meyer lemon juice (about 2 medium lemons), plus thin slices for garnish
- ⅓ cup fresh mint leaves, plus 4 sprigs for garnish
- 4 cups sparkling water, chilled
- Ice, for serving (optional)

In a blender, combine the strawberries, agave, lemon juice, and mint leaves. Blend until completely smooth. Pour in the sparkling water and use a long spoon to mix well.

Divide the lemonade among glasses or transfer it to a pitcher. Add ice, if desired, and garnish with the strawberry halves, Meyer lemon slices, and mint sprigs.

SAND'S GREEN JUICE

I fancy myself a green juice connoisseur because I have them wherever I go, and I can attest that my brother-in-law's is by far the best. His recipe is perfectly balanced among the bitter, sweet, and sour without it tasting too intensely "green"—exactly what a green juice should be. This is a great thirst-quenching, nutrient-packed refreshment, particularly at the start of the day or on an empty stomach, but it can be enjoyed any time you feel like a yummy, revitalizing infusion.

SERVES *2*
TOTAL TIME: *5 minutes*

- 2 medium seedless cucumbers
- 2 medium green apples (or red for a sweeter juice)
- 8 large curly or Tuscan kale leaves, midribs stripped out
- 4 celery stalks
- 1 lemon or lime, peeled and pith removed
- 1½-inch piece fresh ginger
- Handful of fresh parsley leaves

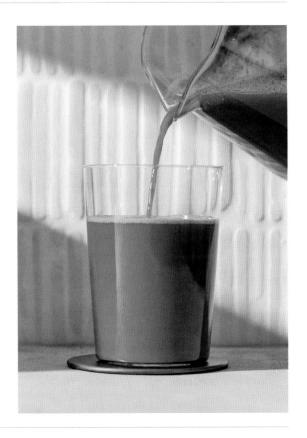

Roughly chop the cucumbers and apples into pieces small enough to fit through your juicer (see Note); no need to peel or core the cucumbers and apples. Pass the cucumbers, apples, kale, celery, lemon or lime, ginger, and parsley through the juicer.

Divide between two glasses and serve. The nutrients will be the most concentrated immediately after the juice is made, but you can refrigerate leftovers in a sealed container for up to 2 days.

NOTE   If you don't have a juicer, blend the ingredients in a high-powered blender and strain through a fine-mesh sieve.

MOON MILKS

If there were ever a magic potion for sleep, these infused milks would absolutely be it. I designed each of these recipes to channel the calming energy of the moon, soothe your senses, and quiet your nervous system, and to introduce you to the incredible world of adaptogens. Adaptogenic herbs are herbs, roots, and plant extracts that, very simply put, help your body adapt to the stresses of life. They bring balance and homeostasis to all your systems, returning them to their ideal chilled-out state. The adaptogens used in the recipes—ashwagandha, crushed rose petals, dried chamomile flowers, and butterfly pea flower powder (also called blue matcha)—can all be found in natural foods stores or online.

Sip, exhale, and let the moon's nurturing energy wash over you.

UNWIND
(CHERRY & ROSE)

SERVES *1*
TOTAL TIME: *10 minutes*

- 1 cup plain unsweetened almond or oat milk
- ¼ cup tart cherry juice
- 1 tablespoon crushed dried rose petals or rose powder
- ½ tablespoon ground cardamom
- Jaggery or coconut sugar

In a small saucepan, bring the milk to a simmer over medium-low heat. Whisk in the cherry juice, rose, and cardamom. Reduce the heat to low and cook until warmed through and the fragrance of cardamom has bloomed, 1 to 2 minutes. Remove the pan from the heat and let the milk cool slightly. Sweeten to taste with jaggery and serve.

CALM
(CHAMOMILE & STAR ANISE)

SERVES *1*
TOTAL TIME: *10 minutes*

- 1 cup plain unsweetened vegan milk
- 1 tablespoon dried chamomile flowers or 1 chamomile tea bag
- 2 whole star anise
- 1 teaspoon date syrup or sweetener of choice
- 1 teaspoon saffron threads (optional)

In a small saucepan, combine the milk, chamomile, star anise, date syrup, and saffron (if using) and bring to a boil over medium-high heat. Immediately reduce to a simmer, then right away increase the heat back to medium-high and bring to a boil once more. (The idea is to let the mixture brew properly without the milk overflowing.) Again, reduce to a simmer before the milk comes over the edge of the pot. Then return to a boil again, reduce to a simmer, and cook for 3 to 5 minutes, until your kitchen smells delightful. Remove the chamomile tea bag (if using) or strain out the chamomile flowers and the star anise and serve.

REST
(LAVENDER & BLUE MATCHA)

SERVES *1*
TOTAL TIME: *10 minutes*

- 1 cup plain unsweetened vegan milk
- 1 teaspoon dried lavender buds or 1 lavender tea bag
- 1 teaspoon honey or date syrup
- ½ teaspoon vanilla extract
- ¼ teaspoon butterfly pea flower powder (also called blue matcha)

In a small saucepan, combine the milk, lavender, honey, vanilla, and butterfly pea flower powder and bring to a boil over medium-high heat. Immediately reduce to a simmer, then right away increase the heat back to medium-high and bring to a boil once more. (The idea is to let the mixture brew properly without the milk overflowing.)

Again, reduce to a simmer before the milk comes over the edge of the pot. Then return to a boil again, reduce to a simmer, and cook for 3 to 5 minutes, until your kitchen smells delightful. Reduce the heat to medium-low and simmer for 3 to 5 minutes. Remove the lavender tea bag or strain out the loose lavender (if using) before serving.

SLEEP
(NUTMEG & ASHWAGANDHA)

SERVES *1*
TOTAL TIME: *10 minutes*

- 1 cup plain unsweetened almond milk
- ½ teaspoon ground turmeric
- ¼ teaspoon saffron threads
- ½ teaspoon ground cinnamon
- ½ teaspoon ashwagandha root powder
- ¼ teaspoon ground nutmeg
- ¼ teaspoon ground cardamom
- ⅛ teaspoon freshly ground black pepper
- 1 teaspoon organic cold-pressed coconut oil
- Jaggery or coconut sugar

In a small saucepan, bring the milk to a simmer over medium-low heat. Add the turmeric, saffron, cinnamon, ashwagandha, nutmeg, cardamom, and pepper, whisking vigorously to break up any clumps.

Add the coconut oil, reduce the heat to low, and cook until the coconut oil is melted and warmed through and the spices' aromas fill your kitchen, 1 to 2 minutes. Remove the pan from the heat and let the milk cool slightly. Sweeten to taste with jaggery or coconut sugar and serve.

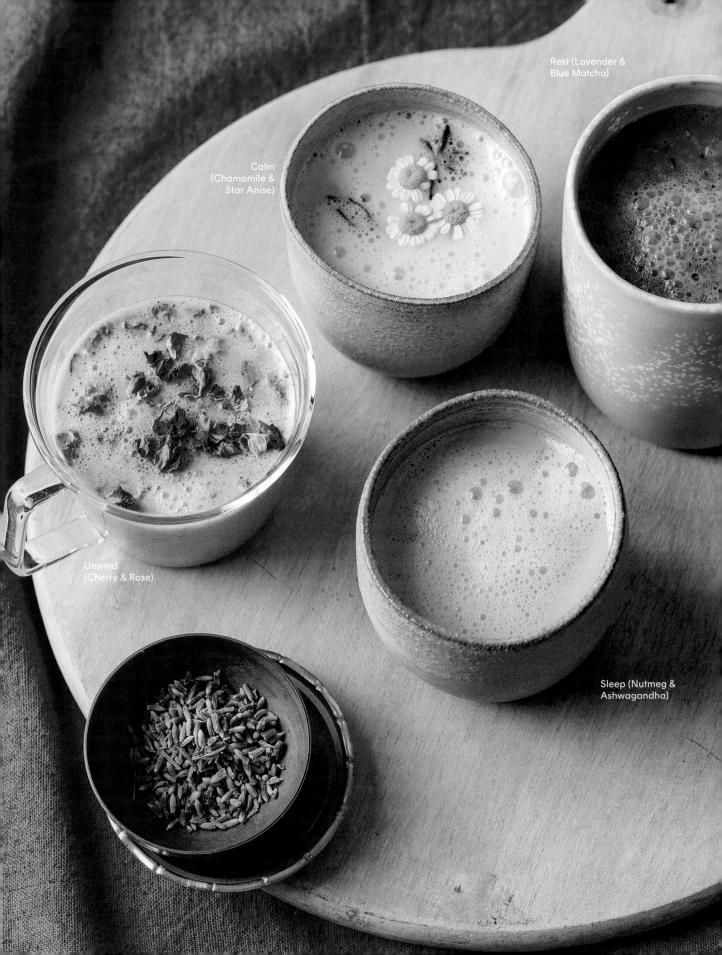

Rest (Lavender &
Blue Matcha)

Calm
(Chamomile &
Star Anise)

Unwind
(Cherry & Rose)

Sleep (Nutmeg &
Ashwagandha)

My 5 a.m.-ish Morning Routine

About ten years ago, when I was first starting down the path of meditation and developing my spiritual practice, I wanted to go *all in*. So I started waking up at 3:45 a.m. to meditate with the monks at a local temple called Bhaktivedanta Manor in Watford, England. The experience was so transformative and miraculous that I kept it up for a year and a half. But eventually I wanted to give myself a *little* more time to sleep in. So I ended up settling into a 5 a.m.-ish wake-up time and a morning routine, which over the years has brought definition and joy to my life.

Getting up early might seem beyond what you can imagine right now, but think about it this way: The time before the sun comes up has the moon's calming, soothing energy, which is powerful for supporting prayer, meditation, and reflection. And I guarantee you that eventually, once you set the habit of getting up earlier and experiencing all the special moments with the world before the sun's go, go, go energy takes over, you'll adjust to it. It's also important to point out that my morning routine is made possible by an intentional, sleep-promoting nighttime routine (see My Mindful and Relaxing *Aaaaaah* Evening Routine, page 256)—the two go very much hand in hand when it comes to resetting your clock to a more natural rhythm.

These are the highlights of my morning routine. I don't always manage to do all of them, but having each of these practices in my toolbox means I can pick and choose as time and mood allows. I invite you to choose any piece or pieces of it that speak to you and build from there.

5 A.M. WAKEY WAKEY

When I first open my eyes in the morning, I'm greeted by spiritual images such as pictures of temples in India that I've hung near my bed to spark thoughts of gratitude. I say a quick prayer (such as "Thank you for this gift of breath and life today") and then roll out of bed. As I put my feet on the ground, I think of a Sanskrit prayer that pays respect to and honors Mother Earth, which translates to "I'm sorry for placing my feet on your head."

ABHYANGA MASSAGE: *Abhyanga* is Sanskrit for "self-massage," and it's a relaxing self-love practice. All you need is high-quality oil—either Ayurvedic medicated oils or household oils like organic sesame, almond, or extra-virgin coconut. Then you rub your body all over with long strokes toward the heart, and circular motions on your joints and belly. The idea is that you're encouraging circulation, releasing any toxins through the lymphatic system that may have stagnated in the body, lubricating your joints, and sending that calm, loving energy through your skin, which is then absorbed by the nervous system to help you feel grounded.

TONGUE SCRAPING AND MARMA MAT: While I'm at the sink brushing my teeth, I'm also accomplishing two vital parts of my morning routine. First, I'm using a tongue scraper, which is exactly what it sounds like—a small U-shaped tool that scrapes the surface of your tongue to clear away bacteria that accumulated overnight, which Ayurveda says can lead to illness. And while I'm brushing and scraping, I'm also standing on my marma mat, an acupressure mat that stimulates the 72,000 nerve endings in my feet that connect to every part of the body. Stimulating these pressure points can relieve pain, fatigue, muscle tension, and stress, in addition to encouraging the movement of lymph fluid, your body's detoxification system. That's what you call efficiency!

GHARSHANA (DRY BRUSHING): By using a stiff bristle brush to make long, gentle strokes over your skin, you're sloughing off old skin cells as well as stimulating your lymphatic system. Lymph fluid lives all over your body and is like a river that removes waste and toxins. So helping it circulate is not only cleansing but also keeps your immune system strong. I like doing this for a couple of minutes before I get into the shower or before bed. Give yourself 2 or 3 minutes to move the brush up your legs and arms (toward the heart, always), as well as in circular motions on your belly.

SHOWER AND GET DRESSED: Nothing fancy here! Just do what feels good and keep it comfy.

TEA: To gently wake up my digestion and introduce much-needed hydration into my body after sleep, I make myself a pot of CCF Detox Tea (page 49).

5:30 A.M. MEDITATION

LIGHT A CANDLE AND BURN SOME INCENSE: Before I settle in for my morning meditation, I set the tone and intention by lighting a candle. In Vedic culture, lighting a candle symbolizes offering an element back to God/the Universe as a thank you for providing us with the elements we need to live and breathe and nourish ourselves throughout the day. As I light my candle, I like to think about how the wick represents our soul and the oil or wax represents all the impurities we accumulate over time, and how the process to purify ourselves is an ongoing effort. It can also be a nice touch to burn your favorite incense, which will begin to draw your senses into your practice.

SETTLE IN: Wherever I've lived, whether in a tiny apartment or a house, I've always had a dedicated space for my morning meditation—even if it's just a little pillow. Your meditation space doesn't have to be fancy, but do try to have a regular place, which helps reinforce the habit. It could be the corner of your bedroom or living room, or outside on your fire escape.

YOGIC BREATHWORK: A few rounds of mindful breathwork help me settle into the practice and calm my mind. I choose from a variety of methods (read about some of my favorites in Tuning In with Your Breath (page 184) and go with whatever feels right in the moment.

MANTRA MEDITATION: I've tried various meditation styles, but my daily practice is mantra meditation. *Man* means "mind" and *tra* is to "transcend," and the idea is to say your mantra out loud, on repeat, during the duration of your meditation (more on that below). Here are a few you could start with:

> **Om,** a simple mantra and a sacred sound considered to be the sound of the Universe and encompassing all other sounds within it.

> **Om Namo Bhagavate Vasudevaya** (ohm nah-mo bah-gah-vah-tay vas-ooo-day-vie-yah), meaning "I offer praise unto the all-pervading divinity present within every heart; who is the embodiment of beauty, intelligence, strength, wealth, fame, and detachment."

> **Hare Krishna Hare Krishna Krishna Krishna Hare Hare Hare Rama Hare Rama Rama Rama Hare Hare,** the mantra I connected with the most after making my way through many others and which I have been chanting daily for more than ten years. *Hare* calls to and invites the feminine divine energy (for men and women), Krishna is the all-attractive divine, and *rama* is the source of all pleasure we seek. But more than the meaning of the words is the vibration that's created. It transcends our physical and mental self and connects us with a higher consciousness, where we can slowly shed our ego and connect with our true nature and self.

When practicing your mantra meditation, remember that it is a deep calling in the spirit of service and a deep exchange between you and your soul. What's most important to me during this time—and what helps me stay absorbed and focused—is to incorporate all of my senses. Chanting activates my ears and my mouth, incense stimulates my sense of smell, meditation beads engage my hands and touch, and whenever possible, I take my practice outside so that I can hear the birds and feel the breeze on my skin. In the beginning, your meditation may only last 5 or 10 minutes. But over time, you'll enjoy sitting for longer and longer. During the past decade, I've worked my way up from 10 minutes to an hour and a half, and I've seen the difference in my life: I feel more focused, clear, creative, and connected. Yes, it can take a while to feel the effects of meditation, and some days the practice feels tougher than others, but the experiences that carry the most meaning can sometimes take the longest to come to fruition. It's like building a relationship with your partner or a friend—it takes time to nurture a deep, meaningful connection with yourself.

7:30 A.M. READING

To transition out of my meditation, I'll read for 10 to 15 minutes. I typically reach for spiritual texts, such as the *Bhagavad Gita*, but I read anything that allows for quiet reflection and begins to stir the mind.

8 A.M. EXERCISE

Ayurveda recommends first moving your body before 10 a.m. in order to get your blood pumping and your endorphins flowing and to stimulate all your physiological systems to transition them from sleep. I like to take at least 30 minutes to get a sweat on, whether it's going out for a run, boxing, getting in a hot yoga flow, or challenging myself to a weight training workout.

10:30/11 A.M. BREAKFAST

Now it's time to nourish and replenish. This is when I introduce my first meal of the day, which tends to be light in order not to overwhelm my digestive flame, which hasn't built to a full roar just yet. I usually reach for my Spiced Stewed Apples (page 64) or a Cake Batter Protein Power Smoothie (page 67). Before I start eating, I say a few words of gratitude for all those who made it possible for this meal to be on my table.

REFLECTION

Instead of diving right into the workday, I try to pause for just a moment to write down any thoughts I've had during the morning or anything I've read that I want to share with other people. It helps me soak up what I've learned, process what's on my mind, and gives me that little extra pep in my step as I come up with my goals for the day. Then on to a cute outfit, my laptop, and whatever the day brings!

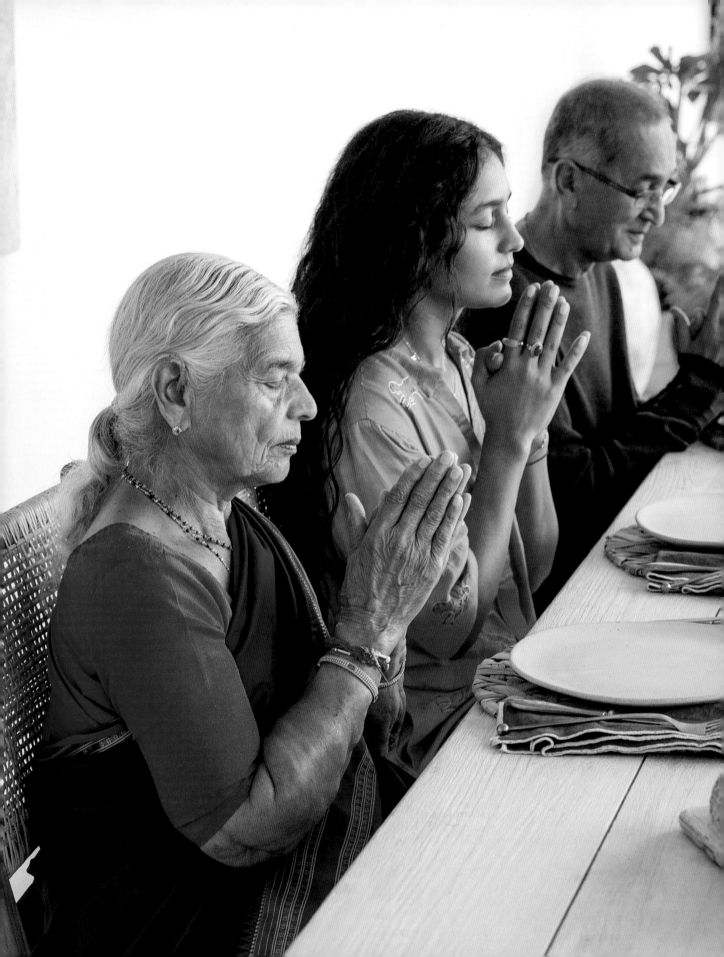

BREAKFAST

These recipes are designed to revitalize your body after it's been at rest for 6 to 8 hours. They are organized in the chapter from lightest to most substantial and include a variety of options—sweet and savory, heavily spiced and subtle, warm and cold—so that you can follow your mood and your appetite. To ease into the day with intention and presence of mind, try this mantra as you prepare your morning meal:

I am so grateful to live another day. Let my hands be used
in service, my eyes see the best in others, my heart be open to receive,
and my words uplift those in need . . .

SPICED STEWED APPLES

From a functional perspective, this dish is pretty hard to beat as a breakfast option—cooked fruit is much easier to digest than raw, and the spice-apple combination can help regulate your blood glucose in the morning, which is important not only for having a steady supply of energy throughout the day but also because repeated spikes can cause damage to your organs, nerves, and blood vessels. But let's be honest, the real reason I make this day after day is because the apples turn juicy and succulent and caramelized as they bubble away in the pan. It's a cozy and satisfying treat that just feels so right after a good night's sleep.

Use the time the apples are gently simmering to ease into your day—stretch, journal, set an intention. Also, when topped with a little vanilla yogurt and a sprinkle of granola, this dish would also make for a lovely, quick dessert.

SERVES *2*
TOTAL TIME: *20 minutes*

- 2 medium apples, such as Braeburn (or other firm, crisp apple), peeled, cored, and diced
- 1 cinnamon stick or ½ teaspoon ground cinnamon
- 2 whole cloves
- Almond butter or sliced almonds (optional), for serving

In a medium saucepan, combine the apples, cinnamon, cloves, and ¾ cup water. Cover and simmer over medium-low heat until the apples are soft, the spices have released their aroma, and only a small amount of water is left on the bottom of the pan, about 10 minutes. If you find not much of the water has evaporated, uncover the pan and increase the heat to medium, stirring occasionally to help the water steam off, about 3 minutes.

Remove the pan from the heat and discard the cinnamon stick and cloves. Let the apples cool slightly before serving. Enjoy this on its own or top with a drizzle of almond butter or sliced almonds.

Store any leftovers in a sealed container in the refrigerator for up to 2 days. Reheat on the stove over low heat until warmed through.

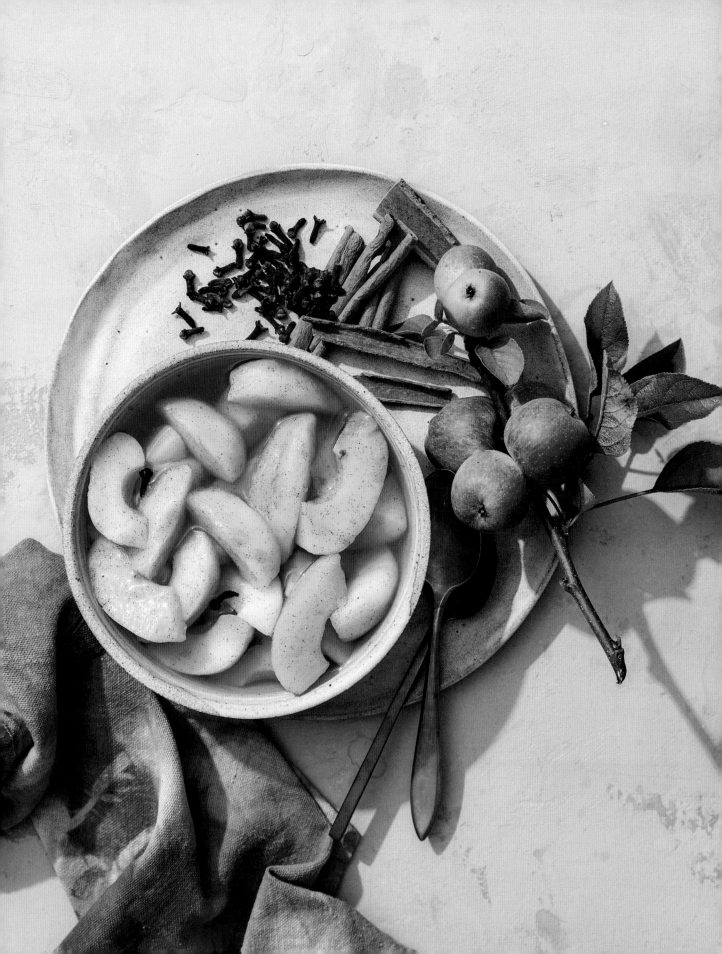

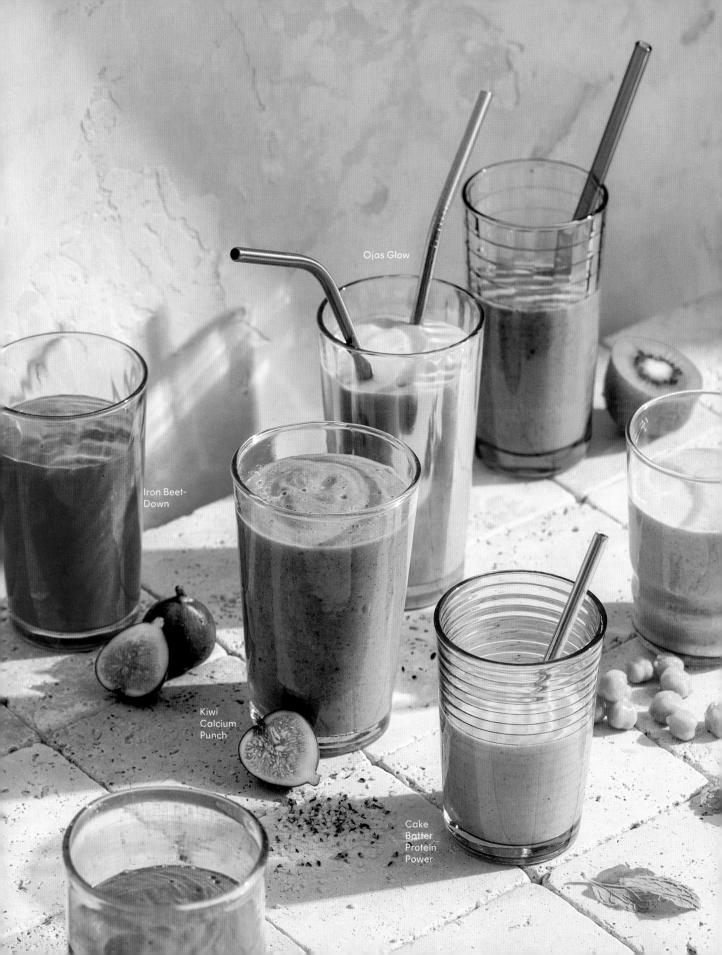

Ojas Glow

Iron Beet-
Down

Kiwi
Calcium
Punch

Cake
Batter
Protein
Power

VEGAN SUPPORT SMOOTHIES

A big question on people's minds when they start eating a plant-based diet is whether they're getting all the nutrients, vitamins, and minerals that they need. While I can tell you that you absolutely can, and have also included a handy chart on pages 28–31 to give you peace of mind, I've also developed four smoothies as your insurance policy for getting enough protein, calcium, iron, and ojas, or vitality. Rotate through them, or choose whichever one speaks to you in the moment. They're the most delicious, nutritious "supplements" you could possibly take.

CAKE BATTER PROTEIN POWER

MAKES *2 smoothies*
TOTAL TIME: *10 minutes*

> 1 cup plain unsweetened oat or almond milk (or a combination)
> ¼ cup cooked or canned chickpeas (rinsed and drained if canned)
> ½ medium banana or peeled avocado (optional)
> 2 tablespoons hemp seeds
> 2 tablespoons unsweetened almond butter
> 1 teaspoon maple syrup
> ¼ teaspoon ground cinnamon

In a high-powered blender, combine the milk, chickpeas, banana or avocado (if using), hemp seeds, almond butter, maple syrup, and cinnamon and blend until completely smooth. Serve immediately.

KIWI CALCIUM PUNCH

MAKES *2 smoothies*
TOTAL TIME: *10 minutes*

> ½ medium avocado, pitted
> 2 medium kiwis, peeled
> 1 cup chopped or torn kale (about ⅓ bunch), any type
> ½ cup plain unsweetened almond milk
> 1 fresh Black Mission fig, stemmed
> 15 fresh mint leaves

Scoop the avocado into a high-powered blender. Add the kiwis, kale, almond milk, fig, and mint leaves and blend until smooth. Serve immediately.

IRON BEET-DOWN

MAKES *2 smoothies*
TOTAL TIME: *10 minutes*

> ½ medium avocado, pitted
> 1 cup plain unsweetened almond milk
> 1 cup raw spinach (optional)
> 1 medium store-bought cooked beet, chopped
> 2 tablespoons hemp seeds
> 1 tablespoon tahini
> 1 Medjool date, pitted

Scoop the avocado into a high-powered blender. Add the almond milk, spinach (if using), beet, hemp seeds, tahini, and date and blend until completely smooth. Serve immediately.

OJAS GLOW

MAKES *2 smoothies*
TOTAL TIME: *10 minutes*

> 1 medium avocado, pitted
> 1 cup unsweetened coconut water
> 1 Medjool date, pitted
> ½ teaspoon ground cinnamon
> ½ teaspoon ground cardamom
> ¼ teaspoon ground ginger

Scoop the avocado into a high-powered blender. Add the coconut water, date, cinnamon, cardamom, and ginger and blend until completely smooth. Serve immediately.

CHAI OATMEAL

Oatmeal for breakfast is certainly nothing new, but it can be quite hard for your body to digest grains in the morning. Digestion-stoking chai spices and rich, fatty milk make oatmeal much gentler on the body—and even more delicious. It really does make you feel like you're eating a cheeky dessert for breakfast.

SERVES *2*
TOTAL TIME: *25 minutes*

- 1 cup quick-cooking oats
- 2 Medjool dates, chopped
- 1 teaspoon chai spice
- ½ teaspoon ground cardamom
- 2 cups plain unsweetened plant-based milk
- Almond butter, toasted pumpkin seeds, sliced almonds, rose petals, or date syrup, for serving

In a medium saucepan, combine the oats, dates, chai spice, cardamom, and ¼ cup water and bring to a simmer over medium heat. Stirring occasionally, cook the oatmeal until it thickens, about 2 minutes. Stir in 1 cup of the milk and cook, stirring, until the oatmeal has thickened again, about 5 minutes. Add the remaining 1 cup milk and continue cooking, stirring occasionally, until thick and creamy, another 5 to 10 minutes.

Divide the oatmeal between two bowls and top as desired with almond butter, pumpkin seeds, almonds, rose petals, and/or date syrup.

MAKE-AHEAD This recipe is quick enough to come together on a busy morning, but you could also prep a batch the night before, stash it in the fridge, and enjoy it the next day.

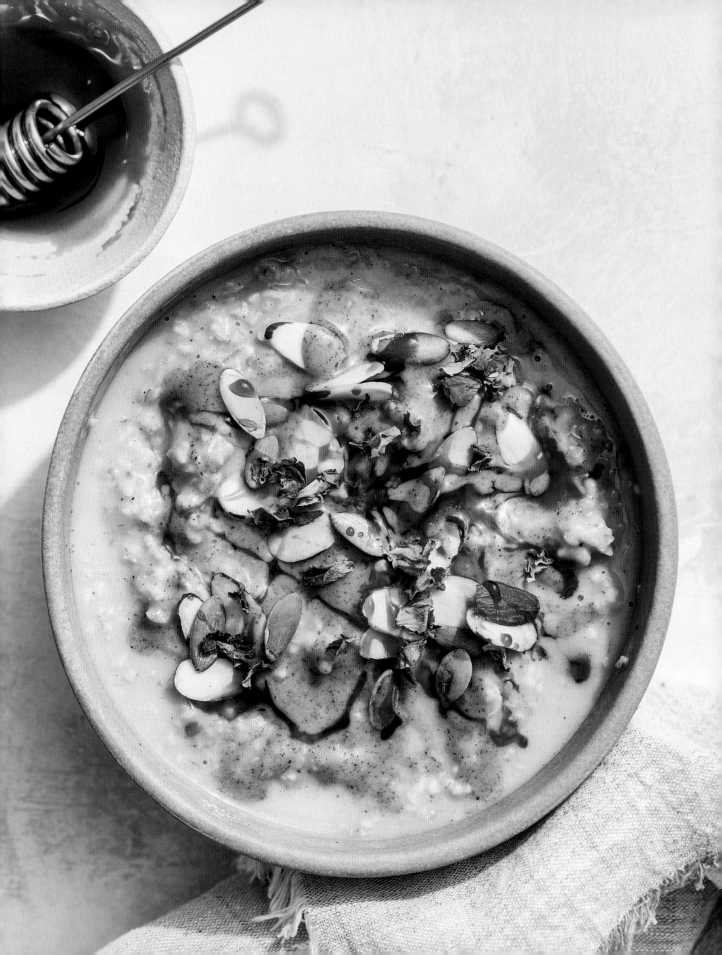

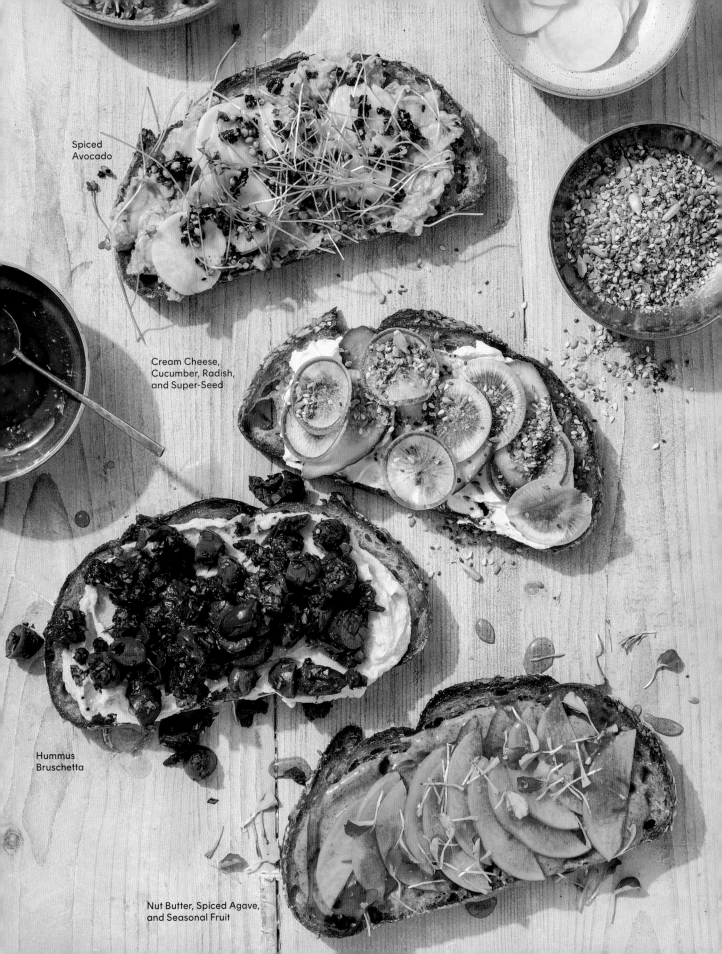

Spiced
Avocado

Cream Cheese,
Cucumber, Radish,
and Super-Seed

Hummus
Bruschetta

Nut Butter, Spiced Agave,
and Seasonal Fruit

LOADED TOAST FOUR WAYS

Sometimes we find beautiful, nourishing morning moments in the simplest of places—including on toast. When I'm not in the mood to cook breakfast, or don't have the time, or just need a hearty, bready meal, I always know that I can make one of these recipes and still feel like I'm giving my body the sustenance it needs to meet the day. The trick is having some of the components prepped in advance so they're ready to grab (such as Cashew/Sunflower Seed Cream Cheese, page 72, and my Perfect Hummus, page 239), combining different flavors and textures to keep it interesting, while also using spices like cumin, coriander, and black pepper, which help kick your digestive fire into gear.

SPICED AVOCADO

SERVES *2*
TOTAL TIME: *10 minutes*

- 2 tablespoons extra-virgin olive oil
- ½ teaspoon crushed whole coriander seeds or powder
- ½ teaspoon kalonji seeds (nigella seeds)
- ¼ teaspoon freshly ground black pepper
- ¼ teaspoon ground cumin
- ¼ teaspoon red chile flakes
- ¼ teaspoon asafoetida
- 2 medium avocados, halved and pitted
- 1 tablespoon fresh lime juice
- ¼ teaspoon sea salt
- 2 thick slices sourdough, ciabatta, or other hearty bread
- Vegan sour cream, for serving (optional)
- 2 tablespoons chopped fresh cilantro leaves or microgreens

In a small skillet, heat 1½ tablespoons of the oil over medium-low heat. Add the coriander, kalonji seeds, black pepper, cumin, chile flakes, and asafoetida and cook until just fragrant, about 30 seconds. Remove the pan from the heat and set aside.

Scoop the avocado flesh into a small bowl. Add the lime juice, salt, and about half of the spice oil and combine with a fork, mashing as you mix.

In a medium skillet, heat the remaining ½ tablespoon oil over medium heat. Add the bread and toast until crispy, 2 to 3 minutes per side.

Transfer the toasts to a plate and spread half of the avocado mixture onto each slice. Drizzle the toasts with the remaining spice oil. If desired, drizzle on some cashew sour cream. Top with the cilantro.

HUMMUS BRUSCHETTA

SERVES *2*
TOTAL TIME: *10 minutes*

- 10 pitted black or green olives (a mix is nice), roughly chopped
- 5 oil-packed sun-dried tomatoes, drained and roughly chopped (it's okay if they're still a little oily)
- 2 tablespoons chopped fresh parsley leaves
- Sea salt and freshly ground black pepper
- 2 thick slices sourdough, ciabatta, or other hearty bread
- ½ cup hummus, homemade (page 239) or store-bought
- Extra-virgin olive oil or chili oil, for drizzling

In a medium bowl, toss together the olives, sun-dried tomatoes, parsley, and salt and pepper to taste. Set aside.

Toast the bread and spread each toast with a thick layer of hummus. Spoon on the olive and sun-dried tomato mixture. Drizzle with olive oil or chili oil and serve.

Recipes Continue

CREAM CHEESE, CUCUMBER, RADISH, AND SUPER-SEED TOASTS

Both the cream cheese and the seed mix can be made ahead, which will help make morning prep even quicker. I also highly recommend using the super-seed mix for any other dish that could use a bit of crunch—salads, soups, or even your oatmeal!

SERVES *2*
TOTAL TIME: *10 minutes*

- ¼ cup Cashew/Sunflower Seed Cream Cheese (recipe follows)
- ¼ cup Super-Seed Mix (recipe follows)
- 2 thick slices sourdough, ciabatta, or other hearty bread
- ½ tablespoon extra-virgin olive oil or chili oil
- 1 Persian or ½ English cucumber, thinly sliced
- 8 to 10 thin watermelon radish slices (optional)
- 8 to 10 thin purple daikon radish slices (optional)
- Flaky salt

Make the cream cheese and seed mix as directed.

Heat a large cast-iron skillet over medium heat. Drizzle both sides of the bread slices generously with olive oil or chili oil and toast each side to your liking in the hot pan.

Spread the toasts with a thick layer of the cream cheese and arrange the sliced cucumber on top, along with the radish and daikon, if using. Sprinkle generously with the seed mix, drizzle with more oil if desired, and top with flaky salt.

Cashew/Sunflower Seed Cream Cheese

While these days it's much easier to find a high-quality vegan cream cheese at the grocery store, it's actually incredibly easy to make, and the homemade version will always be tastier and contain far fewer preservatives than the store-bought kind.

MAKES *2 cups*
TOTAL TIME: *15 minutes, plus soaking time*

- 1 cup raw cashews
- 1 cup sunflower seeds
- ½ cup plain unsweetened almond milk
- 2 tablespoons plain vegan yogurt
- ½ tablespoon nutritional yeast
- ½ tablespoon apple cider vinegar
- 1 teaspoon sea salt

In a medium bowl, combine the cashews and sunflower seeds with enough water to submerge them and soak overnight. (Alternatively, you can soak them in hot water for 1 hour.) Drain, rinse until the water is clear, and drain again thoroughly.

In a high-powered blender, combine the soaked cashews and sunflower seeds, almond milk, yogurt, yeast, vinegar, and salt and blend until completely smooth. Transfer to a sealed container and refrigerate until ready to use, up to 5 days.

Super-Seed Mix

In addition to bringing rich depth of flavor and crunch to any dish, seeds are also high in essential nutrients like omega-3s, healthy fats, and fiber. Nutritional yeast in particular is a complete protein and is loaded with B_{12}. This tasty mix will last for up to a month in your fridge, which means you can add a sprinkle to any of your meals for an extra nutritional boost.

MAKES *about 2 cups*
TOTAL TIME: *5 minutes*

> ½ cup golden flaxseeds
>
> ¼ cup sunflower seeds
>
> ¼ cup chia seeds
>
> ¼ cup white sesame seeds
>
> ¼ cup hemp seeds
>
> ¼ cup plus 1 tablespoon nutritional yeast
>
> ½ teaspoon sea salt

In a large cast-iron skillet, combine the flaxseeds, sunflower seeds, chia seeds, sesame seeds, and hemp seeds and toast over low heat, stirring frequently, until golden brown and fragrant, 3 to 5 minutes. Add the nutritional yeast and salt and remove the pan from the heat. Toss well to combine and store the mixture in a sealed jar in the fridge for up to 1 month.

NUT BUTTER, SPICED AGAVE, AND SEASONAL FRUIT

SERVES *2*
TOTAL TIME: *10 minutes*

> 2 thick slices sourdough, ciabatta, or other hearty bread
>
> ¼ cup crunchy nut butter, such as almond, pistachio, hazelnut, or cashew, plus more if needed
>
> 1 apple, ripe peach, or very ripe persimmon, thinly sliced
>
> Spiced Agave (recipe follows)
>
> Edible flowers, such as sage, for garnish (optional)

Toast the bread and spread each slice with a thick layer of nut butter. Top with the sliced fruit and a drizzle of the spiced agave. If desired, garnish with edible flowers.

Spiced Agave

Spiced agave is delicious drizzled over oats or Spiced Stewed Apples (page 64), stirred into tea, or used as a dip for fresh fruit when you need a quick sweet bite.

MAKES *½ cup*
TOTAL TIME: *5 minutes plus cooling time*

> ½ cup agave nectar or vegan honey
>
> ½ teaspoon ground coriander
>
> 2 whole star anise
>
> ½ teaspoon ground cinnamon
>
> ½ teaspoon ground ginger

In a small saucepan, combine the agave nectar, coriander, star anise, cinnamon, and ginger and cook over medium heat, stirring, until the spices have released their aroma, 3 to 5 minutes. Remove the pan from the heat and set aside to cool completely. The agave can be stored in a sealed container in a cool cupboard for up to 2 weeks.

BUCKWHEAT PANCAKES *with Compote and Sweet Cream*

My older sister, whom I lovingly call Didi, is the baker in our family. She makes the most delicious sweet treats and goodies, and one thing she has perfected over the years is making moist, fluffy pancakes. So when I think about the perfect breakfast, I often dream about a piping-hot stack of her pancakes. I decided to take a shot at making my own version using buckwheat, a flour I absolutely love. It has an earthy, nutty flavor; it's considered a superfood because it's packed with protein and essential amino acids; and it's grain-free and gluten-free, so it feels lighter on your stomach. These pancakes aren't overly sweet, so you can load them up with all the delicious toppings, like fresh compote and sweet cream, maybe a drizzle of almond butter and maple syrup, or perhaps a sprinkle of toasted nuts.

MAKES *about 12 pancakes*
TOTAL TIME: *35 minutes*

COMPOTE

1 cup roughly chopped fresh seasonal fruit, such as peaches, cherries, strawberries, or blackberries

1 teaspoon coconut sugar

¼ teaspoon ground cinnamon (optional)

¼ teaspoon ground ginger (optional)

PANCAKES

1 cup plain unsweetened vegan milk

¼ cup unsweetened applesauce

1 teaspoon vanilla extract

1 tablespoon apple cider vinegar

1 tablespoon extra-virgin coconut oil, melted, plus more for the pan

1 tablespoon maple syrup, plus more for serving

1 cup light buckwheat flour

½ cup almond, oat flour, or all-purpose flour

1 teaspoon baking powder

½ teaspoon baking soda

FOR SERVING

Sweet Cashew Cream (page 263)

Almond or pistachio butter (optional)

Maple syrup (optional)

Toasted nuts (optional)

Mixed fruit, for serving

MAKE THE COMPOTE: In a small pot, stir together the fruit, sugar, cinnamon (if using), and ginger (if using). Bring the mixture to a boil over medium heat. Reduce the heat to a simmer and cook, stirring occasionally, until the fruit is completely cooked and jammy, 3 minutes if you like a looser consistency or 5 minutes if you prefer it thicker. Remove the pan from the heat and set aside.

MAKE THE PANCAKES: In a medium bowl, whisk together the milk, applesauce, vanilla, vinegar, coconut oil, and maple syrup. In a large bowl, sift together the buckwheat flour, almond flour, baking powder, and baking soda. Add the milk mixture to the flour mixture and whisk just until smooth, taking care not to overmix or your pancakes won't be as fluffy.

In a large nonstick skillet, heat about 1 teaspoon coconut oil over medium heat. Add ¼ cup batter per pancake and cook until the top side of each pancake starts to bubble, 3 to 4 minutes. Flip and cook until the second side is matte, another minute or so. Transfer the pancakes to a plate and repeat with the remaining batter.

TO SERVE: Top the pancakes with the compote and drizzle with the cashew cream. If desired, you can also top the pancakes with almond butter, maple syrup, toasted nuts, and/or fresh fruit (or any combination of them!).

NOTE I recommend using light buckwheat flour for this recipe instead of dark. Light buckwheat flour will make the pancakes fluffier and less sticky.

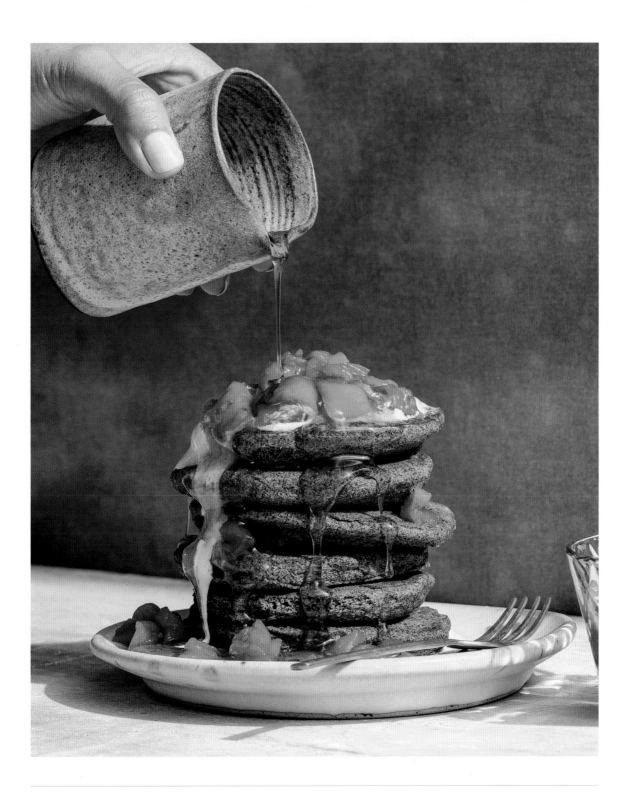

VARIATION *Buckwheat Waffles:* You can also use this batter in a waffle maker for perfect crispy, fluffy waffles (you'll get about 5). Simply preheat the waffle iron, spray or brush with oil, and add about ¾ cup to the iron, making sure it spreads evenly. Cook until the waffle is golden brown, the steam stops rising from the waffle iron, and the waffle lifts easily from the griddle. Serve with the sweet cashew cream and compote.

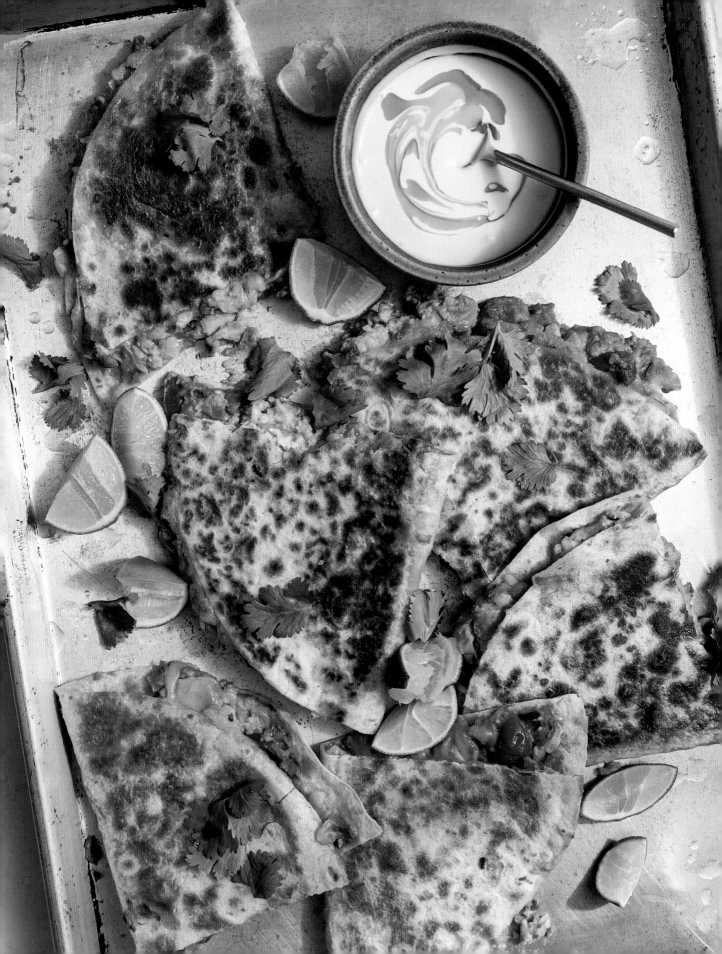

SMASHED CHIPOTLE BEANS AND AVOCADO QUESADILLA

Aside from being one of my all-time favorite Mexican foods, quesadillas are also the perfect quick savory breakfast that will keep you feeling satiated until lunchtime, especially when stuffed with creamy, spiced, protein-packed beans and omega-3-rich avocado. That said, these are just as perfect for lunch, especially topped with your favorite veggies.

SERVES *2 to 4*
TOTAL TIME: *30 minutes*

SMASHED BEANS

- 1 tablespoon avocado oil
- ½ cup finely shredded and chopped cabbage (about ¼ small head)
- ⅛ teaspoon asafoetida
- 1 15-ounce can pinto beans, rinsed and drained
- ½ tablespoon tomato paste
- 1 tablespoon finely chopped jalapeño pepper
- 1 tablespoon taco seasoning (or 1 teaspoon each ground cumin, paprika, and dried oregano)
- ½ teaspoon dried oregano
- ½ teaspoon sea salt
- ¼ teaspoon chipotle powder

AVOCADO SMASH

- 1 medium avocado, cubed
- 1 tablespoon fresh lime juice
- 5 cherry tomatoes, finely chopped
- 1 tablespoon chopped fresh cilantro leaves
- ¼ teaspoon sea salt

QUESADILLAS

- ½ cup vegan sour cream or plain vegan yogurt
- 2 tablespoons vegan mayonnaise
- Olive oil cooking spray or avocado oil
- 2 to 4 of your favorite 8- to 10-inch tortillas
- 1 cup shredded vegan melting cheese
- Hot sauce (optional)

MAKE THE SMASHED BEANS: In a large skillet, heat the oil over medium heat. Add the cabbage and asafoetida and cook, stirring, until soft, 3 to 5 minutes. Add the beans and tomato paste and use a potato masher or the back of a wooden spoon to mash about three-quarters of the beans as you mix them with the cabbage. Add the jalapeño, taco seasoning, oregano, salt, and chipotle powder and cook, stirring, until warmed through and deeply savory smelling, about 2 minutes. Remove the pan from the heat and set aside.

MAKE THE AVOCADO SMASH: In a medium bowl, use a fork to mash and mix the avocado and lime juice. Add the tomatoes, cilantro, and salt and toss gently to combine. Set aside.

MAKE THE QUESADILLAS: In a small bowl, whisk together the sour cream and mayonnaise. Set aside.

Heat a large skillet over medium heat and lightly coat with the olive oil spray or avocado oil. Add a tortilla and toast for about 1 minute per side.

Reduce the heat to low and spread 2 or 3 tablespoons of the smashed beans on one half of the tortilla, followed by 2 tablespoons of the avocado smash and a generous sprinkle of cheese. Fold the tortilla in half and press down gently with a spatula. Increase the heat to medium and cook until the cheese melts and the tortilla is browned and crispy, about 2 minutes per side. Transfer the quesadilla to a plate and repeat with the remaining tortillas and fillings. Remove the pan from the heat.

Cut the tortillas into wedges and drizzle with the sour cream mixture. If desired, serve with your favorite hot sauce.

MAKE-AHEAD Though these are best straight out of the pan, if you have leftovers or want to make them ahead, you can reheat them in a skillet until warmed through.

VEGGIE FRITTATA MUFFINS

For those days when it's nothing but go, go, go, I'm always grateful to have a breakfast option that can be enjoyed while in motion. These muffins are made with protein-rich chickpea flour and can be customized to whatever veg and fresh herbs you like or have on hand (see Note). Plus, they can be enjoyed hot, cold, plain, or slathered in dips. This recipe can also be made into a single quiche (see Variation), which is great for serving company or bringing with you to a picnic—it's a great bring-a-dish dish.

No matter how fast-paced your morning is, I do suggest taking just a moment to pause and say a prayer of gratitude before diving in.

MAKES *12 muffins*
TOTAL TIME: *45 minutes*

- Olive oil cooking spray, sunflower oil, or avocado oil for the muffin tin
- 2 cups chickpea flour (chana lot)
- 1 cup tightly packed chopped spinach
- 2 tablespoons nutritional yeast
- 2 tablespoons fresh lemon juice
- 1 tablespoon Italian seasoning, plus more for topping
- 1 tablespoon sunflower or avocado oil
- 1 teaspoon sea salt
- 1 teaspoon baking powder
- ½ teaspoon baking soda
- ¼ teaspoon asafoetida
- 1 cup finely chopped red bell pepper
- ½ cup finely chopped fresh herbs, such as basil, parsley, or dill (or a combination)
- ½ cup chopped pitted green olives, sun-dried tomatoes, and/or pickled or fresh jalapeño peppers
- ¾ cup crumbled vegan feta cheese
- Muhammara (page 233) or your favorite sauce or dip (see Feeling Saucy, page 231), for serving (optional)

Preheat the oven to 375°F. Lightly coat 12 cups of a standard muffin tin with cooking spray.

In a large bowl, whisk together the chickpea flour, chopped spinach, nutritional yeast, lemon juice, Italian seasoning, oil, salt, baking powder, baking soda, and asafoetida. Add 2 cups water and whisk until the batter is completely smooth. Fold in the chopped bell pepper, herbs, olive mixture, and ½ cup of the feta.

Scoop about ¼ cup of the batter into each cup of the muffin tin, mixing gently between scoops to make sure the vegetables stay well distributed in the batter. Dividing evenly, top the muffins with the remaining ¼ cup feta and a small pinch of Italian seasoning.

Bake until the muffins are set, 25 to 30 minutes. Let the muffins cool in the pan for 5 minutes, then gently remove them and transfer to a wire rack. Serve warm or at room temperature with a sauce or dip, if desired.

NOTE Feel free to swap out the bell pepper and herbs for any other vegetables or herbs you have in the fridge.

FRITTATA QUICHE

MAKES *1 10-inch quiche (serves 6 to 8)*
TOTAL TIME: *1 hour 5 minutes*

- 1 store-bought refrigerated pie crust (or your favorite homemade recipe)
- Muffin batter (from Veggie Frittata Muffins, opposite)
- Thinly sliced tomatoes, for topping
- Italian seasoning, for sprinkling

If using a store-bought pie crust, prebake it at the temperature given on the package for about 5 minutes, until it's warm and pliable. Remove the crust and adjust the oven temperature to 400°F.

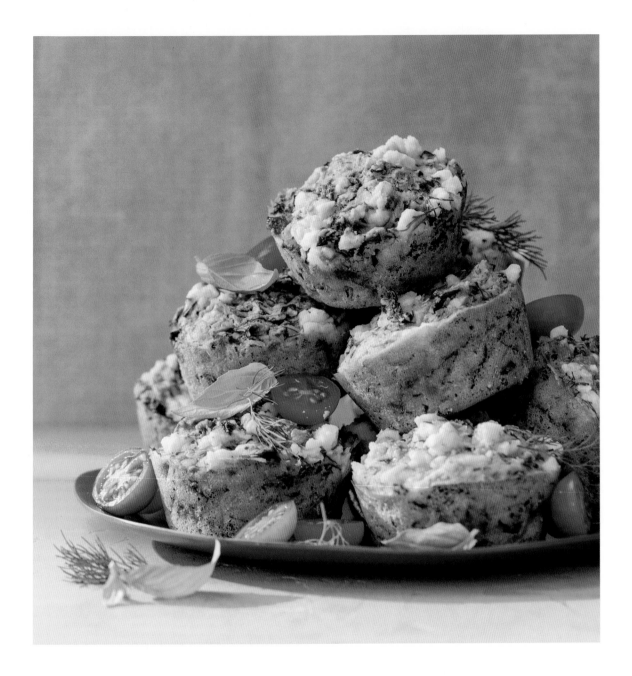

If using a homemade pie crust, roll the dough into a thin 13-inch round. Gently drape the dough over a 10-inch pie plate, slowly working it down as you press it into the bottom and sides, leaving a little extra on the sides to account for shrinking. Use a fork to prick the dough all over the base and sides. Bake until lightly golden brown, about 5 minutes. Set aside to let cool completely.

Meanwhile, make the batter as directed, stirring in the chopped vegetables and herbs and sprinkling the feta on top.

Scrape the filling into the cooled pie crust, top with the tomato slices and sprinkle with a pinch of Italian seasoning. Slide into the oven and bake until the center is set, 40 to 45 minutes.

Serve warm or at room temperature. Store any leftovers in a sealed container. It will last for up to 3 days.

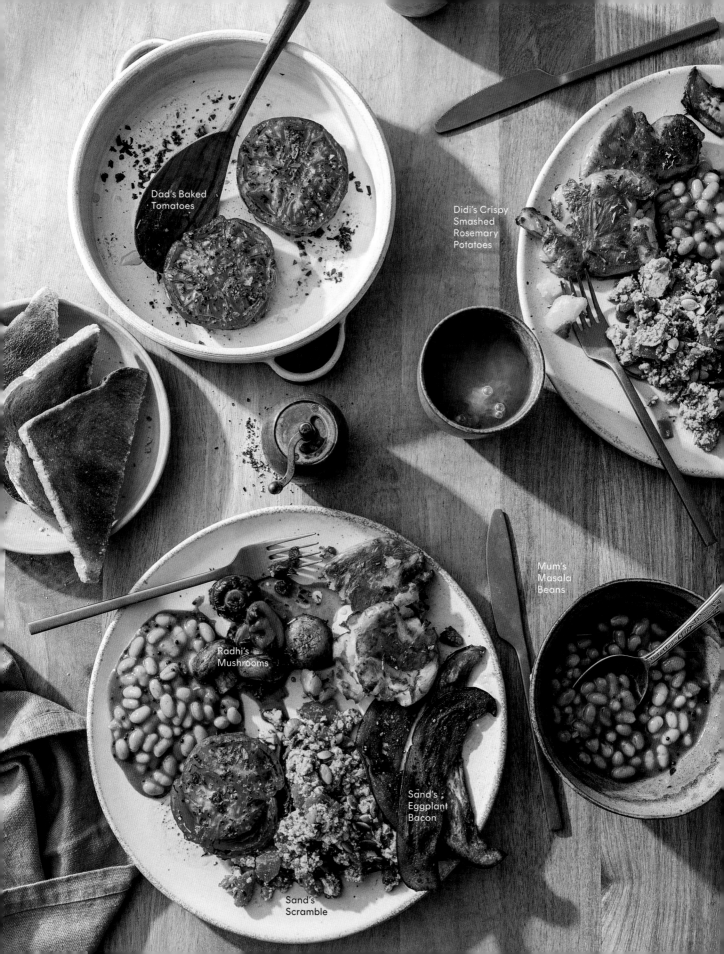

Dad's Baked Tomatoes

Didi's Crispy Smashed Rosemary Potatoes

Mum's Masala Beans

Radhi's Mushrooms

Sand's Eggplant Bacon

Sand's Scramble

MY FAMILY'S INDIAN ENGLISH BREAKFAST

Ask any English person what their favorite breakfast is, and they'll most likely tell you that it's a "fry-up," or a big traditional spread with sausage, beans, toast, and all the fixings. But that doesn't mean that we vegans can't get in on the action! With my brother-in-law's now-famous scramble and sweet-smoky eggplant bacon, my dad's caramelized baked tomatoes, my mum's masala beans, my sister's crispy smashed potatoes, and my herby mushrooms, we cook up a *proper* morning feast. Be sure to serve yours like we do—with plenty of sourdough toast and sliced avocados.

SERVES 6

SAND'S EGGPLANT BACON

TOTAL TIME: *1 hour 10 minutes*

1 medium eggplant

2 tablespoons extra-virgin olive oil

1½ tablespoons maple syrup

1 tablespoon soy sauce

1 teaspoon smoked paprika

½ teaspoon liquid smoke

½ teaspoon freshly ground black pepper

Pinch of sea salt

Trim off both ends of the eggplant and cut it lengthwise into ⅛-inch-thick slabs. A mandoline works well here for getting them nice and thin. Slice each slab lengthwise into 2-inch-wide strips. Set aside.

In a large baking dish, whisk together the olive oil, maple syrup, soy sauce, smoked paprika, liquid smoke, pepper, and salt. Add the eggplant strips to the maple syrup mixture and marinate at room temperature for 30 minutes.

Preheat the oven to 350°F. Line a sheet pan with parchment paper.

Arrange the eggplant strips in an even layer on the prepared pan and drizzle any remaining marinade over the top. Bake until the eggplant strips are browned and crispy, 30 to 40 minutes, turning halfway through.

DAD'S BAKED TOMATOES

TOTAL TIME: *25 minutes*

2 tablespoons extra-virgin olive oil or chili oil

1 tablespoon balsamic vinegar

1 tablespoon finely chopped fresh parsley leaves

½ teaspoon Italian seasoning

½ teaspoon sea salt

¼ teaspoon freshly ground black pepper

4 large tomatoes, such as beefsteak, halved widthwise

Preheat the oven to 450°F. Line a baking sheet with parchment paper.

In a large bowl, whisk together the olive oil, vinegar, parsley, Italian seasoning, salt, and pepper. Gently toss the tomatoes in the mixture.

Arrange the tomatoes cut-side up on the prepared baking sheet. Bake until soft, juicy, and caramelized, 15 to 20 minutes.

Recipes Continue

SAND'S SCRAMBLE

TOTAL TIME: *20 minutes*

- 1 tablespoon extra-virgin olive oil
- 1 14.5-ounce can diced tomatoes
- 1 large beefsteak tomato, finely chopped (optional)
- 2 celery stalks, finely chopped
- 1 tablespoon Italian seasoning
- 1 teaspoon ground turmeric
- 1 teaspoon garam masala or Ground CCF Masala (page 49)
- 1 teaspoon smoked paprika
- 1 teaspoon sea salt
- 1 teaspoon freshly ground black pepper
- 2 12-ounce blocks firm tofu, drained
- ½ cup chopped fresh spinach
- ⅓ cup chopped fresh cilantro leaves
- 1 tablespoon liquid aminos
- 2 teaspoons fresh lemon juice
- Sunflower or pumpkin seeds, for serving

In a large skillet, heat the oil over medium heat. Add the canned tomatoes, fresh tomatoes (if using), celery, Italian seasoning, turmeric, garam masala, smoked paprika, salt, and black pepper. Cook, stirring frequently, until the tomatoes have softened, about 5 minutes.

Crumble in the tofu and cook, stirring constantly, until the liquid evaporates and the scramble thickens slightly, about 5 minutes.

Stir in the spinach, cilantro, liquid aminos, and lemon juice and remove the pan from the heat. Serve topped with the seeds for extra crunch.

MUM'S MASALA BEANS

TOTAL TIME: *10 minutes*

- 1 teaspoon extra-virgin olive oil
- ½ teaspoon brown or black mustard seeds
- 1 small hot Indian or Thai green chile, chopped
- 1 fresh or 10 dried curry leaves, chopped
- ½ teaspoon garam masala or Ground CCF Masala (page 49)
- ¼ teaspoon ground turmeric
- ¼ teaspoon sea salt
- 1 16-ounce can vegetarian baked beans (I like Heinz)

In a medium saucepan, heat the oil over medium-low heat. Add the mustard seeds, cover the pan, and let the seeds warm until they pop, 15 to 30 seconds. Add the chile, curry leaf, masala, turmeric, and salt and cook, stirring, for 1 minute to bloom the spices. Stir in the beans, increase the heat to medium, and bring to a simmer. Cook, stirring, until the flavors have come together, 2 to 3 minutes. Remove from the heat and serve.

DIDI'S CRISPY SMASHED ROSEMARY POTATOES

TOTAL TIME: *1 hour 20 minutes*

- 1½ pounds red, purple, or gold baby potatoes
- 2 tablespoons extra-virgin olive oil or melted unsalted vegan butter, plus more as needed
- 1 tablespoon minced fresh rosemary
- Sea salt
- Freshly ground black pepper
- So Much More Than a Burger Sauce (page 235), ketchup, or dip of choice

Bring a medium pot of water to a boil over medium-high heat. Add the potatoes and a generous pinch of salt. Boil until the potatoes are fork-tender, about 20 minutes. Drain the potatoes and let them steam-dry in a colander.

Meanwhile, preheat the oven to 400°F. Lightly coat a baking sheet with a bit of the olive oil or melted butter. Place a piece of parchment paper on top, flatten the parchment with your hands to distribute the oil, then flip the paper. Set aside.

Transfer the potatoes to the parchment, drizzle with a little more of the oil or butter, and toss to coat. Arrange the potatoes in an even layer. Use a potato masher, spatula, or bottom of a glass to gently flatten the potatoes, trying to keep them in one piece. The thinner they are, the crispier they will get! Let the potatoes sit for 5 minutes to allow any extra moisture to evaporate. Brush the potatoes with the rest of the oil or butter and season with the rosemary, plus a pinch of salt and a few cracks of pepper.

Bake undisturbed until golden and crispy, 30 to 40 minutes.

Serve hot with your dip of choice; we love our So Much More Than a Burger Sauce (page 235; inspired by the sauce at In-N-Out Burger) or ketchup with this!

RADHI'S MUSHROOMS

TOTAL TIME: *15 minutes*

- 1 tablespoon extra-virgin olive oil
- 8 ounces small cremini (chestnut) mushrooms, halved or kept whole
- 1 tablespoon liquid aminos
- 1 teaspoon Italian seasoning
- 1 teaspoon maple syrup
- 1 teaspoon fresh thyme leaves or ½ teaspoon dried thyme
- ¼ teaspoon red chile flakes (optional)
- ⅛ teaspoon asafoetida

In a large skillet, heat the oil over medium heat. Add the mushrooms, aminos, Italian seasoning, maple syrup, thyme, chile flakes (if using), and asafoetida and cook, stirring, until the mushrooms have released their juices and the water evaporates, about 10 minutes. Remove from the heat and serve.

FRENCH TOAST CASSEROLE

When people start moving toward a more plant-based lifestyle, one thing I always hear is that they're sad to leave behind their favorite dishes, especially those that bring them comfort or connect them with their favorite memories. My mum showed me that with just a little creativity and experimentation, you can absolutely re-create those dishes—and make them even *better*. This decadent French toast casserole is the perfect example—it's lusciously custardy, plus it gets a sweet crunch from a maple-y pecan topping.

SERVES 6
TOTAL TIME: *50 minutes*

CASSEROLE

Unsalted vegan butter for the baking dish

2½ cups plain unsweetened almond or oat milk

3 tablespoons maple syrup

2 tablespoons cornstarch or all-purpose flour

2 tablespoons flaxmeal

½ tablespoon vanilla extract

1 14-ounce loaf fresh or day-old sourdough bread, cut into 1-inch cubes

PECAN TOPPING

½ cup chopped pecans

¼ cup almond flour or all-purpose flour

¼ cup coconut sugar

1 tablespoon maple syrup

1 teaspoon ground cinnamon

FOR SERVING

Maple syrup

Sweet Cashew Cream (page 263), vanilla vegan yogurt, or whipped coconut cream

Mixed berries

MAKE THE CASSEROLE: Butter an 11 × 14-inch baking dish and set aside.

In a large bowl, whisk together the milk, maple syrup, cornstarch, flaxmeal, and vanilla. Set aside for 5 minutes.

Scatter the bread cubes in an even layer in the prepared baking dish. Pour the milk mixture over the bread, gently pressing down on any cubes that are poking out. Let sit for at least 15 minutes, or up to overnight in the fridge.

MAKE THE TOPPING: In a medium bowl, toss together the pecans, almond flour, sugar, syrup, and cinnamon. Set aside.

Preheat the oven to 375°F.

Sprinkle the pecan topping evenly over the bread and bake until golden brown on top, about 30 minutes.

Serve warm with maple syrup, cashew cream, and mixed berries.

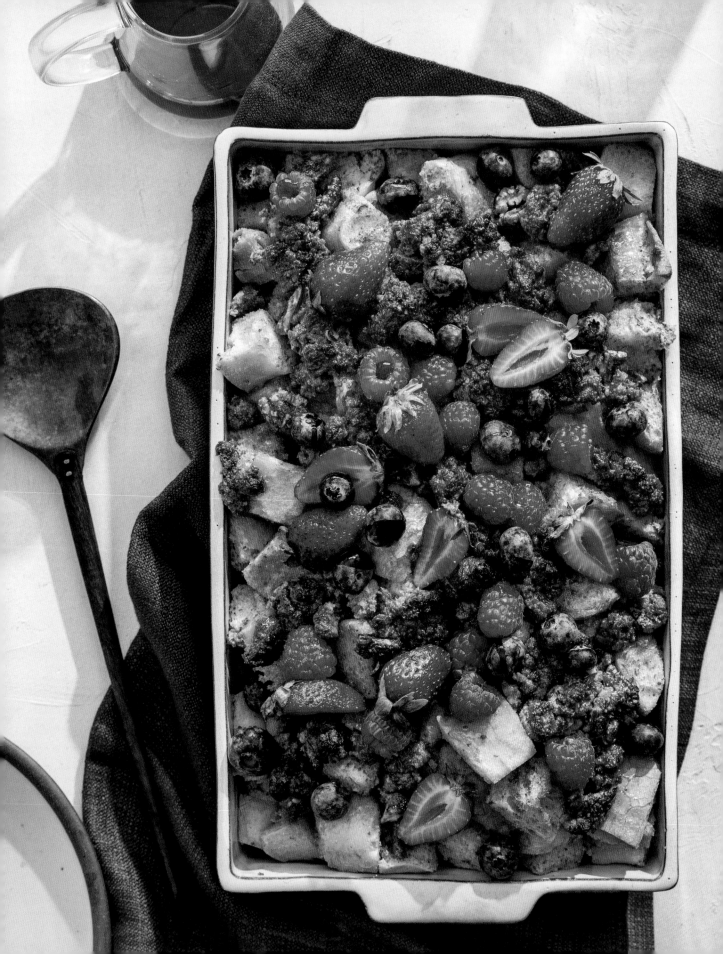

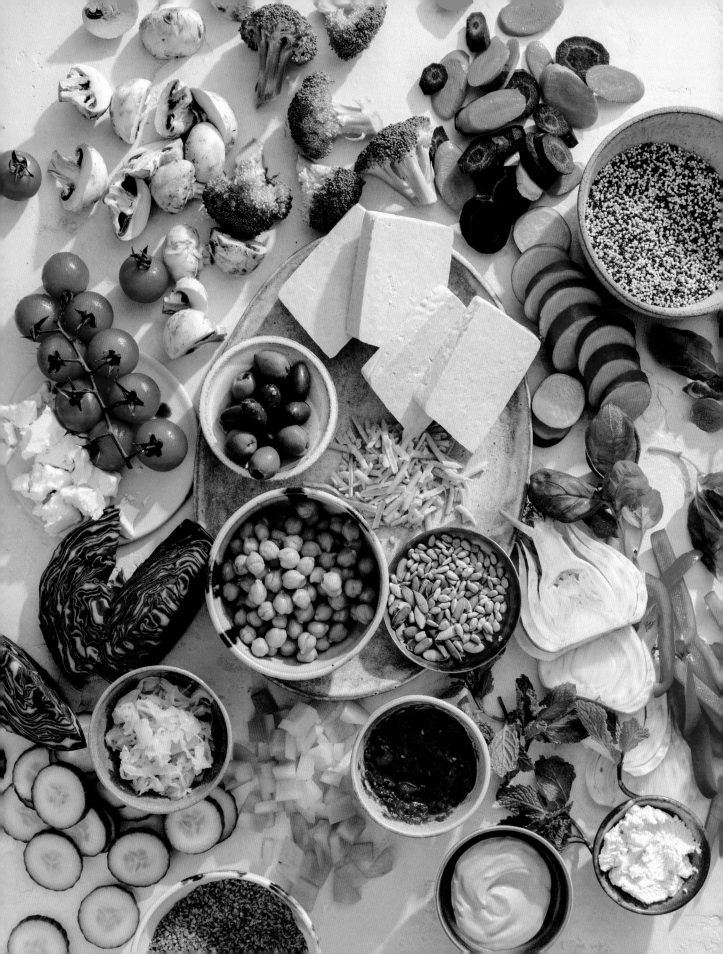

GROUNDING GRAINS

I love grains because not only do they provide energy—our bodies use them most readily as a source of energy—but also because they're comforting to eat: a unique joy unlike any other food there is. These recipes are perfect for midday when your digestive fire is roaring and ready to take on your biggest, most vitalizing meal that will deliver even, sustained fuel—with maximum yumminess, of course.

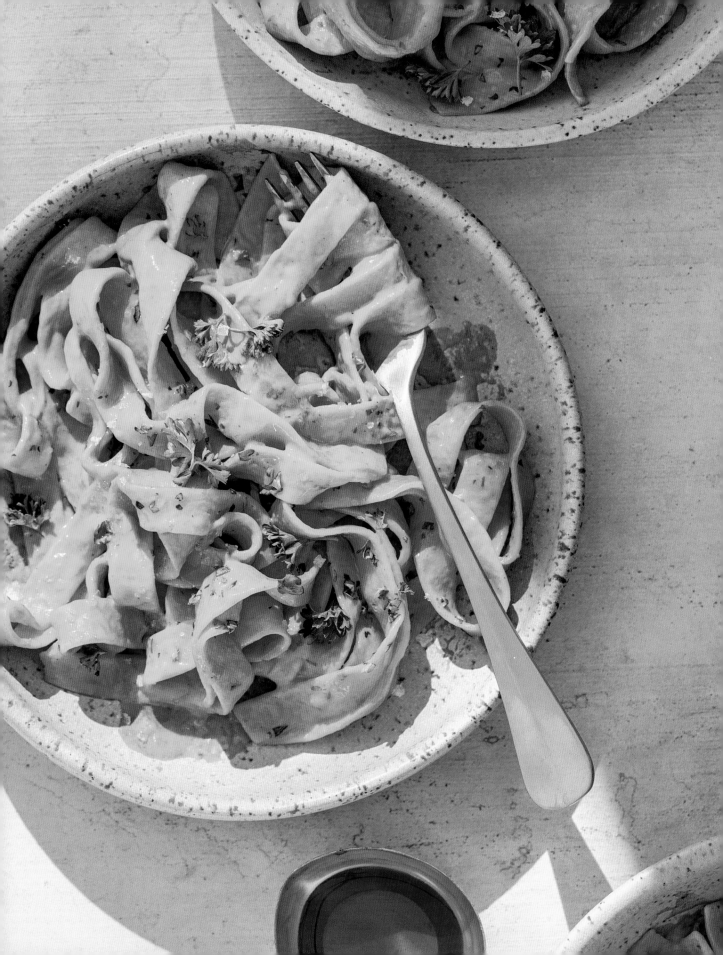

ROASTED RED PEPPER TAGLIATELLE

Consider this an upgrade to your basic marinara pasta dish, almost like Italian and Middle Eastern food had a beautiful baby. The red peppers give the sauce a vibrant orange color and even deeper roast-y flavor, while the tahini lends its signature creamy richness.

SERVES *4*
TOTAL TIME: *35 minutes*

- 3 medium red bell peppers (see Note)
- 1 tablespoon plus 3 teaspoons extra-virgin olive oil
- ½ cup canned full-fat coconut milk
- ½ cup unsweetened almond milk
- ⅓ cup tahini
- 2 tablespoons fresh lemon juice
- 2 tablespoons nutritional yeast
- 1 tablespoon Dijon mustard
- 2 teaspoons yellow miso
- 2 teaspoons paprika
- 1 teaspoon sea salt
- 12 ounces dried tagliatelle pasta
- 2 bay leaves
- ¼ teaspoon asafoetida
- ¼ cup chopped fresh parsley leaves, plus more for serving
- Chili oil, for serving (optional)

Preheat the oven to 425°F. Line a baking sheet with parchment paper.

Coat each pepper with 1 teaspoon of the oil. Set the whole peppers on the prepared baking sheet and roast until each side is charred, 5 to 7 minutes per side, about 20 minutes total. Set aside until the peppers are cool enough to handle. Once cooled, slip off the charred skins and remove the seeds.

In a high-powered blender, combine the roasted red peppers, coconut milk, almond milk, tahini, lemon juice, nutritional yeast, mustard, miso, paprika, and salt and blend until completely smooth.

Cook the pasta according to the package directions.

While the pasta cooks, in a large nonstick pan, heat the remaining 1 tablespoon oil over medium heat. Add the bay leaves and asafoetida and cook, stirring, until the bay leaves are fragrant, about 30 seconds. Add the blended pepper sauce and stir to combine. Reduce the heat to low and simmer until the sauce is warmed through and the flavors have combined, about 5 minutes. Fold in the chopped parsley.

Drain the pasta and add it directly to the sauce, tossing the pasta to coat it evenly. Remove the pan from the heat and top with more chopped parsley and a drizzle of chili oil, if desired. Serve immediately.

Store leftovers in a sealed container in the refrigerator for up to 3 days.

NOTE You could also use 1 cup jarred roasted red peppers. Skip the roasting step and move to the pureeing step.

SPICY INDIAN PASTA

When I was growing up, my cousin Anisha and I spent our school holidays together. I would stay for a few weeks at her house, or she'd come to mine, but wherever we were, we had a ritual of staying up late and making a midnight feast. One of the most memorable things she whipped up was this ridiculously spicy pasta with all kinds of chiles and hot sauce and masala and loads of cheese. We shared so many conversations and laughs (and hot sweats) over that big bowl of pasta that it felt only right that I share this dish with you—and wish you the very same! This dish will easily scale up if you have more people who want to join the fun.

SERVES *2*

TOTAL TIME: *30 minutes*

- 1 cup short fusilli pasta
- 1½ tablespoons extra-virgin olive oil
- 1 cup diced green bell pepper (about 1 large pepper)
- ½ cup finely chopped cabbage (about ½ small head)
- 1 small hot Indian or Thai green chile, sliced
- ½ tablespoon dried oregano
- 1 teaspoon curry powder, garam masala, or Ground CCF Masala (page 49)
- 1 teaspoon sea salt
- ½ teaspoon ground coriander
- ½ teaspoon freshly ground black pepper
- ¼ teaspoon ground turmeric
- ¼ teaspoon asafoetida
- 1 cup canned crushed tomatoes
- ½ cup passata (or more crushed tomatoes)
- ½ cup fresh sweet corn kernels (about 1 ear) or thawed frozen
- 1 tablespoon nutritional yeast
- 1 tablespoon soy sauce
- 2 tablespoons fresh cilantro leaves, for serving
- 2 tablespoons canned full-fat coconut milk or vegan cream, for serving (optional)
- 2 tablespoons shredded vegan cheddar cheese, for serving

Cook the pasta according to the package directions. Drain and set aside.

Meanwhile, in a large skillet, heat the oil over medium heat. Add the bell pepper, cabbage, and green chile and cook, stirring, until the vegetables soften, about 5 minutes. Add the oregano, curry powder, salt, coriander, black pepper, turmeric, and asafoetida and cook, stirring, until the spices are fragrant, about 1 minute.

Reduce the heat to low and add the crushed tomatoes, passata, corn, nutritional yeast, and soy sauce. Cook, stirring occasionally, until the sauce is warmed through and the flavors have combined, about 5 minutes. Add the cooked pasta to the sauce and toss to coat.

Serve warm topped with the cilantro, coconut milk (if using), and cheese.

Store leftovers in a sealed container in the refrigerator for up to 3 days.

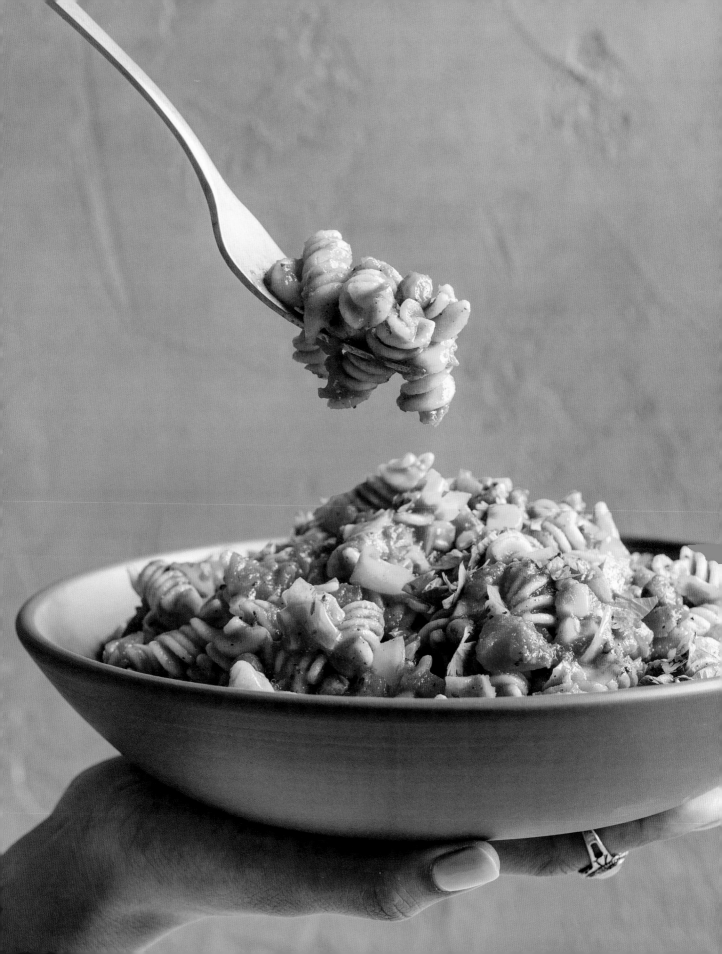

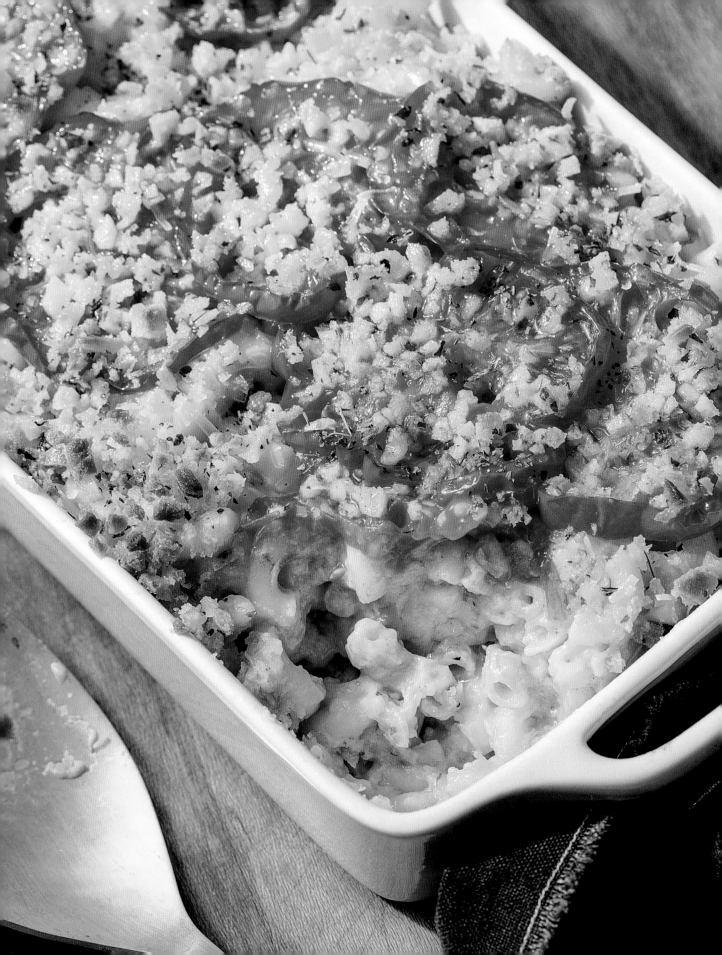

DAD'S MAC 'N' SHEEZE

Whenever my mum would go out of town, my dad would be in charge of mealtime, and his signature dish was this take on mac 'n' cheese. As much as we'd of course miss Mum, we'd always look forward to her leaving because we'd not only get to eat dinner in front of the TV (something we wouldn't usually do if she were home!) but we'd also get to enjoy this indulgent dish with its baked golden crust and rich, creamy center.

SERVES *4*

TOTAL TIME: *45 minutes*

- Olive oil cooking spray or avocado oil
- 2 cups (8 ounces) elbow macaroni
- ⅓ cup unsalted vegan butter
- ¼ cup all-purpose or spelt flour
- 2½ cups plain unsweetened almond or oat milk
- 1¼ cups shredded vegan cheddar cheese
- 2 tablespoons nutritional yeast
- 1 teaspoon sea salt
- ½ teaspoon paprika
- ½ tablespoon yellow English mustard or Dijon mustard
- ¼ teaspoon asafoetida
- ¼ teaspoon freshly ground black pepper
- 2 medium Roma tomatoes or 1 cup cherry tomatoes, sliced
- ¼ cup chopped pickled jalapeños
- 1 tablespoon dried parsley
- 1 cup panko bread crumbs

Preheat the oven to 350°F. Lightly coat a 2-quart baking dish with cooking spray or avocado oil.

Cook the macaroni according to the package directions. Drain and set aside.

In a large saucepan, melt the butter over medium heat. Sprinkle the flour evenly over the butter, whisking constantly until it forms a smooth paste. Reduce the heat to low and continue cooking until golden, 2 to 3 minutes. Add the milk slowly, whisking constantly until smooth and combined. Increase the heat to medium-high and bring the mixture to a boil. Reduce the heat to a simmer and cook, stirring occasionally, until thickened, about 10 minutes.

Whisk in ¾ cup of the cheese, the yeast, salt, paprika, mustard, asafoetida, and black pepper, whisking until smooth. Add the cooked macaroni and toss to coat. Transfer the mixture to the prepared baking dish and top with the remaining ½ cup cheese. Layer on the sliced tomatoes and pickled jalapeños, followed by the parsley and panko.

Bake until the cheese is melted and the bread crumbs are golden, 15 to 20 minutes. Let stand for 5 minutes or so to cool before serving.

Store leftovers in a sealed container in the refrigerator for up to 3 days.

STICKY HOISIN UDON NOODLES

I developed this recipe as a play on Chinese takeout. It's got that signature blend of crunchy stir-fried veg, plus a plummy sweet sauce that clings to the noodles and makes everything sticky and delicious.

SERVES *2*
TOTAL TIME: *20 minutes*

SAUCE

2 tablespoons soy sauce

1½ tablespoons sambal oelek

1 tablespoon molasses

½ tablespoon agave nectar

½ tablespoon cornstarch

½ teaspoon Chinese five-spice powder

NOODLES

8 ounces udon noodles

1 tablespoon toasted sesame oil

1 cup shredded napa cabbage (about ½ small head)

1 cup peeled and julienned carrots (about 2 medium carrots)

1 cup thinly sliced green bell pepper (about 1 large pepper)

1 cup sliced shiitake mushrooms (about 3 ounces)

1 teaspoon grated fresh ginger

⅛ teaspoon asafoetida

1 tablespoon white sesame seeds

2 tablespoons chopped fresh cilantro leaves

MAKE THE SAUCE: In a jar with a tight-fitting lid, combine the soy sauce, sambal, molasses, agave, cornstarch, and five-spice powder. Seal the jar and shake well to combine. Set aside.

MAKE THE NOODLES: In a large pot, cook the noodles according to the package instructions. Drain and set aside.

In a large skillet, heat the sesame oil over medium-high heat. Add the cabbage, carrots, bell pepper, mushrooms, ginger, and asafoetida and cook, stirring constantly, until the vegetables are tender but still crisp, 6 to 8 minutes.

Reduce the heat to low and pour the sauce over the vegetables. Cook, stirring frequently, until the sauce thickens and releases its sweet-savory aroma, about 1 minute. Add the noodles and cook, stirring and tossing to coat, 1 to 2 minutes.

Divide the noodles between two bowls and top with the sesame seeds and cilantro.

Store leftovers in a sealed container in the refrigerator for up to 3 days.

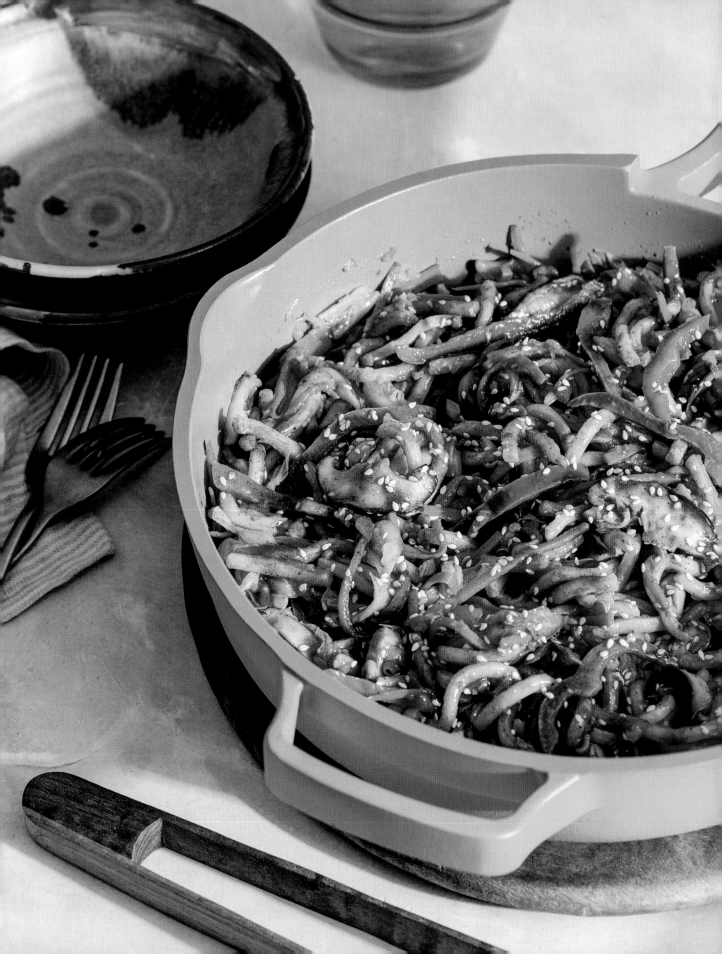

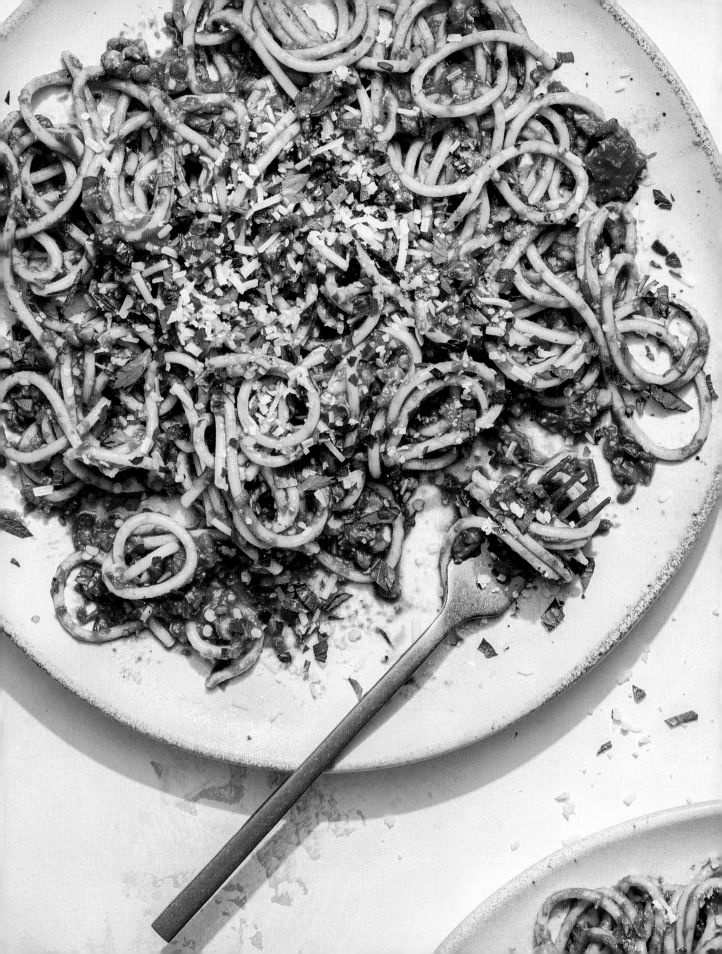

WALNUT-LENTIL BOLOGNESE

I am a firm believer in having a dish for every mood, and this one happens to be completely appropriate for so many of them. Celebrating the end of a productive, satisfying day? Bolognese. Need a comforting hug of a dish because you're feeling a little down? Bolognese. Hungry? Bolognese. My version of the traditional preparation is loaded with hearty walnuts and lentils, veggies, and tons of herbs, which is guaranteed to always be just the thing.

SERVES *2*
TOTAL TIME: *30 minutes*

- 6 ounces pappardelle or spaghetti
- 2 cups finely chopped walnuts
- 1 cup cooked or canned lentils
- ¾ cup peeled and finely chopped carrots (about 1½ medium carrots)
- ⅓ cup finely chopped celery (about 1 stalk)
- 1 tablespoon Italian seasoning
- 1 tablespoon dried parsley
- ½ tablespoon dried oregano
- 1 teaspoon sea salt
- ¼ teaspoon asafoetida
- 2 tablespoons extra-virgin olive oil
- 1 28-ounce can crushed tomatoes
- 2 bay leaves
- 1 teaspoon light brown sugar
- Grated or shaved vegan parmesan, for serving
- Chopped fresh parsley leaves, for serving
- Sliced fresh red chiles or red chile flakes, for serving

Cook the pasta according to the package directions. Reserve ½ cup of the cooking liquid and drain the pasta. Return the pasta to the pot and add just enough of the cooking liquid to coat the pasta (see Note). Set aside.

Meanwhile, in a food processor, combine the walnuts, lentils, carrots, celery, Italian seasoning, parsley, oregano, salt, and asafoetida and pulse until the mixture is coarse and chunky.

In a medium saucepan, heat the oil over medium-low heat. Add the tomatoes, bay leaves, and brown sugar and cook, stirring, until simmering, about 5 minutes. Add the walnut and lentil mixture and cook, stirring, until the flavors have come together and the sauce begins to smell deeply toasty and savory, another 5 minutes. Add the cooked pasta and toss well to coat.

Serve with lots of vegan parmesan, chopped fresh parsley, and sliced red chiles or chile flakes.

Store leftovers in a sealed container in the refrigerator for up to 3 days.

NOTE Many people toss cooked pasta with some oil to keep the noodles from sticking together, but that actually creates a barrier between the flavorful sauce and pasta. Instead, I recommend either just rinsing the pasta with a little cold water or keeping some of the cooking water in the pot with the pasta until you're ready to add the sauce.

MEXICAN LASAGNA

This is real-life cooking at its finest. Instead of the fuss of making individual enchiladas or burritos, you can throw all your favorite ingredients into a baking dish—the tortillas, the filling, the veggies, the sauce, the cheese (so much cheese)—dollop on some sour cream and guac, oooh and some spicy or lime-y crushed tortilla chips, and you're good to go. It's a truly fuss-free feast.

SERVES *4*

TOTAL TIME: *40 minutes*

FILLING

- 1 tablespoon sunflower or avocado oil
- 1 cup finely chopped or shredded cabbage (about ½ small head)
- 1½ cups cooked black beans or 1 15-ounce can, rinsed and drained
- 1½ cups cooked pinto beans or 1 15-ounce can, rinsed and drained
- 1 cup fresh sweet corn kernels (about 2 ears) or thawed frozen
- 3 tablespoons finely chopped pickled or fresh jalapeño (about 1 large pepper)
- 2½ teaspoons taco seasoning (or 1 teaspoon each ground cumin, paprika, and dried oregano)
- 1 teaspoon sea salt

LASAGNA

- Olive oil cooking spray, sunflower oil, or avocado oil
- 4 of your favorite 8- or 10-inch tortillas, cut into 1-inch-wide strips
- 1 cup of your favorite salsa or canned crushed tomatoes
- 1 cup shredded vegan cheddar cheese or a blend of cheddar and mozzarella

FOR SERVING

- Guacamole
- Vegan sour cream
- Tortilla chips (optional)

Preheat the oven to 425°F.

MAKE THE FILLING: In a large skillet, heat the oil over medium heat. Add the cabbage and cook, stirring, until softened, about 5 minutes. Add the black beans, pinto beans, corn, jalapeños, taco seasoning, and salt and cook, stirring occasionally, until the flavors have come together and the seasonings are aromatic, about 5 minutes. Remove the pan from the heat and set the filling aside.

ASSEMBLE THE LASAGNA: Lightly coat an 8-inch square baking dish with cooking spray. Spread about one-third of the tortilla strips in an even layer across the bottom, trying to avoid any gaps. Add half of the bean mixture in another even layer, followed by another one-third of the tortilla strips. Layer with the remaining bean mixture and top with the remaining tortilla strips. Finish with the salsa and cheese.

Bake until hot and bubbling, about 20 minutes.

TO SERVE: Cut the lasagna into squares and serve with the guacamole and sour cream, plus chips, if you like.

Store leftovers in a sealed container in the refrigerator for up to 3 days.

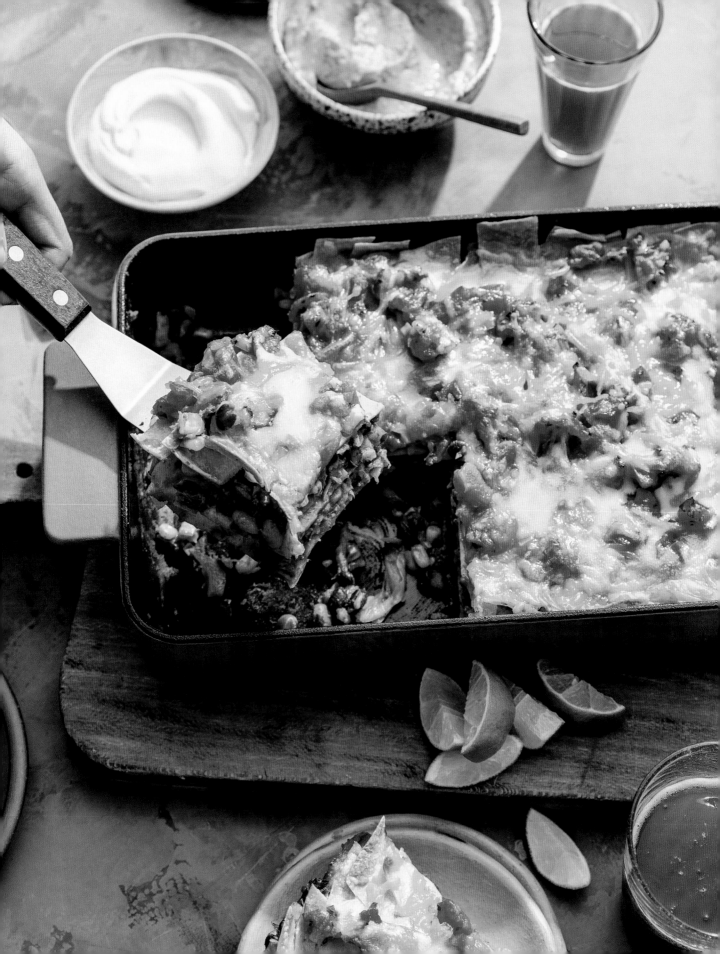

ONE-POT LEMONY SPAGHETTI

For a dish this simple, I've only got three words: creamy, zesty perfection. All the ingredients are tossed in a single pot, so they cook down with the starch from the pasta, which blends with the coconut milk to make the most luxurious—and refreshingly effortless—lemon-scented sauce. I like to top off the pasta with a spoonful of Pistachio Gremolata (page 253), which I keep stashed in the fridge for any time I need a hit of bright, herby crunch. This is an under-30-minute meal, but you'd never guess it.

SERVES *4*
TOTAL TIME: *30 minutes*

- 1 13.5-ounce can full-fat coconut milk
- 2 tablespoons extra-virgin olive oil or vegan butter (or, if you have it, 1 tablespoon chili oil and 1 tablespoon extra-virgin olive oil)
- 3 tablespoons fresh lemon juice
- ½ tablespoon Dijon mustard
- 2 teaspoons yellow miso
- 2 teaspoons sea salt
- ¼ teaspoon asafoetida
- 1 7.7-ounce package brown rice spaghetti or your favorite spaghetti
- Pistachio Gremolata (optional; page 253), for serving

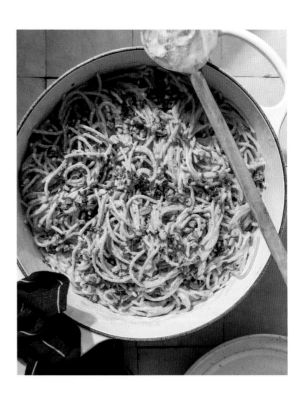

In a large saucepan, combine 2½ cups water, the coconut milk, olive oil, lemon juice, mustard, miso, salt, and asafoetida. Bring the mixture to a boil over high heat and add the spaghetti, gently pushing it down into the pan as it softens. Reduce the heat to medium-low and cook, uncovered, stirring occasionally, until the pasta is cooked and the sauce thickens up, 15 to 20 minutes. Remove the pot from the heat.

Divide the pasta among four bowls. If desired, dollop with the gremolata.

Store leftovers in a sealed container in the refrigerator for up to 3 days.

MAKE-AHEAD If made ahead, gently heat the pasta with a splash of water since it will soak up the sauce as it sits.

THAI CURRY FRIED RICE

I like to think of this dish as being the one-and-done version of Thai curry and rice. It will satisfy your craving for aromatic coconut milk curry with plenty of fresh green heat, and I've simplified the cooking process so that the rice is simmered right in the sauce. The curry gets creamy from that extra starch, while the rice gets to soak up all that extra flavor. Winning all around.

SERVES *2*
TOTAL TIME: *30 minutes*

RICE

- 1 cup canned full-fat coconut milk
- ½ cup chopped green bell pepper
- ⅓ cup chopped fresh cilantro leaves
- 6 fresh makrut or Thai lime leaves (dried will work in a pinch)
- 2 stalks lemongrass, trimmed and roughly chopped
- 1 large green hot chile, such as Thai, roughly chopped
- 2 tablespoons soy sauce
- Juice of ½ lime
- 1 tablespoon minced fresh ginger
- ½ tablespoon coconut sugar
- 1 teaspoon coriander seeds
- 1 teaspoon cumin seeds
- 1 teaspoon sea salt
- ⅓ cup jasmine rice

VEGETABLES

- 1 tablespoon sunflower or avocado oil
- 1 cup thinly sliced zucchini half-moons (about 1 medium zucchini)
- ½ cup peeled and julienned carrot (about ½ medium)
- ½ cup thinly sliced green bell pepper (about ½ large)
- ½ cup chopped fresh broccoli florets (about ⅓ small head)

MAKE THE RICE: In a high-powered blender, combine the coconut milk, bell pepper, cilantro, lime leaves, lemongrass, green chile, soy sauce, lime juice, ginger, sugar, coriander, cumin, and salt and blend until completely smooth.

Transfer the sauce to a medium saucepan and bring to a low boil over medium-high heat. Reduce the heat to low, stir in the rice, cover, and simmer the mixture until the rice is tender, about 15 minutes. Remove from the heat and set aside.

MAKE THE VEGETABLES: In a large nonstick skillet, heat the oil over medium heat. Add the zucchini, carrot, bell pepper, and broccoli and cook, stirring, until just tender and still crisp, about 6 minutes. Add the rice and its sauce and cook, stirring to coat, until all is warmed through, another 2 minutes.

Remove the pan from the heat and serve warm.

Store leftovers in a sealed container in the refrigerator for up to 3 days.

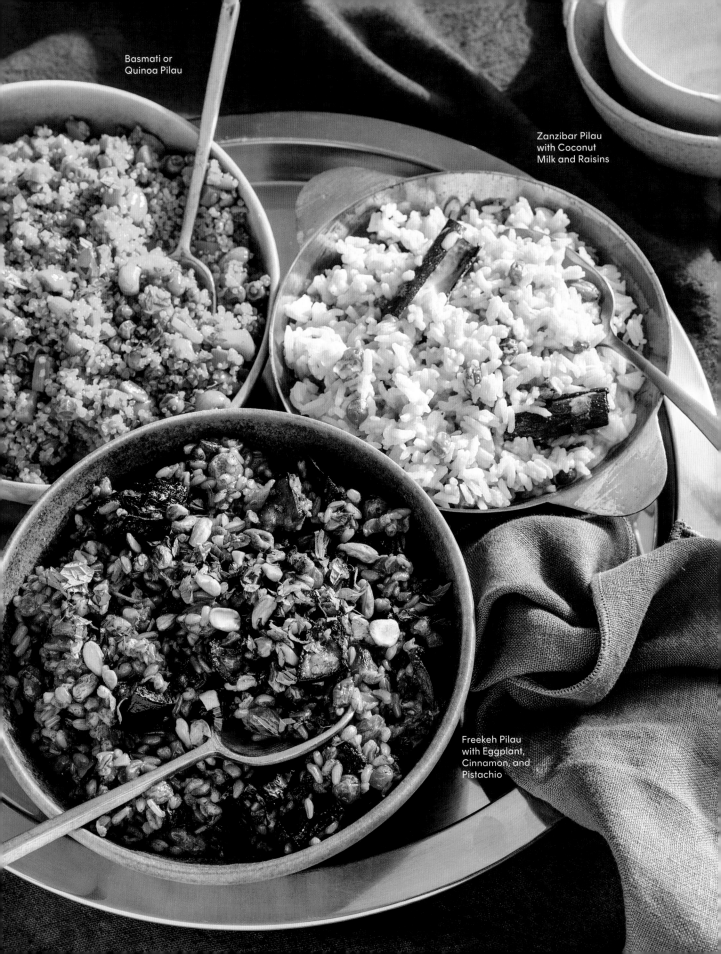

Basmati or
Quinoa Pilau

Zanzibar Pilau
with Coconut
Milk and Raisins

Freekeh Pilau
with Eggplant,
Cinnamon, and
Pistachio

PILAU THREE WAYS

To me, a pilau—or pilaf, depending on where you're from—is your "gourmet" rice dish. It's usually a spiced rice or grain, sometimes mixed with nuts and/or veggies, and is most often served on its own, ideally with a dollop of Raita (page 246) or Chutney (page 243). I love pilau because it's so easy and comes together quickly, and yet you get layered flavors and textures that make for a really satisfying dish on its own or with more cooked veggies or curries spooned over the top. I've included three of my favorite recipes because I wanted to show you just how creative you can get, plus introduce you to different types of grains that you can work into your rotation.

ZANZIBAR PILAU WITH COCONUT MILK AND RAISINS (THE FRUITY ONE)

SERVES *2 as a main or 4 as a side*
TOTAL TIME: *25 minutes*

- 1 tablespoon unsalted vegan butter
- 3 green cardamom pods, pressed gently with the side of a knife
- 1-inch cinnamon stick
- 1 bay leaf
- 1 whole clove
- ½ cup basmati rice, rinsed and drained
- ½ cup canned full-fat coconut milk
- 1 tablespoon golden raisins
- ¼ teaspoon sea salt

In a medium saucepan, melt the butter over medium-high heat. Add the cardamom, cinnamon, bay leaf, and clove and cook, stirring, until the spices release their aroma, about 1 minute. Add the rice, coconut milk, raisins, salt, and ½ cup water and bring to a boil. Cover, reduce the heat to low, and simmer for 15 minutes. Remove the pan from the heat and let rest, covered, for 5 minutes.

Discard the cardamom pods, cinnamon stick, bay leaf, and clove. Fluff the rice with a fork and serve.

Store leftovers in a sealed container in the refrigerator for up to 3 days.

BASMATI OR QUINOA PILAU (THE GOLDEN ONE)

SERVES *2 as a main or 4 as a side*
TOTAL TIME: *20 minutes*

- 1 tablespoon unsalted vegan butter
- ¼ cup chopped cashews
- 1 teaspoon cumin seeds
- 1 whole star anise
- ¼ teaspoon ground turmeric
- ¼ teaspoon sea salt
- ½ cup peeled and diced carrots (about ½ medium carrot)
- ½ cup petite fresh, canned and drained, or frozen and thawed peas
- ½ cup basmati rice or quinoa, rinsed and drained
- Chopped fresh cilantro leaves, for serving

In a medium saucepan, melt the butter over medium-high heat. Add the cashews, cumin seeds, star anise, turmeric, and salt and stir for 30 seconds to release the oils of the nuts and spices. Stir in the carrots, peas, rice or quinoa, and 1 cup water and bring to a boil. Reduce the heat to low, cover, and cook until the grains have absorbed the water, about 15 minutes.

Serve hot and top with chopped fresh cilantro.

Store leftovers in a sealed container in the refrigerator for up to 3 days.

Recipes Continue

FREEKEH PILAU WITH EGGPLANT, CINNAMON, AND PISTACHIO (THE FREEKY ONE)

SERVES *2 as a main or 4 as a side*
TOTAL TIME: *50 minutes*

EGGPLANT

- 2½ cups 1-inch pieces eggplant (about 1 medium eggplant)
- 1½ tablespoons extra-virgin olive oil
- 1 teaspoon paprika
- ½ teaspoon ground cinnamon
- Pinch of sea salt

FREEKEH

- 2 tablespoons extra-virgin olive oil
- ¼ cup raw pistachios, chopped
- 3 tablespoons golden raisins
- 2 bay leaves
- 1 teaspoon ground coriander
- 1 teaspoon paprika
- ½ teaspoon ground cumin
- ½ teaspoon ground cinnamon
- ½ teaspoon sea salt
- ¼ teaspoon ground turmeric
- 1 cup cracked freekeh, rinsed and drained
- ½ cup fresh parsley leaves, chopped, plus 1 tablespoon for garnish
- ¼ cup fresh mint, chopped, plus 1 tablespoon for garnish
- ¼ cup chopped unsalted roasted pistachios, for garnish

COOK THE EGGPLANT: Preheat the oven to 400°F. Line a baking sheet with parchment paper.

In a medium bowl, toss the eggplant with the olive oil, paprika, cinnamon, and salt. Spread out the eggplant on the prepared baking sheet and bake for 8 minutes. Toss the eggplant and return to the oven until crisped along the edges and juicy inside, another 7 to 8 minutes. Set aside to cool.

WHILE THE EGGPLANT BAKES, MAKE THE FREEKEH: In a medium saucepan, heat the olive oil over low heat. Add the raw pistachios, raisins, bay leaves, coriander, paprika, cumin, cinnamon, salt, and turmeric and cook, stirring, until fragrant, about 1 minute. Add the freekeh and 2 cups water and bring the mixture to a boil. Cover, reduce the heat to low, and simmer for 15 minutes.

Remove the pan from the heat and let it sit, covered, for 5 minutes.

Discard the bay leaves and stir in the parsley, mint, and roasted eggplant. Serve garnished with the roasted pistachios and more parsley and mint.

Store leftovers in a sealed container in the refrigerator for up to 3 days.

JAY'S MEXICAN RICE

My husband, Jay, as much as he is a man of many talents, has never cooked in his life. He just doesn't enjoy it. But for kicks, one day we decided to switch roles, which meant he was in charge of our meals while I went to his office and pretended to boss everyone around. I had just seen a Mexican-flavored rice dish in a magazine that sounded tasty and simple to make, so I gave him the recipe and wished him luck. It turned out so surprisingly well that I've included a version of it in this book. Although, he never did make it for me again . . . A one-hit wonder.

SERVES *4*

TOTAL TIME: *1 hour 5 minutes*

- 1 cup short-grain brown rice
- 1 cup canned diced tomatoes or your favorite salsa
- 2 tablespoons sunflower or avocado oil
- 1 cup chopped bell pepper (about 1 large; I like to use a mix of colors, but any color will do)
- 1 cup finely chopped cabbage (about ½ small head)
- 1 bay leaf
- ¾ cup cooked or canned black beans (rinsed and drained if canned)
- ½ cup chopped jalapeño peppers (2 medium peppers)
- ¼ cup fresh sweet corn kernels (from 1 ear), or thawed frozen
- 2 tablespoons taco seasoning (or 2 teaspoons each paprika, ground cumin, and dried oregano)
- 1 tablespoon tomato paste
- 1 teaspoon raw organic sugar
- ½ teaspoon sea salt
- ¼ teaspoon asafoetida
- ½ tablespoon fresh lime juice
- ¼ cup chopped fresh cilantro

In a medium saucepan, combine the rice, 1 cup water, and ½ cup of the tomatoes (or salsa). Bring the mixture to a boil over medium-high heat. Reduce the heat to low, cover, and simmer until the rice is cooked and has absorbed all of the liquid, 45 to 50 minutes. Remove the pan from the heat, fluff the rice with a fork, and cover again while you prep the filling.

In a large skillet, heat the oil over medium-low heat. Add the bell peppers, cabbage, and bay leaf, stirring frequently, until soft, about 5 minutes. Stir in the remaining ½ cup tomatoes (or salsa), the beans, jalapeños, corn, taco seasoning, tomato paste, sugar, salt, and asafoetida. Add the cooked rice and gently mix everything together.

Drizzle the lime juice over the rice, top with the cilantro, and serve hot.

Store leftovers in a sealed container in the refrigerator for up to 3 days.

RAINBOW NOODLE STIR-FRY

This is a go-to staple for me almost every week. It's not only a supremely delicious dish with a rich, creamy satay sauce but you can also use up all the veggies you have in the fridge—just spiralize or grate every last one and chuck 'em into the stir-fry. It's especially great for those days when you maybe haven't had as many veggies as you'd like, and nobody's sad when there's a tasty sauce and noodles involved.

SERVES *2 to 4*
TOTAL TIME: *20 minutes*

FOR THE NOODLES

- 1 tablespoon toasted sesame oil
- 1 tablespoon minced or grated fresh ginger
- 1/8 teaspoon asafoetida
- 1½ cups shredded green cabbage
- 1 cup shredded red cabbage
- 1½ cups thinly spiralized zucchini
- 1½ cups spiralized carrots
- 2 ounces flat or thin ramen, or curly rice noodles

FOR THE SAUCE

- ¼ cup liquid aminos
- 2½ tablespoons unsweetened peanut or almond butter
- 2 tablespoons agave nectar or maple syrup
- 1 tablespoon rice vinegar
- 1 tablespoon sambal oelek
- Black sesame seeds, for serving
- Chopped fresh cilantro leaves, for serving

Heat the sesame oil in a large wok or skillet over high heat. Add the ginger and asafoetida and cook for just a few seconds. Add the green and red cabbage and cook, stirring, until the cabbage has broken down a bit, about 2 minutes. Add the zucchini and carrots and cook, stirring constantly, for 5 minutes. Reduce the heat to medium and continue cooking until the vegetables are tender but still crisp, 3 to 5 minutes more. Remove the wok from the heat and set aside.

Cook the rice noodles according to the package directions. Drain and set aside.

MAKE THE DRESSING: In a jar with a lid or in a blender, combine the aminos, nut butter, agave nectar, rice vinegar, and sambal oelek. Shake or blend until well combined and smooth.

Assemble the noodles: Toss the noodles with the vegetables in the pan until combined. Add the sauce and toss once more. Set the pan over high heat and cook, tossing and mixing, until the noodles are well coated and warmed through, about 2 minutes.

Divide among 2 to 4 bowls and top with black sesame seeds and chopped cilantro.

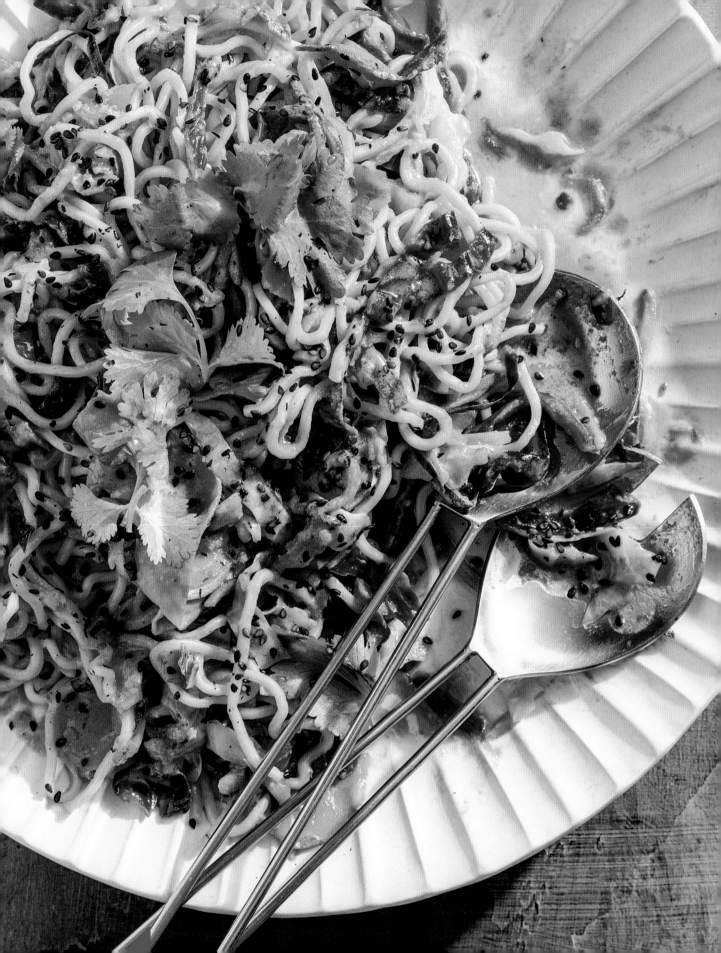

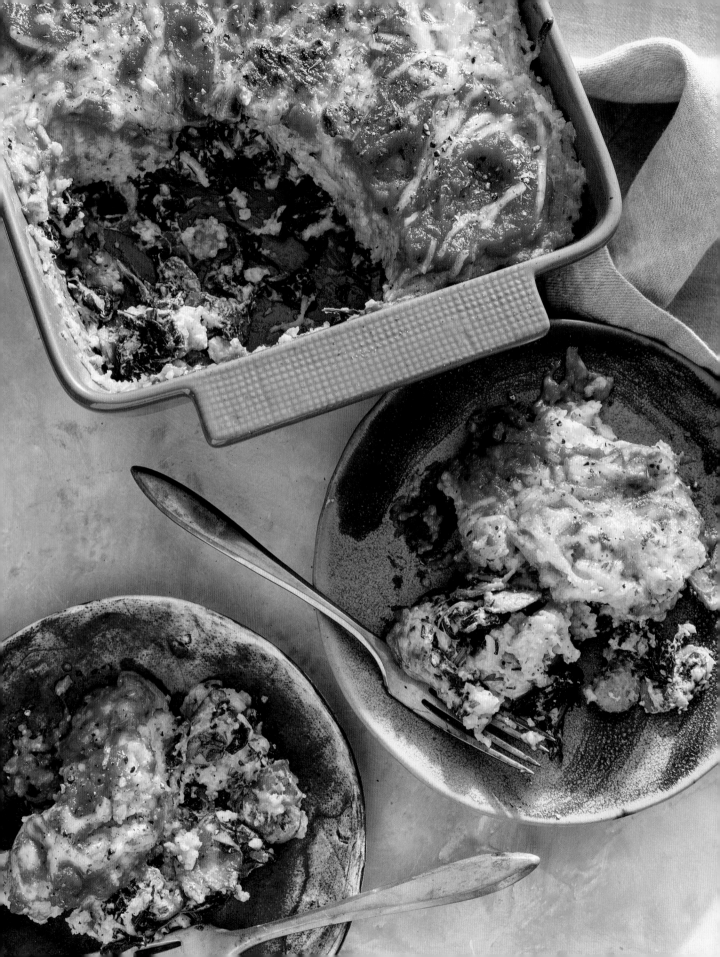

POLENTA BAKE *with Creamy Mushrooms and Chili-Spiked Tomato Sauce*

It doesn't get homier or more comforting than a casserole, especially when it's topped with soft, buttery polenta that's gone crispy around the edges and smothered in a chili-infused tomato sauce. You just cut yourself a slab and dig right in. Sure, it's not the prettiest dish, but we love it anyway.

SERVES *4 to 6*
TOTAL TIME: *50 minutes*

POLENTA

1 cup plain unsweetened vegan milk, such as almond

½ cup medium-ground cornmeal

1 tablespoon nutritional yeast

½ tablespoon Italian seasoning

½ tablespoon dried parsley

¾ teaspoon sea salt

¼ teaspoon freshly ground black pepper

2 tablespoons vegan parmesan cheese (optional)

SAUCE

2 tablespoons extra-virgin olive oil

2 cups cherry tomatoes, halved, or 1 14.5-ounce can crushed tomatoes

1 tablespoon chili oil

1 bay leaf

¼ teaspoon sea salt

¼ teaspoon freshly ground black pepper

FILLING

1 tablespoon unsalted vegan butter

8 ounces white mushrooms, sliced

2 bay leaves

1 teaspoon fresh thyme leaves or ¼ teaspoon dried

½ teaspoon sea salt

⅛ teaspoon asafoetida

4 cups packed fresh spinach leaves (about 32 ounces)

⅓ cup chopped fresh parsley leaves

1 tablespoon nutritional yeast

4 ounces vegan cream cheese

1 cup shredded vegan mozzarella

MAKE THE POLENTA: In a medium saucepan, combine the milk and 1½ cups water. Bring to a boil over high heat and slowly stir in the cornmeal. Stir in the nutritional yeast, Italian seasoning, dried parsley, salt, and pepper. Reduce the heat to medium-low and cook, stirring occasionally, until the polenta is smooth and soft, 20 to 25 minutes. If the polenta is thickening too quickly, add a splash of water to the pan. Stir in the parmesan (if using) and remove the pot from the heat. Cover to keep warm.

MAKE THE SAUCE: In a large skillet, heat the olive oil over medium-low heat. Add the tomatoes, chili oil, bay leaf, salt, and pepper and cook, stirring occasionally, until the tomatoes begin to take on some color, 10 to 12 minutes. Stir and mash the tomatoes a bit with your spoon to create a chunky sauce consistency. Remove the pan from the heat and set aside.

Preheat the broiler to 400°F.

MAKE THE FILLING: In a large skillet, melt the butter over low heat. Add the sliced mushrooms, bay leaves, thyme, salt, and asafoetida. Cook, stirring occasionally, until the mushrooms are soft and the herbs release their fragrance, about 5 minutes. Add the spinach, parsley, and nutritional yeast and cook until the spinach wilts, about 5 minutes.

Discard the bay leaves. Stir in the cream cheese and ½ cup of the mozzarella. Cook, stirring, until creamy and combined, 1 to 2 minutes.

Transfer the filling mixture to a 7 × 11-inch heatproof baking dish. Spread the polenta over the filling in an even layer. Top the polenta with generous dollops of the sauce and the remaining mozzarella. Broil until the cheese melts and the sauce is bubbling, 5 to 6 minutes.

Serve warm. Store leftovers in a sealed container in the refrigerator for up to 3 days.

How to Make a RAINBOW GRAIN BOWL

This is your secret weapon for making quick and easy but deeply satisfying and nourishing meals, particularly ones that please all the senses. All you need to do is assemble any combination of veggies, protein, and grains. Then pick a dressing or sauce (called Drizzles and Dollops below), and maybe some crunchy bits or other exciting sprinkles. Then dive right into that beautifully balanced bowl.

The trick for keeping it fresh, and for loading your plate with different colors, flavors, and textures, is to change up how you prepare the vegetables: grill, steam, boil, and sauté; or if using raw veg, use a blend of grating, spiralizing, cubing, and slicing.

SERVES *1*

⅓ cup Grain

1 Vegetable from each color category (as many as you like!)

½ cup Protein

¼ cup Crunchy Bits, or to taste

2 tablespoons Plant-Based Dairy Sprinkle

Salty Bits, to taste

Herbs, to taste

1 to 2 Drizzles and Dollops, to taste

TO MAKE A BASIC RAINBOW BOWL: Choose from the lists of categories opposite.

GRAINS

Brown rice

Bulgur wheat

Farro

Freekeh

Quinoa

VEGGIES

RED

Radicchio

Red bell peppers

Red cabbage

Red chard

Tomatoes

YELLOW

Corn

Golden beets

Rutabaga

Summer squash

Yellow bell peppers

GREEN

Arugula

Asparagus

Avocado

Broccoli

Brussels sprouts

Cabbage

Celery

Cucumbers

Edamame

Green bell pepper

Hearty greens (kale, Swiss chard, spinach, mustard greens)

Okra

Snow peas

Tomatillos

Watercress

Zucchini

PURPLE

Beets

Japanese sweet potatoes

Purple carrots

Purple cauliflower

Radishes

Red cabbage

ORANGE

Carrots

Orange bell peppers

Sweet potatoes

Winter squash

WHITE

Cauliflower

Fennel

Mushrooms

Parsnips

Potatoes

Turnips

PROTEINS

Beans

Lentils

Tempeh

Tofu

CRUNCHY BITS

Corn nuts

Nuts (such as chopped walnuts, pecans, pistachios, almonds, cashews, and Brazil nuts)

Seeds (such as lotus seeds, sunflower seeds, pumpkin seeds, sesame seeds, and hemp seeds)

Tortilla chips or strips

Caraway Croutons (page 253)

Cheesy Curried Crispy Kale (page 254)

"Popcorn" Pumpkin Seeds (page 255)

Super-Seed Brittle (page 255)

Chili Croutons (page 253)

Thyme Crostini (page 254)

Pistachio Gremolata (page 253)

PLANT-BASED DAIRY SPRINKLES

Cheddar

Cream cheese

Feta

Gouda

Mozzarella

Ricotta

Sour cream

SALTY BITS

Capers

Olives

Sauerkraut

Sun-dried tomatoes

Pickled Carrot and Apple (page 251)

Pickled Turmeric and Ginger (page 249)

Pink Pickled Turnips and Beets (page 249)

FRESH HERBS

Basil

Cilantro

Curly or flat-leaf parsley

Dill

Mint

DRIZZLES AND DOLLOPS

FRESH AND BRIGHT

Cavolo Nero Pesto (page 200)

Corn Salsa with a Kick (page 240)

Green Goddess Dressing (page 171)

Herby Vinaigrette (page 166)

Mango Salsa (page 240)

Zhoug (page 211)

SPICED AND SULTRY

Creamy Sambal Dressing (page 180)

Curried Cashew Dressing (page 172)

Muhammara (page 233)

Paprika Vinaigrette (page 179)

Spiced Yogurt with Charred Tomatoes (page 245)

Zucchini "Baba Ghanoush" (page 194)

ZIPPY AND ZINGY

Citrus Vinaigrette (page 169)

Raita (page 246)

Soy-Ginger Dressing (page 170)

Tzatziki (page 246)

Yogurt Mint Sauce (page 245)

CREAMY AND DREAMY

Beet, Pine Nut, and Feta Dip (page 236)

Butternut, Bean, and Sun-Dried Tomato Dip (page 238)

Creamy Sambal Dressing (page 180)

Curried Cashew Dressing (page 172)

Perfect Hummus (page 239)

Red Lentil Daal Dip (page 123)

Tahini Drizzle (page 241)

Zucchini "Baba Ghanoush" (page 194)

Prayers

When you sit down to eat, whether alone or with others, it is a chance to connect. And not just with yourself or with those you care about but also with a higher purpose. Prayer or sharing words in union can encourage a collective consciousness and create a sacred space. I don't necessarily mean that in a religious way. Rather, I believe it is an opportunity to acknowledge that this moment in time is made possible by many small miracles—from the food that nourishes our bodies to the company of people we love to simply being alive—and to say thank you. That can be to God, the Universe, Mother Earth, or any higher power that speaks to you. You can say any prayer that comes to your heart, but if you are looking for guidance or a place to start, here are some beautiful offerings I turn to during mealtimes—or any time throughout the day when I feel I need them.

PURIFICATION PRAYER

This prayer for purification comes from the Ayurvedic idea of asatmya-indriyartha-samyog. It's a Sanskrit notion that "uncontrolled," misused, or overstimulated senses can be at the root of our anxieties, impatience, need for instant gratification, and, ultimately, poor health. The prayer is my way of hitting the reset button, calming my senses from all that has been bombarding them from the moment I wake up. Food that is offered and purified with these words is called prashad.

I offer this food to the divine within me. Food that is meditated on, created with love, and offered with heart can not only cleanse me physically but purify my senses and uplift me emotionally, mentally, and spiritually, too. My body is a sacred vessel harnessing eternal joy, knowledge, and love. This food, when offered, becomes sacred and nourishes the deepest parts of me.

GRATITUDE PRAYER

This prayer shares appreciation for everything and everyone—from the food on your plate to your higher power for creating it to the work and care that made the meal possible.

Thank you for the nourishment we are about to receive that has come to us through so many different vessels. The vegetables, grains, legumes, spices, and herbs that combine together to bring balance and flavor; the farmer who grew, watered, and cared for these ingredients; the soil for maintaining and supporting the roots; the sun for providing light and warmth for them to grow; the moon for infusing flavor into them; Mother Earth for endlessly providing; the hands that cooked these ingredients with love; and, ultimately, the Universe and God for creating all that we need to exist. Please let this food deeply nourish my body, mind, and soul so that I can continue to be an instrument of love, compassion, and healing in this world. What I take in, I will give out to others. I receive this food with immense gratitude.

PRAYER OF AWARENESS AND PRESENCE

This prayer brings presence into the moment. It's lovely when you're about to eat, but it's also especially meaningful before you begin cooking a meal. Remember, the consciousness and intention with which you prepare a meal—even if it's just for yourself!—infuses that food with positive vibrations. That elevated frequency is healing not only for you as the vessel but also for anyone else who enjoys that food.

May I remember the cooking, eating, and sharing of this meal in divine consciousness, to be fully present and aware that the food itself is a blessing, the process of creating this meal is a blessing, and the nourishment I receive is a blessing. Therefore, may the preparation be done with presence and the cooking infused with devotion, served with love, and eaten with joy.

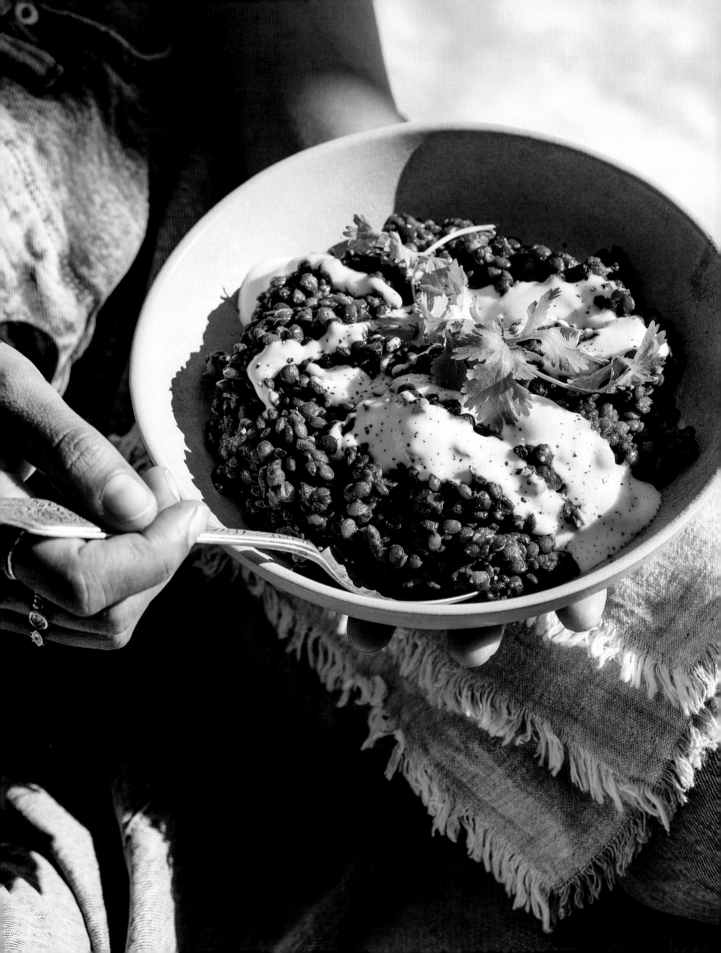

LENTILS, BEANS, PROTEINS, AND CURRIES

These dishes are your nurturers, your fortifiers, and your belly fillers. Many of them are recipes that I grew up eating and a few my grandmothers and their grandmothers before them prepared for their families. They can be enjoyed alone, or paired with a rice dish and a Hero Veg (see page 187) for a wholesome, balanced meal.

NOTE   These recipes will work with either dried or canned beans and lentils, but I highly recommend dried because they not only taste so much better but are also more nutritionally dense. It just takes an easy extra step—soaking them overnight or in hot water for a few hours—but the payoff is so worth it. I use a 90 percent rule: 90 percent of the time I make legumes from scratch, and for the rest I use a shortcut. But depending on where you're at, that might be 50/50 or even 10/90—go at your own pace! Like anything, after preparing dried legumes for the first few times—including soaking them in advance, which makes them easier to digest—you will hardly notice the extra step. It gets easier and easier until it becomes a practice.

SPLIT MOONG DAAL *with Dill*

What mashed potatoes is to Western countries, daal is for me (and a lot of other Indians). Whenever I come back from traveling or want cozy comfort food, the first thing I think of is a bowl of daal and rice. Moong daal is known as the queen of all lentils in Ayurveda because it has the most nutrient value (it's rich in alkaline minerals such as calcium, magnesium, and potassium) and is the easiest to digest—making it a great starter lentil if you've had issues digesting them in the past. The spices I added here are quite simple because I love the flavor of the lentils themselves, and while I use fresh dill, any fresh herb would be delicious. Pair this with basmati rice or any of the pilaus (pages 103–4), or enjoy it with some yogurt and a Hero Veg (page 187) and call it a meal.

SERVES *4*

TOTAL TIME: *35 minutes, plus soaking time*

- 1 cup yellow moong daal (split moong beans), soaked in water for at least 1 hour or overnight, rinsed, and drained
- 1 tablespoon vegan butter or avocado oil
- 1 teaspoon cumin seeds
- ½ teaspoon brown or black mustard seeds
- 10 fresh or dried curry leaves
- 1 tablespoon minced fresh ginger
- ⅛ teaspoon asafoetida
- ¼ cup chopped fresh dill
- 1 teaspoon Ground CCF Masala (page 49)
- ¾ teaspoon sea salt
- Lime wedges, for squeezing

In a large deep pot, bring 3 cups water to a simmer over medium heat. Add the moong daal and cook until very tender and creamy, about 20 minutes.

While the lentils cook, in a small skillet, heat the oil over medium heat. Add the cumin seeds and mustard seeds and cook, stirring, until they pop and brown, about 1 minute. Add the curry leaves, ginger, and asafoetida and cook, stirring, until fragrant, about 1 minute. Remove the pan from the heat.

Add the toasted spice mixture, dill, CCF masala, and salt to the lentils and cook, stirring occasionally, until the flavors have come together, about 5 minutes.

Divide among bowls and serve with the lime wedges for squeezing.

Leftovers can be stored in a sealed container in the refrigerator for up to 3 days.

CARAMELIZED FENNEL *with Chickpeas and Spinach*

I'm taking this opportunity to show off a discovery I made, which is that when you sauté fennel in asafoetida, it ends up tasting like caramelized onions. Folding these rich, golden fennel slices into a tahini-enriched sauce with lots of greens is just a divine way to enjoy these ingredients and have an exciting new chickpea curry experience.

SERVES *2*
TOTAL TIME: *15 minutes*

- 1 packed cup fresh spinach leaves
- ¼ cup tahini (see Note)
- 2 teaspoons ground cumin
- ⅛ teaspoon asafoetida
- ½ teaspoon sea salt
- 1 tablespoon extra-virgin olive oil
- 1 cup very thinly sliced or grated fennel (about 1 medium head)
- ½ teaspoon minced hot Indian or Thai green chile
- 1 15-ounce can chickpeas, rinsed and drained
- ½ tablespoon cornstarch or tapioca starch (optional)

In a high-powered blender, combine the spinach, tahini, and 1 cup water and blend until smooth. Set aside.

In a large skillet, stir the cumin and asafoetida over medium-low heat until the seeds smell nice and toasty, about 30 seconds. Add the salt and oil and let it heat until it just begins to shimmer, about 1 minute. Add the fennel and green chile and cook, stirring, until the fennel softens and turns golden, about 10 minutes.

Stir in the chickpeas and the spinach mixture, bring it to a simmer, and cook, stirring, until everything has heated through and the flavors have married.

The sauce should be thick enough to coat the vegetables. If it needs thickening, in a small bowl, whisk the cornstarch with 1 tablespoon water until smooth. Stir the slurry into the vegetables and cook, stirring occasionally, until thickened, about 4 minutes.

Remove the pan from the heat and serve warm.

Leftovers can be stored in a sealed container in the refrigerator for up to 3 days.

NOTE   The consistency of tahini can vary widely, so if yours is on the looser side, I've included how you can use a quick cornstarch or tapioca starch slurry to thicken it up so it will hug the vegetables well.

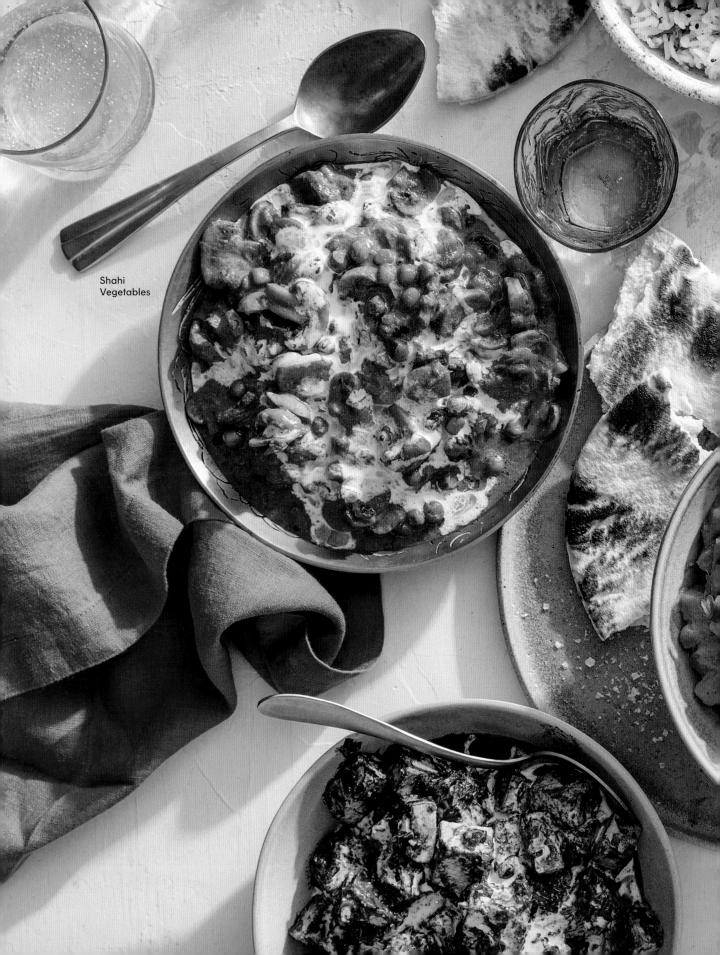

Shahi
Vegetables

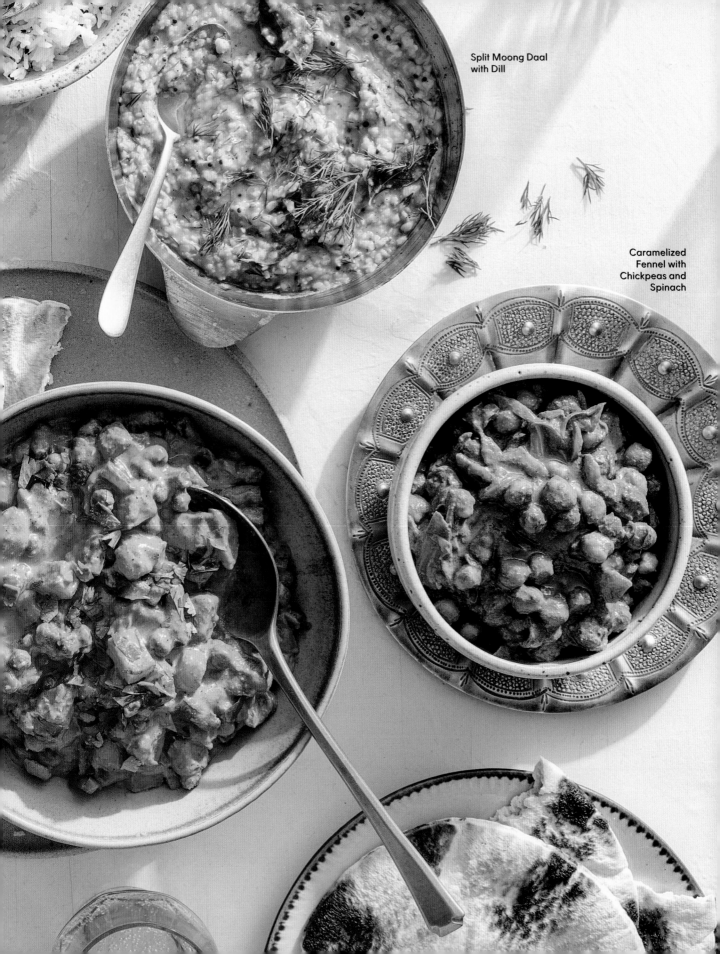

Split Moong Daal
with Dill

Caramelized
Fennel with
Chickpeas and
Spinach

SHAHI VEGETABLES

VEGGIES IN CREAMY MASALA TOMATO SAUCE

This Hyderabadi dish features a blend of veggies simmered in a bold, creamy, rice-filled masala tomato sauce that gets a punch of heat from a blend of fresh and dried chiles. The ingredient list might look a little . . . extensive, but the recipe isn't much more than a quick blender sauce that infuses the sautéed bell peppers, green beans, carrots, and potatoes with maximum flavor. You can also look at this as an opportunity to expand your spice drawer and palate. But don't worry if you don't have every single one of these seasonings; a good garam masala goes a long way.

SERVES 6

TOTAL TIME: *30 minutes, plus soaking time*

VEGETABLES

- 1 cup chopped green or red bell peppers
- 1 cup fresh or frozen green peas (5 ounces)
- 1 cup trimmed and roughly chopped green beans (4 ounces)
- 1 cup 2-inch pieces peeled carrots (about 2 medium)
- 1 cup ½-inch cubed Yukon Gold potatoes (about 1 medium) or quartered baby potatoes (about 5 baby potatoes)
- ½ teaspoon sea salt

SAUCE

- 1½ tablespoons avocado oil
- 1 teaspoon cumin seeds
- 1 teaspoon grated fresh ginger
- 1 teaspoon finely chopped hot Indian or Thai green chile
- 2 bay leaves
- 1 small cinnamon stick
- ½ tablespoon garam masala or Ground CCF Masala (page 49)
- 2½ teaspoons sea salt
- ½ teaspoon ground coriander
- ½ teaspoon ground Kashmiri red chile or chile powder
- ¼ teaspoon asafoetida
- ¼ teaspoon ground cardamom
- ¼ teaspoon ground turmeric
- 1 tablespoon sambal oelek (optional)
- 1 14-ounce can crushed tomatoes
- ½ cup cashews, soaked in hot water for 30 minutes

FOR SERVING

- Yogurt Mint Sauce (optional; page 245)
- Hot cooked white or brown rice or Proper Good Naan (page 156)

MAKE THE VEGETABLES: In a large skillet, bring ½ cup water to a simmer over medium heat. Reduce the heat to medium-low and add the bell peppers, peas, green beans, carrots, potatoes, and salt. Cover and simmer, stirring frequently, until the vegetables are tender, about 8 minutes. If the pan gets too dry before then, add a splash more water. Remove the pan from the heat and set aside.

MAKE THE SAUCE: In a large skillet, heat the avocado oil over medium heat. Add the cumin seeds and cook, stirring, until they pop, about 1 minute. Add the ginger, green chile, and bay leaves and cook, stirring, for 30 seconds until aromatic. Reduce the heat to low and add the cinnamon stick, garam masala, 1 teaspoon of the salt, the coriander, Kashmiri chile, asafoetida, cardamom, turmeric, and sambal (if using) and cook, stirring constantly, until the spices release their oils and fragrance, about 1 minute. Remove the pan from the heat and set aside.

In a high-powered blender, combine the tomatoes, soaked cashews, the remaining 1½ teaspoons salt, and ½ cup water and blend until smooth. Add the sauce to the spice mixture in the pan and return to medium heat. Cook, stirring, until the flavors have melded, 2 to 3 minutes.

Add the cooked vegetables to the sauce and toss to combine. Reduce the heat to low and cook, stirring occasionally, until the vegetables have soaked up some of the sauce and the flavors have married, about 5 minutes.

TO SERVE: Divide the mixture among bowls. If desired, drizzle with the yogurt sauce. Enjoy on its own or with rice or naan.

Leftovers can be stored in a sealed container in the refrigerator for up to 3 days.

NOTE I love that once you have the base of the sauce, it's easy to customize it. One of my favorite variations is North Indian dum aloo (see Variation below), which is made with baby potatoes instead of the combination of vegetables. Seeing as this sauce would be delicious on just about anything, you can do no wrong here.

VARIATION *Dum Aloo:* Instead of all the vegetables, start with 1½ pounds baby potatoes and cook them in a large pot of boiling water until the potatoes are fork tender, about 10 minutes, depending on the size of the potatoes. Drain, cut the potatoes into halves or quarters, and set aside while you prepare the sauce as directed. Add the potatoes to the sauce and simmer as you would the mixed vegetables.

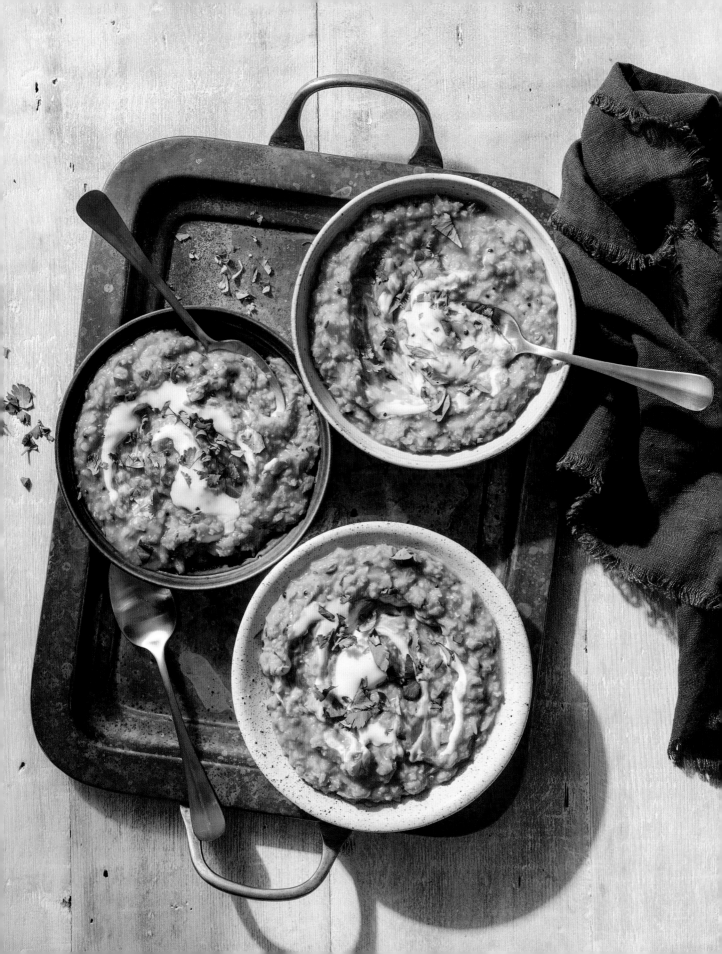

RED LENTIL DAAL *(My Go-To Lentils)*

Also known as masoor daal, this dish is exceptionally easy to make and just as delicious. All the ingredients go into one pot, and the lentils cook quite quickly, which means you're never more than a few minutes away from a soothing, creamy, nourishing bowl of daal. And as an added bonus, that means you're also only a few minutes away from a hearty, flavorful dip, because that's what this daal becomes when tossed in a blender. I serve it with toasted naan sliced into little soldiers or pita, usually drizzled with a bit of yogurt. What can I say, it's just *daal*icious.

SERVES *4*

TOTAL TIME: *40 minutes*

- 1 tablespoon sunflower or avocado oil
- 1 teaspoon brown or black mustard seeds
- 2 teaspoons cumin seeds
- 15 fresh or dried curry leaves, chopped
- ½ to 1 tablespoon curry powder, garam masala, or Ground CCF Masala (page 49)
- 1 teaspoon minced hot Indian or Thai green chile
- ½ teaspoon finely grated fresh ginger
- ¼ teaspoon asafoetida
- 2 tablespoons tomato paste
- 1 cup finely chopped mixed vegetables, such as cauliflower, zucchini, or green beans (optional)
- 1½ cups red lentils, thoroughly rinsed and drained
- 1 teaspoon sea salt
- 1 cup canned full-fat coconut milk
- 1 tablespoon sambal oelek (optional)
- 2 tablespoons chopped fresh cilantro leaves
- 2 tablespoons plain vegan yogurt

In a large deep pot, heat the oil over medium heat. Add the mustard and cumin seeds and cook, stirring constantly, until they pop, about 1 minute. Add the curry leaves, curry powder, green chile, ginger, and asafoetida and cook, stirring, until fragrant, about 2 minutes. Add the tomato paste and stir until just combined.

If you're adding mixed vegetables, add them now and cook, stirring, until just tender, about 3 minutes.

Add the lentils, salt, and 3 cups water. Bring to a boil, reduce the heat to a simmer, and cover. Cook until the lentils are soft and tender, about 10 minutes.

Stir in the coconut milk and sambal (if using), cover, and cook until the mixture is super creamy, 10 to 12 minutes. If the mixture becomes too thick, add up to ¼ cup water.

Serve topped with the chopped cilantro and a swirl of yogurt.

Store leftovers in a sealed container in the refrigerator for up to 3 days.

NOTE The amount of curry powder, garam masala, and CCF masala you use will depend on how fresh or potent your spices are.

VARIATION *Red Lentil Daal Dip:* Add any amount of the daal to a high-powered blender and puree until smooth. Add a little extra water to thin the dip, if needed. Scoop into a bowl and top with the cilantro and yogurt. Serve with naan, pita, or your favorite dipping crackers or vegetables.

MOONGLETTES

SAVORY LENTIL PANCAKES

If moong daal (split and peeled mung beans) were a person, they would be the kindest, warmest individual who gave the greatest cuddles. They're balancing and gentle on the belly, and they have the most grounding, earthy flavor. Which is why I was very excited to use them to show you that there's more to lentils than just daal. These veggie-packed savory pancakes—or "moonglettes," as I like to call them—manage to be both fluffy and crisp and would be the perfect addition to a lazy Sunday breakfast spread with all sorts of chutneys, or as a meal in their own right. Just remember to soak the moong daal before you go to bed the night before.

SERVES *4*

TOTAL TIME: *15 minutes plus soaking time*

- 1 cup moong daal (split moong beans)
- 2 tablespoons white rice flour
- 1½ teaspoons sea salt
- 1 teaspoon Ground CCF Masala (page 49)
- ¼ teaspoon ground turmeric
- ¼ teaspoon baking soda
- ⅛ teaspoon asafoetida
- Olive oil cooking spray or avocado oil
- ½ cup peeled and grated carrots (about 1 medium)
- ¼ cup fresh cilantro leaves
- White sesame seeds, for sprinkling
- Cilantro-Mint Chutney (page 243) or Hyderabadi Chutney (page 243), for serving

Soak the moong daal at room temperature overnight or for at least 6 hours. Drain and rinse the moong daal until the water runs clear.

In a high-powered blender, combine the soaked moong daal, rice flour, salt, CCF masala, turmeric, baking soda, asafoetida, and ¼ cup water and blend until completely smooth.

Heat a cast-iron skillet over medium-high heat. Reduce the heat to medium, lightly coat the pan with cooking spray or avocado oil, and ladle ¼ to ⅓ cup of the batter into the pan. Use the bottom of the ladle to spread the batter to 5 or 6 inches in diameter. Cook until the top of the pancake looks dry and starts to bubble, about 3 minutes.

Sprinkle on about 1 tablespoon of the grated carrots, 1 teaspoon of the cilantro leaves, and a pinch of sesame seeds. Spray the top of the pancake with a bit more oil, then use a spatula to carefully flip it over. Cook until the first side is golden, another 2 to 3 minutes.

Serve immediately or transfer the cooked pancakes to a plate under foil or to a baking sheet in an oven set at the lowest heat to keep warm. Repeat with the remaining batter. Serve warm with the chutney of your choice.

NOTE   If you have leftover moonglettes, you could either gently warm them in a pan to soften them up, or you could chop them into bite-size pieces and sauté them with a sprinkling of your favorite spices until crispy. They become delicious little bites you can dip into sauces.

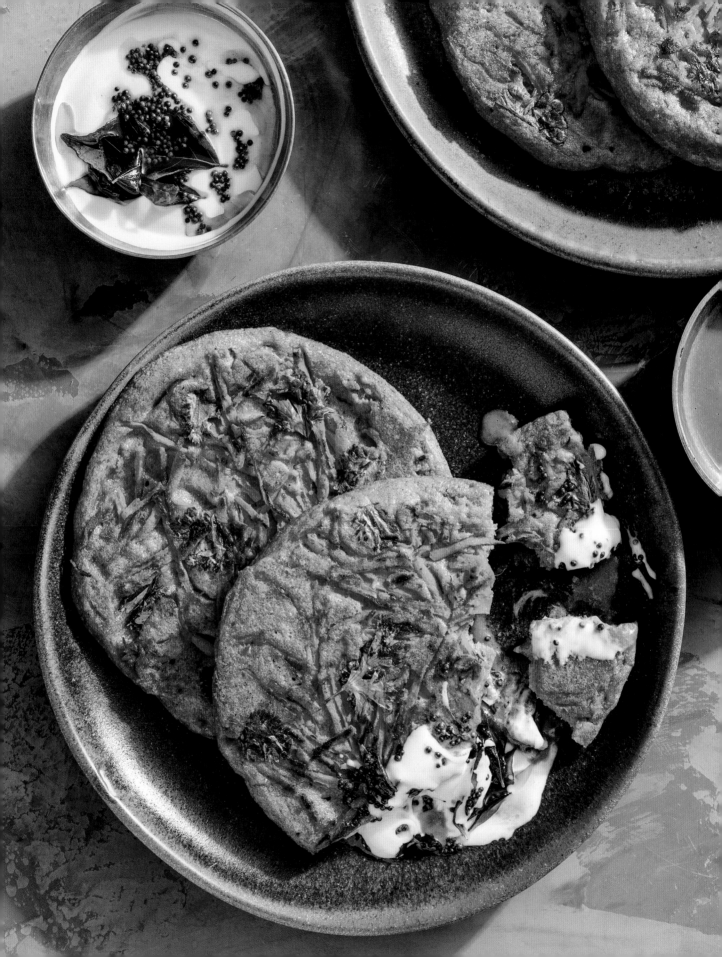

BAKED FALAFEL PITA SANDWICHES

In the past, I've tried getting creative and have made falafel from all sorts of things like lentils and different bean varieties, but nothing beats a good ol' chickpea falafel. Even when baked (because I avoid deep-frying whenever possible), these are light on the inside and crispy on the outside—no stodgy falafel here! And I've stuffed them full of fresh herbs, just like the ones I used to order on repeat from my favorite spot, Taim, when I lived in New York. For this recipe, I've also given you my secret to making the best-ever pita sandwich or wrap. Since it can be difficult to get all the good stuff in every bite, I mix up all the fillings and sauces before stuffing them into the pita. Just like that—saucy all the way through!

SERVES *4 to 6*

TOTAL TIME: *45 minutes, plus soaking time*

FALAFEL

- 1 cup dried chickpeas (see Note)
- ½ teaspoon baking soda
- Olive oil cooking spray or avocado oil
- ½ cup chopped fresh cilantro leaves
- ½ cup chopped fresh parsley leaves
- ¼ cup chopped fresh dill or mint leaves, or a combination
- 2 tablespoons extra-virgin olive oil
- 1 teaspoon sea salt
- 1 teaspoon ground cumin
- 1 teaspoon paprika
- 1 teaspoon ground sumac
- ½ teaspoon baking powder
- ⅛ teaspoon asafoetida

SANDWICHES

- 2 cups chopped romaine lettuce (about ⅓ medium head)
- 2 cups chopped Roma tomatoes (about 3 small) or cherry tomatoes (about 25)
- 2 cups chopped seedless cucumbers (about 1½ medium)
- 1 cup chopped Pink Pickled Turnips and Beets (page 249) or store-bought pickled peppers or turnips
- Tahini Drizzle (page 241)
- Perfect Hummus (page 239)
- Zhoug (page 211)
- 6 to 8 wraps or pitas

In a large bowl, combine the chickpeas, baking soda, and enough water to cover. Soak the chickpeas for at least 6 hours or up to overnight in the refrigerator. Rinse and drain the chickpeas and set aside.

Position an oven rack in the middle of the oven and preheat the oven to 400°F. Line a baking sheet with parchment paper and lightly coat the parchment with cooking spray or brush with avocado oil.

In a food processor or high-powered blender, combine the drained chickpeas, cilantro, parsley, mint, olive oil, salt, cumin, paprika, sumac, baking powder, and asafoetida. Pulse until the mixture is coarsely pureed.

Using a small ice cream scoop (about 2 tablespoons), scoop the batter into balls and place them on the prepared baking sheet about 1 inch apart.

Lightly coat the falafel with cooking spray and bake for 15 minutes. Use a spatula to gently turn the falafel, then bake for another 15 minutes, until the falafel are golden brown and feel dry to the touch.

MEANWHILE, START TO ASSEMBLE THE SANDWICHES: In a medium bowl, toss the lettuce, tomatoes, cucumber, and pickles with a few tablespoons of each of your sauces of choice, until combined. Set aside.

Toast the wraps or pitas in a medium skillet over medium heat, until warm. Stuff each with a scoop of the salad and a couple falafel and drizzle with additional sauce as desired.

Leftover falafel and salad can be stored separately in sealed containers for up to 2 days.

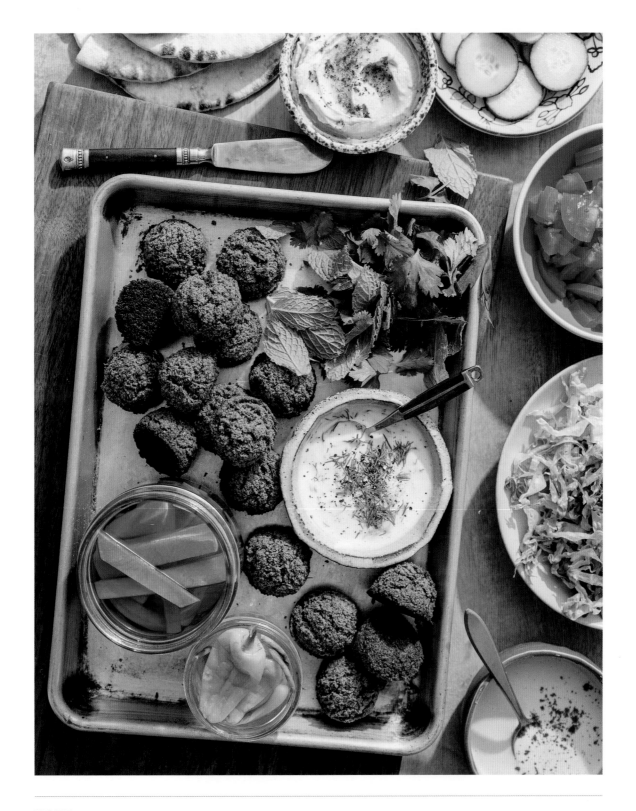

NOTE   You can use canned chickpeas here; just skip the soaking step. The falafel is also great broken up over salads. Or serve them on their own and go wild with the dipping!

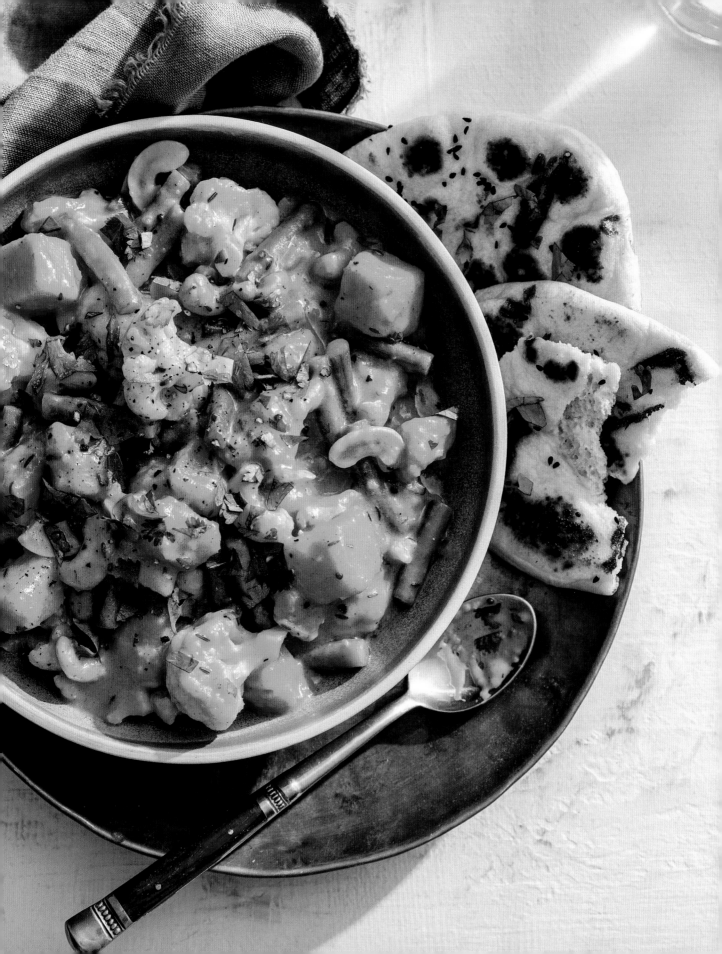

SWEET POTATO, CAULIFLOWER, GREEN BEAN, AND CASHEW CURRY

I once went through a period during which I was making this once a week—and I still come back to the recipe again and again. I just love how, for a very quick, very easy curry, it still feels substantial. The greens combined with the richness of sweet potato, cauliflower, coconut milk, and cashews plus all the spices are deeply delicious and nourishing. And then there's the lemongrass-like fresh curry leaves, which are not only aromatic and flavorful but also antimicrobial (by removing any unwanted interlopers from your gut) and blood purifying (by helping the liver and kidneys remove toxins from the body). Just be sure to chew them to get all their benefits.

SERVES *4*

TOTAL TIME: *40 minutes*

- 1 tablespoon extra-virgin olive oil
- 1 teaspoon cumin seeds
- ½ teaspoon brown or black mustard seeds
- 15 fresh or dried curry leaves
- 1 teaspoon grated fresh ginger
- ½ teaspoon minced hot Indian or Thai green chile
- ½ tablespoon Ground CCF Masala (page 49)
- 1 teaspoon sea salt
- 1 teaspoon garam masala or additional Ground CCF Masala (page 49)
- ¼ teaspoon ground turmeric
- ⅛ teaspoon asafoetida
- 3 cups 1-inch cubes peeled sweet potatoes (about 3 medium)
- 1 cup cauliflower florets (about ¼ medium head)
- ¼ cup cashews
- 8 ounces French or regular green beans, cut into thirds (about 2 cups)
- 1 cup canned full-fat coconut milk
- ½ tablespoon cornstarch, potato starch, or tapioca starch (optional)
- Chopped fresh cilantro leaves, for serving

In a large saucepan, heat the oil over medium heat. Add the cumin seeds and mustard seeds and cook until they pop, about 1 minute. Add the curry leaves, ginger, and green chile and cook, stirring, for just about 10 seconds to release the oils and aromas from the spices. Stir in the CCF masala, salt, garam masala, turmeric, and asafoetida and cook until just combined and aromatic, about 30 seconds.

Add the sweet potato, cauliflower, cashews, and ½ cup water and bring to a simmer. Cover, reduce the heat to medium-low, and simmer, stirring frequently, until the sweet potato just begins to soften, 3 to 5 minutes. Add the green beans, cover, and cook until all the vegetables are tender, about 2 minutes longer. If the mixture looks too dry, add a few splashes of water.

Stir in the coconut milk and simmer, uncovered, until the flavors have come together and the sweet potatoes are tender, 10 to 12 minutes.

For a thicker sauce, whisk together the cornstarch and 1 tablespoon water until smooth. Stir the mixture into the curry and cook, stirring, until the curry has thickened, 2 to 4 minutes.

Divide the curry among bowls and top with cilantro.

Leftovers can be stored in a sealed container in the refrigerator for up to 3 days.

MOMMA'S RICH AND CREAMY THREE-BEAN RED PEPPER CURRY

This is another recipe passed down from my sweet momma bear. It has a fortifying, wholesome blend of black-eyed peas, black chickpeas, and kidney beans in a tomato-y, gingery, coconut milky sauce. But what really puts it over the top is a surprising secret ingredient that gives it savory, umami flavor: peanut butter.

SERVES *4*
TOTAL TIME: *40 minutes*

- ½ tablespoon sunflower or avocado oil
- 1 teaspoon cumin seeds
- 20 fresh or dried curry leaves
- ½ teaspoon grated fresh ginger
- ½ teaspoon ground turmeric
- ¼ teaspoon asafoetida
- ¼ teaspoon minced hot Indian or Thai green chile (optional)
- 1 cup roughly chopped red bell pepper (about 1 large pepper)
- 1½ cups canned crushed tomatoes
- 1 13.5-ounce can full-fat coconut milk
- 1 cup canned black-eyed peas, rinsed and drained
- 1 cup canned black chickpeas (see Note), rinsed and drained
- 1 cup canned kidney beans, rinsed and drained
- 1 tablespoon unsweetened peanut butter
- ½ tablespoon garam masala or Ground CCF Masala (page 49)
- 1 teaspoon sea salt
- 1 teaspoon ground coriander
- 1 tablespoon cornstarch
- 2 tablespoons chopped fresh cilantro leaves

In a large skillet, heat the oil over medium heat. Add the cumin seeds and cook until they pop, about 1 minute. Add the curry leaves, ginger, turmeric, asafoetida, and green chile (if using) and cook, stirring, until the spices release their oils and become fragrant, about 2 minutes.

Add the bell pepper and cook, stirring, until softened, about 5 minutes. Stir in the tomatoes and coconut milk, reduce the heat to low, and cook, stirring, until the flavors have come together, about 5 minutes.

Add the black-eyed peas, black chickpeas, kidney beans, peanut butter, garam masala, salt, and coriander. Increase the heat to medium and cook, stirring frequently, until the beans are very soft and the flavors have married, about 10 minutes.

In a small bowl, whisk together the cornstarch and 1 tablespoon water until smooth. Add the mixture to the curry and cook until thickened, about 5 minutes.

Divide the curry among bowls and top with the chopped cilantro.

Leftovers can be stored in a sealed container in the refrigerator for up to 3 days.

NOTE Black chickpeas, called kala chana, have a much nuttier flavor than white chickpeas and also hold their shape much better when they're boiled. Plus, they're high in fiber, iron, and calcium. But in a pinch, feel free to use white chickpeas, which are no slouches in the health department. They're also a rich source of vitamins, minerals, and gut-nourishing fiber.

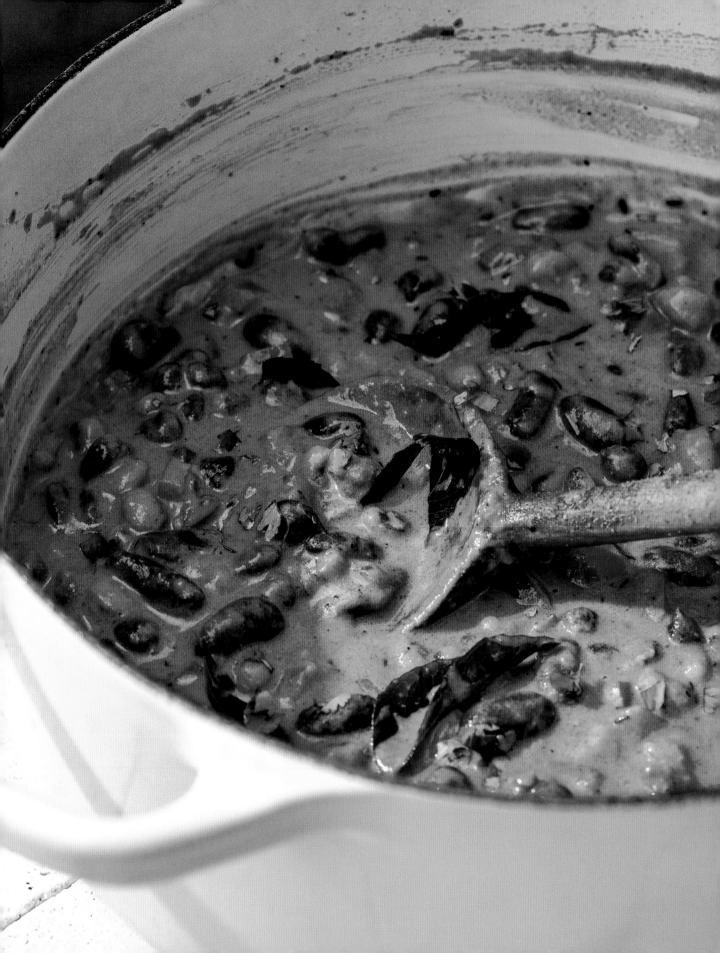

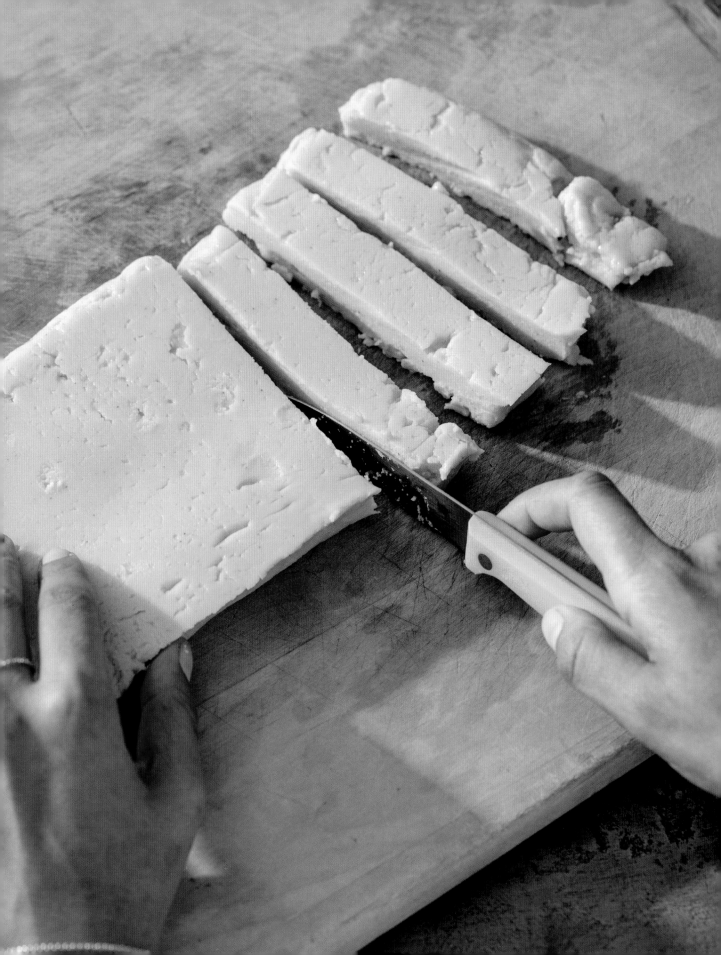

MAGIC PROTEIN "PANEER"

If you were to ask Indians around the world what their favorite dish is, I'd bet on it having paneer in it. I don't blame them—it's a cheese with a magical texture that's soft yet firm, and it has a very mild flavor that absorbs whatever saucy goodness it's tossed with. So when my family went vegan, we definitely had this "Oh no! We'll never eat paneer again!" moment. Then one day my mum was making a dish called khandvi, where you heat chickpea flour with water, spread it thin so it can thicken like (delicious) Play-Doh, then roll it up to eat. By mistake, my mum let it start cooling before she spread it flat, so she cubed it up instead and tossed it into a curry. When we ate it, we thought *for sure* it was paneer. Now we throw this happy accident into any dish we'd normally enjoy with paneer—and have tricked a number of people since.

Chickpea flour is naturally high in protein and low in fat (which paneer is not), and it has a rich flavor. You can include this paneer in curries, marinate it and bake it like tofu, use it in place of jackfruit or cauliflower in wraps, or spice it up and treat it like scrambled eggs to heap onto toast.

MAKES *2½ cups or 35 to 40 ½-inch cubes*
TOTAL TIME: *35 minutes*

- 1 cup besan or gram flour (see Note)
- 1 teaspoon sea salt

In a large bowl, whisk the flour with 2 cups water until very smooth.

Transfer the mixture to a deep heavy-bottomed pot over medium-low heat. Whisking constantly, cook until the mixture becomes rather thick, like polenta, 10 to 15 minutes. Taste to check the texture—it should not feel "floury" in your mouth. (But also, don't judge the texture or flavor based on this one tiny bite; it will change a lot after some time in the fridge!)

Quickly transfer the mixture to a nonstick sheet pan. Use a silicone spatula or oil your hands to press it into the pan. It doesn't need to fit the pan perfectly—it can press up against one side of the pan and you can simply push it into a rectangle about ½ inch thick.

Refrigerate until fully set, about 10 minutes. Cut the "paneer" into ½-inch cubes and store in a sealed container in the refrigerator for up to 1 week.

NOTE I use besan or gram, essentially brown chickpea flour, for this recipe because it's finer and milder in flavor than white chickpea chana lot. Also, if you don't have a nonstick baking sheet, you can line a regular baking sheet with parchment paper.

BHARAZI

CREAMY PIGEON PEAS WITH GINGER AND CILANTRO

My mum grew up in Uganda, so many of the dishes she made for us were subtly influenced by the food she had experienced there, including this traditional East African recipe. The combination of pigeon peas, coconut milk, spices, and fresh cilantro makes for a gorgeously creamy, gingery dish that feels as warming as its sunshine-yellow color. Just serve it over some basmati rice and feel the love.

SERVES *4*

TOTAL TIME: *25 minutes*

- 1 tablespoon sunflower or avocado oil
- 2 small green chiles, such as Thai, finely chopped
- 1 tablespoon finely grated fresh ginger
- 1 cup grated or very thinly sliced cabbage (about ½ small head)
- 1 teaspoon ground turmeric
- 3 cups cooked or canned pigeon peas (rinsed and drained if canned)
- 1 13.5-ounce can full-fat coconut milk
- ½ teaspoon sea salt
- ¼ teaspoon asafoetida
- ½ tablespoon cornstarch
- ½ cup chopped fresh cilantro leaves, plus more for serving
- 1 lemon, halved

In a large saucepan, heat the oil over medium heat. Add the chiles and ginger and cook, stirring, until fragrant, about 30 seconds. Add the cabbage and turmeric and cook, stirring, for 2 minutes. Reduce the heat to low and add the peas, coconut milk, salt, and asafoetida. Let the mixture simmer gently for 15 minutes.

In a small bowl, whisk together the cornstarch and 2 tablespoons water. Stir the cornstarch mixture into the curry, along with the chopped cilantro. Add a generous squeeze of lemon juice over the top.

Serve sprinkled with more cilantro.

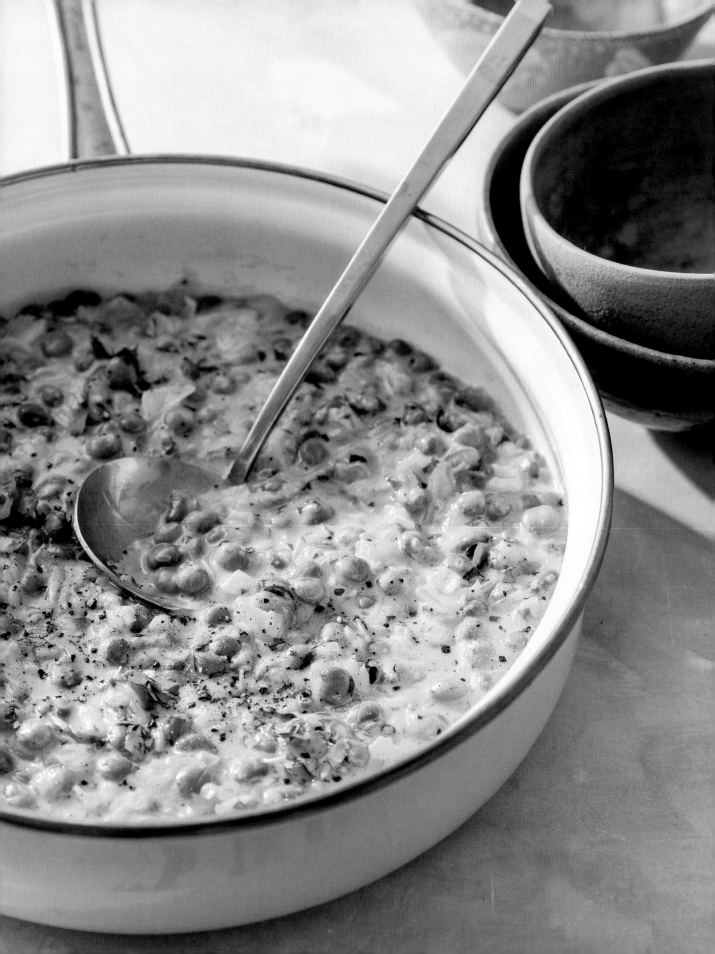

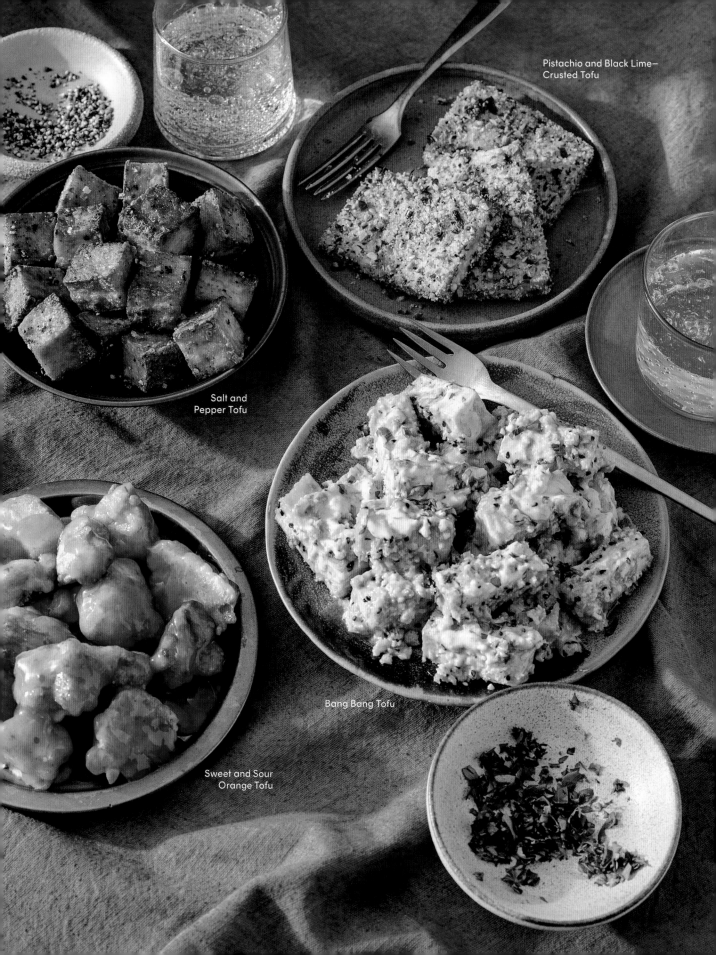

Pistachio and Black Lime–Crusted Tofu

Salt and Pepper Tofu

Bang Bang Tofu

Sweet and Sour Orange Tofu

CRISPY TOFU FOUR WAYS

Tofu gets a bad rap because people assume that it's soggy and bland (which fine, yes, it is—if you eat it straight out of the package, which no one would ever reasonably do). But when you crisp it up, its mild flavor becomes the perfect canvas for all kinds of saucy, spiced combinations. These four variations will scratch the itch whenever you happen to have a block of tofu in your fridge and you need a quick protein-rich dish. You could serve these on their own or heaped over rice, stuffed into tacos, sprinkled on salads, or next to your favorite Hero Veg (pages 187–211). You can also easily scale up these recipes if you want additional servings.

BANG BANG TOFU

SERVES *4 as a side or 2 as a main*
TOTAL TIME: *25 minutes*

1 16-ounce block extra-firm tofu

SAUCE

½ cup vegan mayonnaise

1½ tablespoons sambal oelek

1 tablespoon agave nectar

1 teaspoon rice vinegar

¼ teaspoon sea salt

⅛ teaspoon asafoetida

CRISPY TOFU

Olive oil cooking spray or avocado oil

½ cup panko bread crumbs

2 tablespoons cornstarch

1 tablespoon black sesame seeds

¼ teaspoon asafoetida

¼ teaspoon sea salt

Chopped fresh parsley, for serving

Press the tofu as directed in Pressing Tofu (page 139).

MEANWHILE, MAKE THE SAUCE: In a large bowl, whisk together the mayonnaise, sambal, agave nectar, rice vinegar, salt, and asafoetida. Set aside.

MAKE THE CRISPY TOFU: Preheat the oven to 400°F. Line a baking sheet with parchment paper and lightly coat the parchment with cooking spray or brush with avocado oil.

In a wide, shallow bowl, stir together the panko, cornstarch, sesame seeds, asafoetida, and salt.

Cut the tofu into 1-inch cubes. Working in batches so as not to crumble the tofu, toss the cubes in the panko mixture until each cube is fully coated. Arrange the tofu on the prepared baking sheet and spray with more oil.

Bake the tofu until browned and crispy, about 15 minutes, giving them a toss halfway through.

Transfer the crispy tofu to the sauce and toss well to coat. Sprinkle with chopped parsley and serve immediately.

SALT AND PEPPER TOFU

SERVES *4 as a side or 2 as a main*
TOTAL TIME: *30 minutes*

1 16-ounce block extra-firm tofu

2 tablespoons sunflower or avocado oil

1½ tablespoons liquid aminos, tamari, or soy sauce

1 teaspoon light brown sugar (optional)

¾ teaspoon freshly ground black pepper

⅛ teaspoon sea salt

2 tablespoons cornstarch

Press the tofu as directed in Pressing Tofu (page 139).

Meanwhile, prepare the marinade: In a medium bowl, whisk together 1 tablespoon of the oil, 1 tablespoon of the liquid aminos, the brown sugar (if using), ½ teaspoon of the pepper, and the salt.

Recipes Continue

Unwrap the tofu and cut it into ½-inch cubes. Add the tofu to the marinade and toss well to coat. Set aside to let the tofu soak at room temperature for 10 minutes.

Use a slotted spoon or kitchen spider to transfer the tofu to a large bowl, shaking off any excess marinade. Sprinkle the cornstarch and the remaining ¼ teaspoon black pepper over the tofu. Toss carefully to coat to avoid crumbling the tofu.

In a large nonstick skillet, heat the remaining 1 tablespoon oil over medium-low heat. Add the tofu cubes and cook undisturbed, letting them sizzle and crisp, about 2 minutes. Continue cooking and flipping the tofu until crispy on all sides (a thin metal spatula works well for this). Drizzle the remaining ½ tablespoon liquid aminos over the tofu, carefully toss to coat, and stir-fry for just another minute.

Remove the pan from the heat. Serve immediately.

PISTACHIO AND BLACK LIME-CRUSTED TOFU

SERVES *4 as a side or 2 as a main*
TOTAL TIME: *30 minutes*

Olive oil cooking spray or avocado oil

1 16-ounce block extra-firm tofu

¼ cup liquid aminos

¾ cup vegan mayonnaise

1½ teaspoons Dijon mustard

¼ teaspoon asafoetida

½ cup finely chopped unsalted roasted pistachios (you could pulse them in a food processor or high-powered blender)

½ cup plain dried bread crumbs

2 teaspoons dried parsley

1 teaspoon ground black lime (see Note)

½ teaspoon red chile flakes

So Much More Than a Burger Sauce (page 235) or, to upscale it, Spiced Apple and Golden Raisin Chutney (page 244), for dipping

Preheat the oven to 425°F. Line a baking sheet with parchment paper and lightly coat the parchment with spray or oil.

Press the tofu as directed in Pressing Tofu (page 139).

Meanwhile, set up a dredging station with three shallow bowls: Pour the liquid aminos into one bowl. In a second bowl, whisk together the mayonnaise, mustard, and asafoetida. In the third bowl, combine the pistachios, bread crumbs, parsley, black lime, and chile flakes.

Unwrap the tofu. Cut the tofu into 8 slices ½ inch thick. Cut each slice in half if you prefer smaller pieces. Dip a slice in the aminos to coat on each side. Dip into the mayo mixture and then the pistachio mixture, gently pressing the tofu into the mix to coat all over. Set the tofu on the prepared baking sheet and repeat with the remaining tofu slices.

Lightly coat the tofu with cooking spray or brush with avocado oil and bake the tofu slices until the bread crumbs are crisp and golden brown, about 20 minutes, flipping halfway through (a thin metal spatula works well for this).

Serve the crispy tofu with sauces for dipping, if desired.

NOTE   Black limes are sun-dried limes that were originally used in Middle Eastern cooking. They bring a seductive smoky-citrus note to a dish. You can find whole black limes as well as ground black limes in international markets or online. Use this versatile ingredient to add a bright, tart depth of flavor to pretty much anything you're cooking.

SWEET AND SOUR ORANGE TOFU

SERVES *4 as a side or 2 as a main*
TOTAL TIME: *25 minutes*

CRISPY TOFU

- 1 16-ounce block extra-firm tofu
- ⅓ cup all-purpose flour
- ¼ cup cornstarch
- ½ teaspoon sea salt
- ¼ teaspoon freshly ground black pepper
- 2 tablespoons sunflower or avocado oil

SAUCE

- 1 cup freshly squeezed orange juice (about 3 large oranges)
- 2 tablespoons soy sauce
- 2 tablespoons rice vinegar
- 2 tablespoons agave nectar
- 1 tablespoon toasted sesame oil
- 1 tablespoon sambal oelek
- ¼ teaspoon finely grated fresh ginger
- ¼ teaspoon freshly ground black pepper
- ⅛ teaspoon asafoetida
- 1 tablespoon cornstarch

MAKE THE CRISPY TOFU: Press the tofu as directed in Pressing Tofu (at right).

Meanwhile, in a shallow bowl, whisk together the flour, cornstarch, salt, pepper, and ½ cup water.

Unwrap the tofu, tear it into 1-inch pieces, and add the pieces to the batter.

Set a wire rack in a sheet pan. In a large skillet, heat the oil over medium-low heat until it shimmers. Working in batches if needed, shake off any excess batter and add the tofu pieces to the hot oil. Cook undisturbed until the underside is golden brown, about 2 minutes. Turn the tofu pieces (a thin metal spatula works best for this) and cook, continuing to turn, until they're evenly crisp on all sides, 1 or 2 minutes per side. Transfer the crispy tofu to the wire rack (this will keep the tofu from steaming and getting soggy as it sits, and the baking sheet will catch any excess oil). Repeat with the remaining tofu. Remove the skillet from the heat and allow it to cool slightly.

MAKE THE SAUCE: Carefully wipe out the pan to remove as much of the excess oil as possible. Add the orange juice, soy sauce, vinegar, agave, sesame oil, sambal, ginger, black pepper, and asafoetida and whisk to combine.

In a small bowl, mix the cornstarch with 1 tablespoon water until it forms a slurry. Whisk the slurry into the sauce. Place the pan over medium heat and cook while whisking until it thickens, about 5 minutes.

Add the crispy tofu to the sauce and gently toss to coat. Serve immediately.

Pressing Tofu: The Secret to Extra-Crispy Results

There's a direct connection between the crispiness of tofu and its deliciousness, which is why it's worth getting it right for these recipes.

Luckily, it's very simple:

1. Wrap an extra-firm tofu block in a few layers of paper towel or a clean kitchen towel and set it on a plate.

2. Place something heavy on top of the tofu, like a cutting board topped with a skillet, and let sit for 30 minutes to release the excess liquid. (Alternatively, you could use a tofu press, if you have one.)

You could also freeze the tofu overnight to enhance the texture. It transforms from slippery cube to chewy and firm. And when it's thawed, the tofu becomes a porous sponge that can soak up even more of your marinade or sauce.

KITCHARI *(aka The Belly Cuddle)*

Kitchari means "mixture" and it is an age-old recipe Indian mums and dads reach for whenever someone's feeling a little under the weather. It's warm, mildly flavored, and easy to digest—basically like a little hug for your belly. In Ayurveda, kitchari is considered the mother of all dishes because the combination of split and peeled mung beans and rice makes a complete protein, and the ingredients are thought to cleanse the stomach and digestive system, as well as help nourish, replenish, and reset your body during seasonal changes. (The reason why it's the foundation of a staple Ayurvedic cleanse, which you can read more about in Kitchari Reset, page 142.) As a kid, I'd always get so mad whenever I had to eat kitchari because I always thought of it as what you eat when you're sick, or as a meal that felt too "boring," but now I regularly treat myself to a warm, nourishing bowlful.

SERVES *4 to 6*

TOTAL TIME: *25 to 40 minutes, plus soaking time*

- 1 cup moong daal (split moong beans)
- 1 cup basmati rice (or ½ cup quinoa and ½ cup basmati rice)
- 2 cups chopped mixed fresh or frozen and thawed vegetables, such as green beans, zucchini, or carrots (a great opportunity to clean out your crisper!)
- 1 cup packed fresh spinach leaves, chopped
- 1 tablespoon extra-virgin olive oil
- 1 teaspoon cumin seeds
- 1 teaspoon brown or black mustard seeds
- ¼ cup canned full-fat coconut milk (optional)
- 10 fresh or dried curry leaves
- 1 teaspoon Ground CCF Masala (see page 49)
- 1 teaspoon garam masala or additional ground CCF masala
- 2 teaspoons finely grated fresh ginger
- ½ teaspoon ground turmeric
- 1 teaspoon sea salt
- Cilantro-Mint Chutney (page 243), for serving
- Plain vegan yogurt, for serving

In a medium bowl, combine the moong daal and enough water to cover. Soak in the refrigerator for at least 2 hours or overnight.

Drain the lentils through a fine-mesh sieve and add the rice. Rinse them under running water until the water runs clear.

In a large pot, combine the rinsed moong daal, rice, and 6 cups water. Cover partially and cook over medium heat for 10 minutes. Add the chopped vegetables, partially cover again, and cook until the vegetables, moong daal, and rice have bonded and become friends—the texture will be mushy and soupy, 20 to 25 minutes. About 5 minutes before the mixture is done cooking, stir in the spinach.

Meanwhile, in a large skillet, heat the olive oil over medium heat. Add the cumin and mustard seeds and cook, stirring, until they pop, 1 to 2 minutes. Add the coconut milk (if using), curry leaves, CCF masala, garam masala, ginger, turmeric, and salt and cook, stirring, until soft and fragrant, about 2 minutes. Transfer the mixture to the daal-rice mixture and stir to incorporate.

Add more water, if desired, to loosen the consistency and serve with the chutney and yogurt.

Leftovers can be stored in a sealed container in the refrigerator for up to 3 days.

NOTE I like adjusting the consistency of this to suit my mood—sometimes I like it thick and creamy, while other times I prefer it looser and soupier. I've noted where you can add more water to make this to your and your body's liking.

RADHI DEVLUKIA-SHETTY

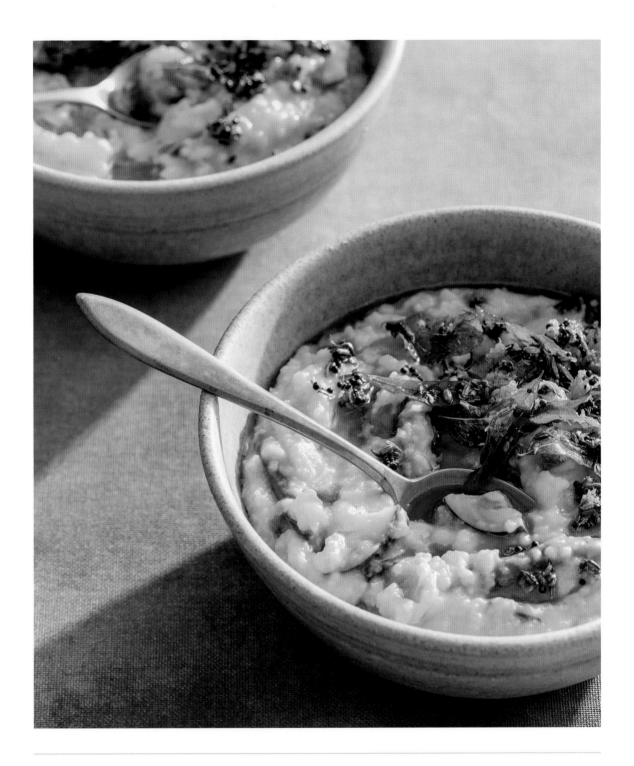

VARIATION *Pressure Cooker Kitchari:* To make this in an electric pressure cooker, add the rinsed moong daal and rice, chopped vegetables, coconut milk (if using), and 6 cups water to the pot. Close, seal, and cook on high for 8 minutes. Let the pressure release naturally for 10 minutes, then manually release any remaining pressure. Meanwhile, make the sautéed spiced mixture as directed (minus the coconut milk, which is already in the pot). When the daal-rice mixture is done, stir in the spinach and the toasted spice mixture. Add more water, if desired, to loosen the consistency and serve with the chutney and yogurt.

Kitchari Reset

Our bodies very much want to sync with nature, so during seasonal transitions, just like Mother Nature, we go through significant changes. You might notice when the seasons change how you feel a little heavier and sluggish, or maybe get the sniffles, a cough, or seasonal allergies as your body adjusts. To help support your body through these shifts, Ayurveda recommends a kitchari reset.

This brief mono-diet—meaning you'll enjoy the same simple (but delicious and flavorful) foods for most of your meals—is about paring back the variety of what you're tasking your digestive system with so that it has an opportunity to rest and restore, while also deeply nourishing your body (particularly your gut) with essential nutrients. Kitchari (page 140), with its blend of easy-to-digest rice, split moong beans, and stewed veggies, is the perfect way to deliver that nutrition without taxing the digestive system.

You can follow this protocol for 3 to 5 days, or start with just one day until you feel more comfortable. Once you see how incredible you feel, I'm willing to bet you'll want to sign on for longer—which is completely fine seeing as you're not doing anything but enjoying whole, plant-based meals.

BENEFITS OF THE RESET

- Improved digestion

- Regular elimination (aka helps you poop if you're not going daily . . . which you should be!)

- Boosted energy levels and mood

- Improved mental clarity (aka less of a foggy head)

- Better sleep quality

- Strengthened digestion and absorption of nutrients

- Generally feeling like the best version of you!

HOW TO DO IT

Traditionally for this protocol, kitchari is eaten three times a day. However, if you want some variety, you can mix it up with some simple veggie soups (the fewer ingredients, the better). Zucchini, Fennel, and Mint Soup (page 223) or Curried Butternut Squash Soup (page 228) would be particularly nice, as well as Spiced Stewed Apples (page 64). I'm recommending these foods in particular because they're so nourishing as well as easy on the digestive system. Here's what your menu will look like:

- **BREAKFAST**
  Spiced Stewed Apples (page 64) or Kitchari (page 140)

- **LUNCH**
  Soup or Kitchari

- **DINNER**
  Soup or Kitchari

- **WATER**
  3 liters warm or hot water throughout the day

TIPS

- Try to eat with your hands to reconnect with your food.

- Keep at least 3 hours between your meals.

- Try to eat your evening meal before 7 p.m. (or at least 3 hours before you sleep)

- Avoid snacking between meals. I once read in an Ayurvedic textbook: "When we eat a meal, our body is using that for fuel. Only when the food is fully digested does it allow our body to start using the fat in our body as fuel. Fat is where the toxins hide and reside." Ideally, we want to get into that state as often as possible to be able to get the most out of this cleanse!

- If you do get hungry, have a small piece of fruit or more stewed apples.

- Get to bed by 10 p.m. so the body can use the evening to do what it is meant to be doing . . . resting and detoxing!

- Try to make time for self-care rituals that enhance this detox process, such as abhyanga massage (page 58), a bath, and gharshana (dry brushing, page 59).

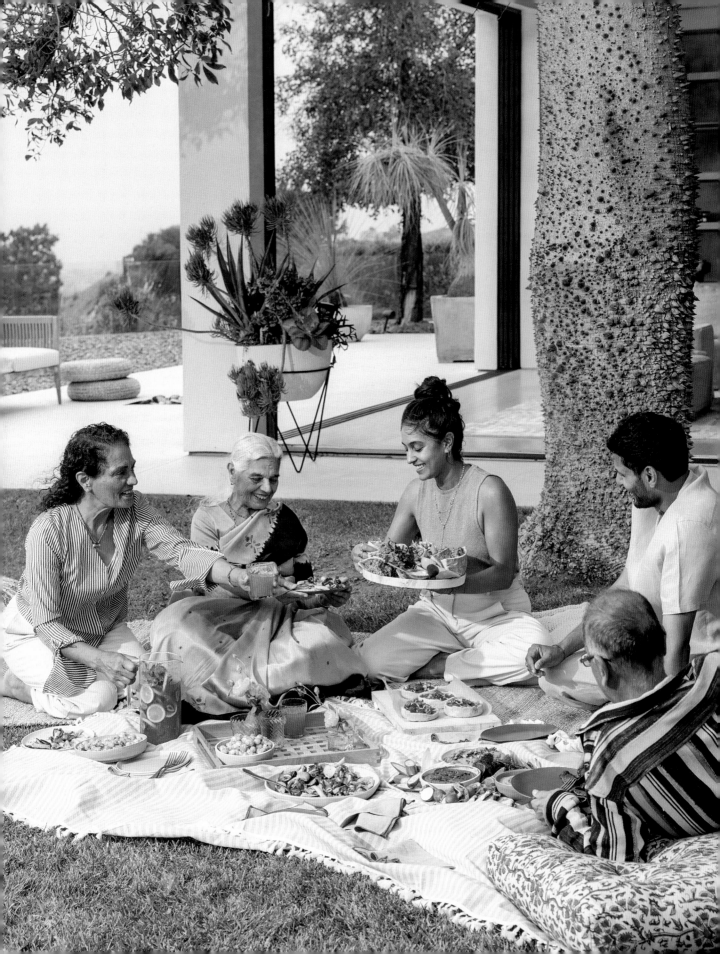

BREAD IS LIFE

With a few exceptions, in Ayurveda, there is no such thing as a wholly "bad" food; Ayurveda doesn't judge. Rather, the practice guides you to ask your body whether you're eating the foods it needs at the right time and in the right way. We need carbohydrates at the peak of our day when we're burning through energy. And what more enjoyable, more satisfying way to enjoy them than with breads? I've dedicated this chapter to my younger self and the bravery it took to say, "I'd rather treat this body with love than with fear." Without her, I'd never know the truth: Bread is life.

THE EVERYTHING SANDWICH

When we were children, my sister and I were allowed to go to the corner shop once a week to buy crisps (what Americans call potato chips). After carefully making our selections, we'd go home and create an epic sandwich stuffed with the crisps, along with pretty much every condiment we had in the fridge (my love for sauces started young!). This approach to sandwich making has stayed with me, and of all the elaborate meals I've made for family and friends, it's this "dish" that stands out. Even my dad asks me to make it for him every time I'm home in London. It's a super-saucy, deeply flavorful mix of herbaceous pesto, creamy mayo, spicy jalapeños, salty sun-dried tomatoes, and some fresh greens, plus a cheeky drizzle of ketchup (because who doesn't like ketchup?). Don't be surprised if you see me open a sandwich shop and this one's on the menu.

MAKES *1 sandwich*
TOTAL TIME: *15 minutes*

Extra-virgin olive oil, for toasting

1 6-inch ciabatta roll or piece of focaccia, halved, or 2 slices of your favorite bread

2 tablespoons vegan mayonnaise or vegan cream cheese

2 tablespoons Perfect Hummus (page 239)

2 teaspoons Cavolo Nero Pesto (page 200) or store-bought basil pesto

1 teaspoon sambal oelek

1 teaspoon spicy English or Dijon mustard

3 to 5 slices vegan cheese or ¼ to ½ cup shredded vegan cheese

3 or 4 oil-packed sun-dried tomatoes, chopped

2 tablespoons chopped pitted green or black olives

5 to 6 slices pickled jalapeño peppers, chopped

½ cup arugula

Ketchup (optional, but strongly advised)

Your favorite potato chips (optional, but strongly advised)

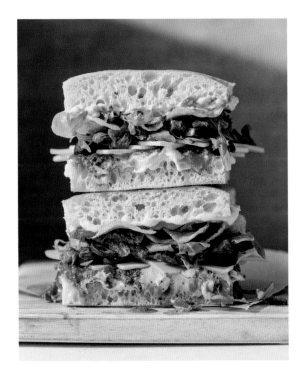

Brush olive oil on both sides of each slice of bread. In a large skillet, toast the bread over medium heat on both sides. (You could also do this under a low broiler or in a toaster, but without the oil.) Let cool.

Spread mayo over both slices of bread, followed by a layer each of hummus and pesto. Spread the sambal on one piece of bread and the mustard on the other. Layer on the cheese, sun-dried tomatoes, olives, and jalapeños. Top with the arugula. If desired, add a squirt of ketchup and a handful of potato chips. Devour immediately.

SPICY BEAN BURGERS *with Caramelized "Onions"*

Because I grew up a vegetarian, the burgers I ate were always made with lentils or beans and tons of spices. So when all those mock meat burgers appeared in markets with the promise that they tasted "meaty," it just wasn't something I could get used to or enjoy. I'd so much rather have a big, crispy breaded patty filled with smoky, spicy flavor and fresh ingredients. And don't go thinking this one's going to fall apart on you—which I get; I've been there—this burger can go the distance. Plus, we're dressing it with a creamy vegan sauce (inspired by In-N-Out Burgers), a fresh corn salsa, and my famous caramelized "onions," which are actually made from cabbage (you'd never know, though—they fooled every single person who tried them at a London food festival). All to say, you need this burger in your life.

SERVES *6*

TOTAL TIME: *1 hour*

BURGERS

Olive oil cooking spray or avocado oil

2 tablespoons avocado oil, plus more as needed

1 cup shredded cabbage

½ cup peeled and finely grated carrot

½ cup finely diced green bell pepper

1½ teaspoons ground cumin

1 teaspoon sea salt

½ teaspoon asafoetida

1 tablespoon tomato paste

1 15-ounce can black beans, rinsed and drained

1 15-ounce can kidney beans, rinsed and drained

½ cup plain fine bread crumbs

⅓ cup chopped fresh cilantro

10 slices pickled jalapeño peppers, chopped

1 tablespoon nutritional yeast

2 teaspoons dried parsley

1 teaspoon chipotle powder

½ teaspoon dried oregano

CARAMELIZED CABBAGE

2 tablespoons avocado oil

2 cups finely shredded cabbage (about ½ small head)

1 teaspoon sea salt

½ teaspoon liquid aminos

¼ teaspoon asafoetida

ASSEMBLY

Burger buns, pita, or sandwich thins, toasted

Mustard, So Much More than a Burger Sauce (page 235) or ketchup, vegan mayonnaise

Vegan cheddar cheese slices (optional)

Corn Salsa with a Kick (page 240)

Sliced tomatoes

Sliced pickles

Lettuce leaves

MAKE THE BURGERS: Preheat the oven to 350°F. Line a baking sheet with parchment paper and lightly coat with the cooking spray or brush with avocado oil.

In a large skillet, heat the oil over medium heat. Add the cabbage, carrot, bell pepper, cumin, salt, and asafoetida and cook until the cabbage starts to sweat and soften, about 10 minutes. Stir in the tomato paste and remove the pan from the heat.

Transfer the vegetable mixture to a food processor or high-powered blender and add 1 cup of the black beans plus all of the kidney beans, bread crumbs, cilantro, jalapeños, nutritional yeast, parsley, chipotle powder, and oregano. Pulse until just combined and evenly mixed but not pureed.

Transfer the vegetable-bean mixture to a large bowl and add the remaining ½ cup black beans. Gently mix until combined; you don't want the mixture to get too mushy.

Recipe Continues

Lightly oil your hands with some avocado oil and use a ⅓-cup measure to form the mixture into patties. Arrange them on the prepared baking sheet and bake until warmed through and browned on each side, 20 to 25 minutes, gently turning halfway through (a thin metal spatula works well here). Transfer the burgers to a wire rack and set aside.

MEANWHILE, MAKE THE CARAMELIZED CABBAGE: In a medium skillet, heat the oil over medium heat. Cook, stirring, until the cabbage begins to soften, about 3 minutes. Add the salt, liquid aminos, and asafoetida and cook, stirring frequently, until the cabbage is soft and caramelized on the edges and has a deep, savory aroma, 5 to 7 minutes. Remove the pan from the heat and set aside.

ASSEMBLE THE BURGERS: Toast the buns, then spread them with mustard, tangy vegan sauce or ketchup, and mayo as desired. Top with a warm burger patty and a slice of cheese, if desired. Add a layer of the caramelized cabbage and corn salsa. Follow with your choice of sliced tomatoes, pickles, and/or lettuce. Top with the other half of the bun and serve.

NOTE You could also grill these burgers, or make them on the stovetop in a grill pan or skillet. To grill, cook over medium-high heat for 1 to 2 minutes per side, until nicely charred and warmed through. To make them on the stovetop, cook them over medium heat for 2 minutes per side.

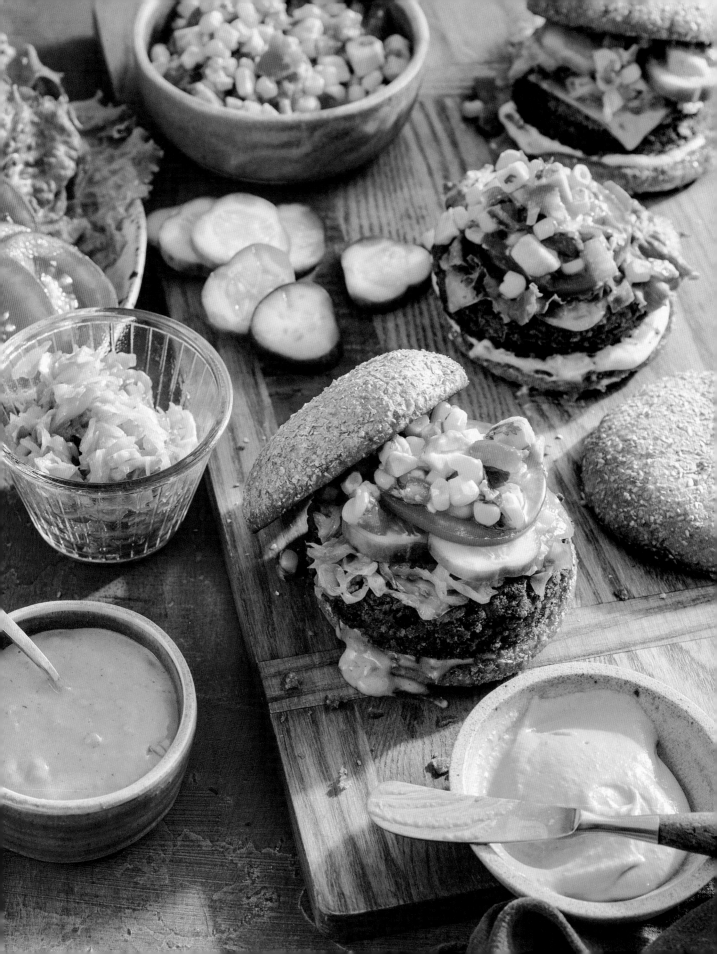

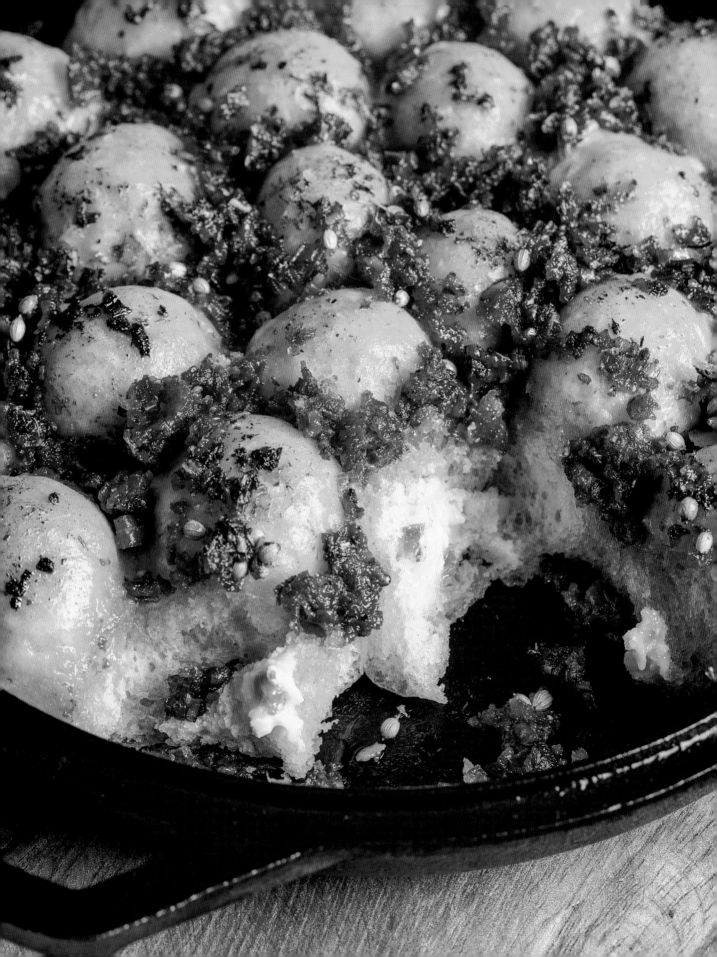

CHEESY BREAD TWO WAYS

These feel like the Saturday Night Dream: bread and cheese. It brings me back to the days of hanging out with my family and sharing a Pizza Hut deep-dish pizza. Does it get better than (a plant-based version of) that with a gooey jalapeño filling plus either a cheesy, tomato-y masala topping or a drizzle of herbed butter? No. No, it doesn't. With a side of dip (obviously) and salad, it's the perfect meal. It's also a fun dish to make with kids or a meditative little project for a weekend afternoon.

SERVES 6
TOTAL TIME: *35 minutes*

DOUGH

- 1 cup warm water
- 2 teaspoons active dry yeast
- 1 teaspoon raw organic sugar
- 3 cups spelt flour, plus more for dusting
- 2 tablespoons extra-virgin olive oil

JALAPEÑO-CHEESE FILLING

- 1½ cups shredded vegan mozzarella, at room temperature
- 4 ounces vegan cream cheese or vegan ricotta
- ¼ cup chopped pickled or fresh jalapeño peppers
- Extra-virgin olive oil, for rolling

ASSEMBLY

- Masala Topping (optional; recipe follows) or Herb Butter (optional; recipe follows)
- Olive oil cooking spray or avocado oil
- Marinara sauce or So Much More Than a Burger Sauce (page 235), for dipping (optional)

MAKE THE DOUGH: In a medium bowl, combine the warm water, yeast, and sugar and stir to combine. Set aside and let the yeast proof for 5 minutes, until you see a thick layer of foam form on the top.

In a large bowl with a wooden spoon or your hands (or in a stand mixer fitted with the dough hook), combine 1 cup of the flour, 1 tablespoon of the olive oil, and the yeast mixture. Gently mix the dough as you continue adding the flour ½ cup at a time. The dough will be a bit sticky.

Dust a work surface with flour and turn out the dough. Knead for about 4 minutes, until it forms a smooth ball. Cover the dough lightly with a towel and set aside for 5 minutes.

MAKE THE JALAPEÑO-CHEESE FILLING: In a medium bowl, combine the mozzarella, cream cheese, and jalapeños. Use a fork to mash everything together.

Use the olive oil to lightly coat your hands and pinch off about 1 teaspoon of the filling. Roll the mixture into a little ball and set aside on a plate. (Prepping the filling like this makes it easy to pop into the dough.) Repeat with the remaining cheese mixture. Freeze the cheese balls while you prepare the other components, if using, at least 10 minutes.

ASSEMBLE THE BREAD: Make either the masala topping or herb butter.

Lightly coat a large (12-inch) cast-iron skillet or a 13 × 9-inch baking dish with cooking spray or brush with avocado oil.

Recipe Continues

Pinch off a tablespoon-size piece of the dough and flatten it a bit in your palm. Press one of the frozen cheese balls in the center. Pinch off a second tablespoon-size piece of dough and flatten it slightly on top of the cheese ball. Roll the filled dough in your hands to make a ball.

FOR THE MASALA VERSION: Dip the ball in the masala mixture, rolling it around a bit if needed to coat it thoroughly. Place the dough ball in the prepared pan. Repeat with the remaining dough, cheese balls, and masala, nestling them closely in the pan.

FOR THE HERB BUTTER VERSION: Just stuff and roll the balls and place them in the baking dish (the herb butter is added after they are baked).

FOR BOTH VERSIONS: Cover the pan with a cloth and let the bread rise for about 45 minutes, until doubled in size.

Preheat the oven to 350°F.

Bake the bread until the top is crisp and golden, about 20 minutes.

FOR THE HERB BUTTER VERSION: Melt the butter in a small pan over medium-low heat. When the bread is done baking, pour the herb butter all over the warm bread.

Serve immediately with dipping sauce, if you like.

NOTE For the ultimate cheat, you can use store-bought pizza dough instead of making your own. You can also press the dough into a large cast-iron pan, layer on the cheesy jalapeño topping, then add the masala or butter and bake it like a pizza.

Herb Butter
MAKES *¼ cup*
TOTAL TIME: *5 minutes*

- 4 tablespoons (2 ounces) unsalted vegan butter, at room temperature or melted
- 1 teaspoon dried oregano
- 1 teaspoon dried basil
- ¼ teaspoon sea salt
- ⅛ teaspoon asafoetida

In a medium bowl, mash together the butter, oregano, basil, salt, and asafoetida.

Masala Topping
MAKES *a scant 1 cup*
TOTAL TIME: *10 minutes*

- ¼ cup extra-virgin olive oil
- 1½ tablespoons garam masala or Ground CCF Masala (page 49)
- 1 tablespoon dried oregano
- 1 tablespoon minced hot green chile, such as Thai
- ½ tablespoon Italian seasoning
- 1 teaspoon sea salt
- ¼ teaspoon asafoetida
- ¼ teaspoon ground turmeric
- 3 tablespoons tomato paste
- ¼ cup grated vegan parmesan cheese
- ¼ cup grated vegan cheddar cheese

In a medium skillet, heat the oil over low heat. Add the garam masala, oregano, green chile, Italian seasoning, salt, asafoetida, and turmeric and warm gently, stirring occasionally, until the spices release their fragrance, about 2 minutes. Add the tomato paste and cook, stirring, until the color deepens and the tomatoes smell deeply savory, about 3 minutes. Remove the pan from the heat and stir in the parmesan and cheddar.

NAAN (OR ROTI) PIZZA FOUR WAYS

My mum often used naan as a base for pizza. We frequently had it left over, and then all she needed to do was slather and sprinkle on a few toppings and dinner or lunch was made. I now prefer the slightly sour tang of the fermented naan to pizza crust, so I see no reason to mess with a good thing. Here are four variations on this super-simple concept that each pack a ton of flavor while requiring very little prep once you have the naan made (and even less if you use store-bought naan!). Make just one or make all four and call it a party.

NOTE   My Proper Good Naan (page 156) is perfect for these recipes and will yield 6 large pizzas, but feel free to use store-bought naan—either 12 small or 6 large—or store-bought pizza dough. If using the small naan, divide the topping ingredients accordingly.

CURRIED CRISPY KALE, MANGO CHUTNEY, AND RICOTTA

MAKES *6 naan pizzas*
TOTAL TIME: *40 minutes*

- 6 large naan, homemade (page 156) or store-bought
- 1 12-ounce jar of Indian mango chutney or 1½ cups Spiced Apple and Golden Raisin Chutney (page 244), pureed in a blender
- 8 ounces vegan ricotta or vegan cream cheese
- 1 4-ounce jar brined capers, drained
- 4 small hot Indian or Thai green chiles (optional), finely chopped
- Cheesy Curried Crispy Kale (page 254), for serving

Preheat the oven to 450°F. Line two baking sheets with parchment paper.

Spread the naan with a generous layer of the chutney, followed by dollops of the ricotta or cream cheese. Sprinkle the capers and chopped chiles (if using) on top.

Bake until the cheese melts, 10 to 12 minutes. Top with the crispy kale, slice, and serve.

GORGEOUSLY GREEN

MAKES *6 pizzas*
TOTAL TIME: *25 minutes*

- 6 large naan, homemade (page 156) or store-bought
- 1 cup Cilantro-Mint Chutney (page 243), Cavolo Nero Pesto (page 200), or store-bought basil pesto
- 1 cup thinly sliced fennel (about 1 small bulb)
- 1 cup thinly sliced zucchini (about 1 medium zucchini)
- 1 cup canned quartered artichokes, drained
- ½ cup thinly sliced red radishes (about ½ bunch)
- 2 cups shredded vegan parmesan or mozzarella, or ricotta

Preheat the oven to 450°F for at least 15 minutes before using. Line two baking sheets with parchment paper.

Spread the naan generously with the chutney or pesto and top with the fennel, zucchini, artichokes, and radishes. Sprinkle the cheese on top.

Bake until the cheese melts, 10 to 12 minutes. Slice and serve hot.

Recipes Continue

TANDOORI JACKFRUIT

MAKES *6 pizzas*
TOTAL TIME: *30 minutes, plus marinating time*

- 1 14-ounce can brined jackfruit, drained
- 1½ cups pizza sauce, homemade (from Spicy Pineapple Supreme Naan Pizzas, at right) or store-bought
- 2 tablespoons Tandoori Marinade (from Tandoori Tacos, page 159)
- 6 large naan, homemade (page 156) or store-bought
- 1 medium green bell pepper, thinly sliced
- Magic Protein "Paneer" (page 133)
- 2 to 3 cups shredded vegan mozzarella cheese
- Chopped fresh cilantro leaves, for serving

Tear the jackfruit into 1-inch pieces. Remove any hard parts, and squeeze out excess liquid with your hands. Place the jackfruit in a large bowl and add the pizza sauce and tandoori marinade. Toss well to coat the jackfruit. Set aside to marinate for at least 20 minutes or up to overnight.

Preheat the oven to 450°F for at least 15 minutes before using. Line two baking sheets with parchment paper.

Place the naan on the prepared baking sheets and spread 3 to 4 tablespoons of pizza sauce–marinade mixture onto each naan. Top as desired with the marinated jackfruit, sliced green pepper, and paneer. Sprinkle the mozzarella on top.

Bake until the cheese melts, 10 to 12 minutes. Top with chopped cilantro, slice, and serve.

For Extra-Gooey Cheese

Be sure to preheat your oven for at least 15 minutes, because getting it nice and hot is the key to getting that oh-so-crucial vegan cheese pull.

SPICY PINEAPPLE SUPREME

MAKES *6 pizzas*
TOTAL TIME: *35 minutes*

PIZZA SAUCE
- 1 tablespoon extra-virgin olive oil
- 2 bay leaves
- ⅛ teaspoon asafoetida
- 2 cups tomato puree or passata (16 ounces)
- 1 teaspoon dried oregano
- ½ teaspoon sea salt

ASSEMBLY
- 6 large naan, homemade (page 156) or store-bought
- 2 to 3 cups shredded vegan mozzarella cheese
- 1 cup fresh sweet corn kernels (from about 2 ears), or canned or thawed frozen
- 1 cup sliced jalapeño peppers
- 1 cup sliced black olives
- 1 cup chopped pineapple
- 2 green bell peppers, thinly sliced
- 1 tablespoon extra-virgin olive oil or chili oil

MAKE THE PIZZA SAUCE: In a medium saucepan, heat the oil over medium-low heat. Add the bay leaves and asafoetida and cook, stirring, until fragrant, about 1 minute. Stir in the tomato puree, oregano, and salt. Reduce the heat to low and simmer, stirring occasionally, until the flavors come together and the sauce has thickened, about 10 minutes. Remove the pan from the heat.

Preheat the oven to 450°F for at least 15 minutes before using. Line two baking sheets with parchment paper.

ASSEMBLE THE PIZZAS: Place the naan on the lined baking sheets and spread 3 to 4 tablespoons of sauce onto each naan. Top the pizzas as desired with the cheese, corn, jalapeño, olives, pineapple, and green pepper.

Bake until the cheese melts, 10 to 12 minutes. Drizzle a bit of extra-virgin olive oil or chili oil to finish, slice, and serve.

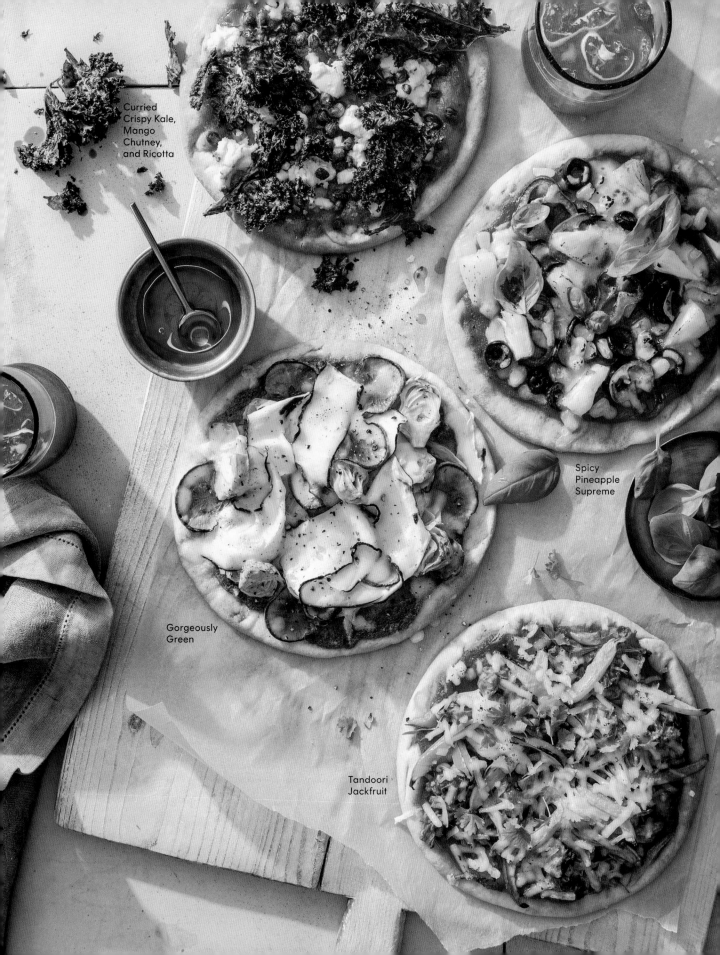

Curried Crispy Kale, Mango Chutney, and Ricotta

Spicy Pineapple Supreme

Gorgeously Green

Tandoori Jackfruit

PROPER GOOD NAAN

In traditional Indian culture, a good wife was assessed by the roundness of her roti, a type of flatbread, and how well she could make them. But ain't no one got time for that these days, so I'm calling this the Modern Woman's (or Man's) Bread. Naan is roti's more popular, less rounded or perfect but fluffier cousin, and is equally essential to an Indian meal because you use it to scoop up all the different components—vegetables, daal, rice, yogurt, chutney—like the most eco-friendly, delicious cutlery there is. This recipe will earn you naan that is doughy and tangy (and profoundly better than anything you could buy from the store), that's not difficult to make, and that certainly doesn't define who you are—unless you want it to!

MAKES *twelve 7-inch naan*

TOTAL TIME: *30 minutes (plus 45 minutes to 1 hour to rise)*

- 3 cups all-purpose flour, plus more for dusting
- ½ teaspoon baking powder
- 1 teaspoon sea salt
- 1 teaspoon raw organic sugar
- ½ tablespoon instant yeast
- 1 cup plain vegan yogurt
- 1 tablespoon avocado oil, plus more for kneading
- Topping options: vegan butter, kalonji seeds (aka nigella seeds), fresh cilantro leaves, chopped fresh hot Indian or Thai green chiles

In a large bowl, whisk together the flour, baking powder, salt, sugar, and yeast. Add the yogurt and combine with a fork until the dough is shaggy and the fork becomes difficult to move in the dough. Add 3½ tablespoons of water, 1 tablespoon at a time, using your hands to gently knead the water into the dough.

Lightly dust a clean work surface with flour. Turn out the dough, lightly oil your hands, and knead the dough for 4 to 5 minutes. (Alternatively, you could do this in a stand mixer fitted with the dough hook.) It will start out quite sticky, but as you continue kneading it will become soft, elastic, and pliable.

Oil a large bowl, place the dough in the bowl, and cover with a clean kitchen towel. Let the dough rest in a warm place until it rises and just about doubles in volume, 45 minutes to 1 hour. If your home is drafty, you can let the dough rise in an unheated oven.

Punch down the air in the dough. Turn it back out onto a work surface and divide it into 12 equal portions (about 2 ounces each). Roll the dough pieces into smooth balls by using your fingers as a "cage" over each ball and moving your hand in circles for a few seconds. Cover the finished dough balls with a kitchen towel to keep them from drying out and repeat with the remaining dough.

Heat a large cast-iron skillet over medium-low heat.

Using a rolling pin, roll each piece of dough into an oval shape. The dough will keep pulling and bouncing back, but keep rolling outward and creating even thickness all around, just shy of ¼ inch, or a little thicker if you like.

Place a naan in the hot skillet and cook until bubbles begin to form on the top, 30 to 45 seconds, then flip. The naan should start to puff up; you can gently press down with a spatula or your hand on any areas that don't puff to help encourage them. (It may sound strange, but it works!) Cook on the second side for another 30 seconds. Repeat with the remaining dough. (Or if not making all the naan at once, store any remaining dough in a sealed container in the fridge for up to 1 day.)

Top the warm naan with any combination of butter, kalonji seeds, cilantro, or green chiles. You can also store leftover cooked naan in the freezer for up to 1 month. Let them thaw before rewarming them in the oven or in a pan.

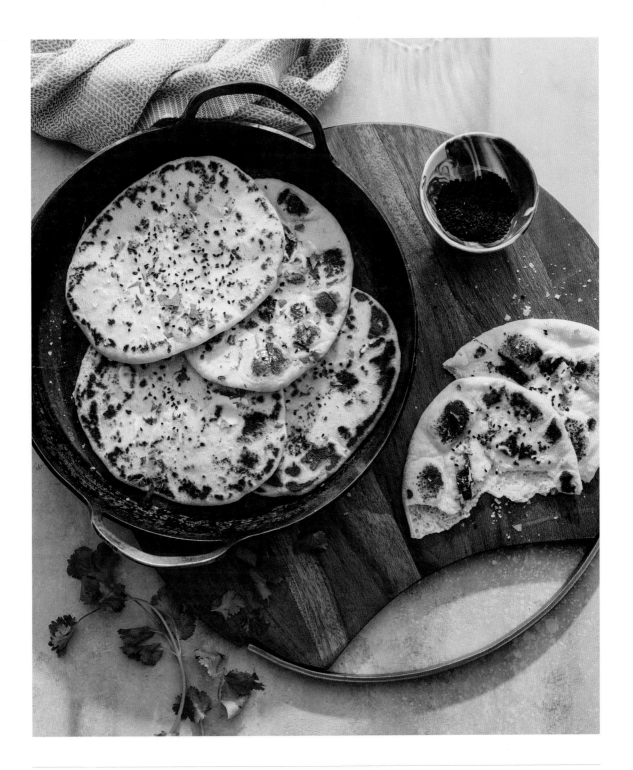

NOTES If you want a nicely browned tandoori naan experience, hold the fully cooked naan with tongs directly over the flame and toast on either side for a few seconds. Or increase the flame to medium or medium-high and keep the naan in the pan until it's browned to your liking.

For especially soft naan, wrap the cooked naan between kitchen towels or foil once they're out of the pan. Conversely, if you prefer them crispy, place the cooked naans on a wire rack.

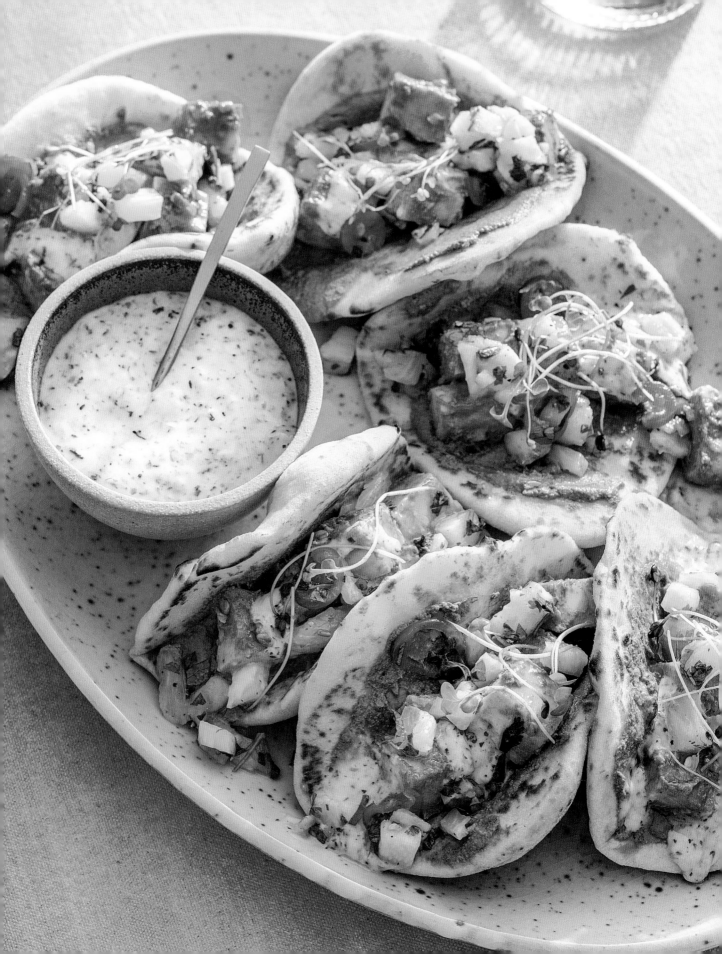

TANDOORI TACOS

I first created this recipe for Omnom, a restaurant in London, but now I make it at home all the time, especially when company comes for dinner. (It scales up really nicely.) It always blows people's minds because they can't believe how delicious the tandoori spices are when combined with the meaty texture of the Magic Protein "Paneer" (page 133) or jackfruit (both work perfectly in this recipe). And when bundled in naan and heaped with minty yogurt, cilantro-mint chutney, and sweet and spicy mango salsa, it's pretty much a party in your mouth. You'd be very right to serve this dish at a summer barbecue.

SERVES *2*
TOTAL TIME: *35 to 40 minutes*

TANDOORI MARINADE

- ¼ cup plain vegan yogurt
- ¼ cup tomato paste
- 1 tablespoon extra-virgin olive oil
- 1 tablespoon dried fenugreek leaves
- ½ tablespoon garam masala or Ground CCF Masala (page 49)
- 1 teaspoon smoked paprika
- 1 teaspoon sea salt
- 1 teaspoon ground coriander
- ¼ teaspoon ground turmeric
- ⅛ teaspoon asafoetida

TACOS

- 2½ cups cubed Magic Protein "Paneer" (page 133) or 1 14-ounce can brined jackfruit, or cauliflower florets
- Olive oil cooking spray or avocado oil
- 4 to 6 small naans, homemade (page 156) or store-bought, pita, or your favorite tortillas
- Cilantro-Mint Chutney (page 243), for serving
- Yogurt Mint Sauce (page 245), for serving
- Mango Salsa (page 240), for serving
- Shredded lettuce or microgreens, for serving

MAKE THE MARINADE: In a large bowl, whisk together the yogurt, tomato paste, oil, fenugreek, garam masala, smoked paprika, salt, coriander, turmeric, and asafoetida.

FOR THE TACOS: Make the protein paneer as directed. Or if using jackfruit, drain and tear in bite-size pieces. Toss the protein paneer or jackfruit in the marinade and let sit for 1 hour. (If you're short on time, the dish will still turn out great if you skip the marinating period!)

Preheat the oven to 400°F. Line a baking sheet with parchment paper and lightly coat the parchment with cooking spray or brush with olive oil.

Spread the marinated paneer or jackfruit over the prepared baking sheet and bake until charred and crispy, shaking the pan once or twice during baking, 10 to 15 minutes total.

To assemble, spread each naan with a thick layer of cilantro-mint chutney, a scoop of the tandoori paneer or jackfruit, followed by a generous drizzle of yogurt sauce and a scoop of salsa. Top with shredded lettuce or microgreens for some crisp freshness and serve.

STUFFED PITA FOUR WAYS

Pita sandwiches have been my go-to whenever I've needed a quick but satisfying meal. Over the years I've rotated among a couple variations, depending on the mood and the occasion, such as a chopped salad in summertime and cheesy sweet corn if it's a cheese emergency (which it often is). I've since added more to my repertoire—roasted butternut squash and chickpea shawarma and protein-packed tofu tikka—and they're such a great tool in your feed-me-fast toolbox. They also make a great picnic meal or packed lunch—just stuff the pita and hit the road.

CHOPPED SALAD

MAKES *2 sandwiches*
TOTAL TIME: *10 minutes*

- ½ cup quartered cherry tomatoes
- ½ cup chopped unpeeled seedless cucumber
- ½ cup chopped bell pepper (choose your favorite color!)
- ½ cup chopped Little Gem lettuce
- ¼ cup mixed pitted olives (optional)
- ¼ cup chopped fresh mint leaves
- ¼ cup chopped fresh parsley leaves
- 1 tablespoon Lemon Vinaigrette (recipe follows)
- 2 tablespoons Perfect Hummus (page 239)
- 2 tablespoons shredded vegan cheese
- 2 tablespoons sweet chili sauce (optional)
- 1 tablespoon Cavolo Nero Pesto (page 200) or store-bought basil pesto
- 1 tablespoon ketchup
- 1 teaspoon spicy English or Dijon mustard
- 2 pitas, toasted and sliced widthwise into pockets

In a large bowl, combine the tomatoes, cucumber, bell pepper, lettuce, olives (if using), mint, and parsley. Add the dressing, hummus, cheese, chili sauce (if using), pesto, ketchup, and mustard.

Divide the salad mixture among the pitas and serve.

MAKE-AHEAD   You can toss together all the salad vegetables and store them undressed for up to 2 days.

Lemon Vinaigrette

This dressing is a versatile, all-purpose vinaigrette that would be delicious with pretty much any salad, bowl, or roasted veg.

MAKES *½ cup*
TOTAL TIME: *5 minutes*

- ¼ cup extra-virgin olive oil
- ¼ cup fresh lemon juice (from 2 lemons)
- 1 teaspoon agave nectar
- ½ teaspoon sea salt
- ¼ teaspoon freshly ground black pepper
- ⅛ teaspoon asafoetida

In a small bowl, whisk together the olive oil, lemon juice, agave, salt, black pepper, and asafoetida. Store in a jar in the fridge for up to 5 days.

Recipes Continue

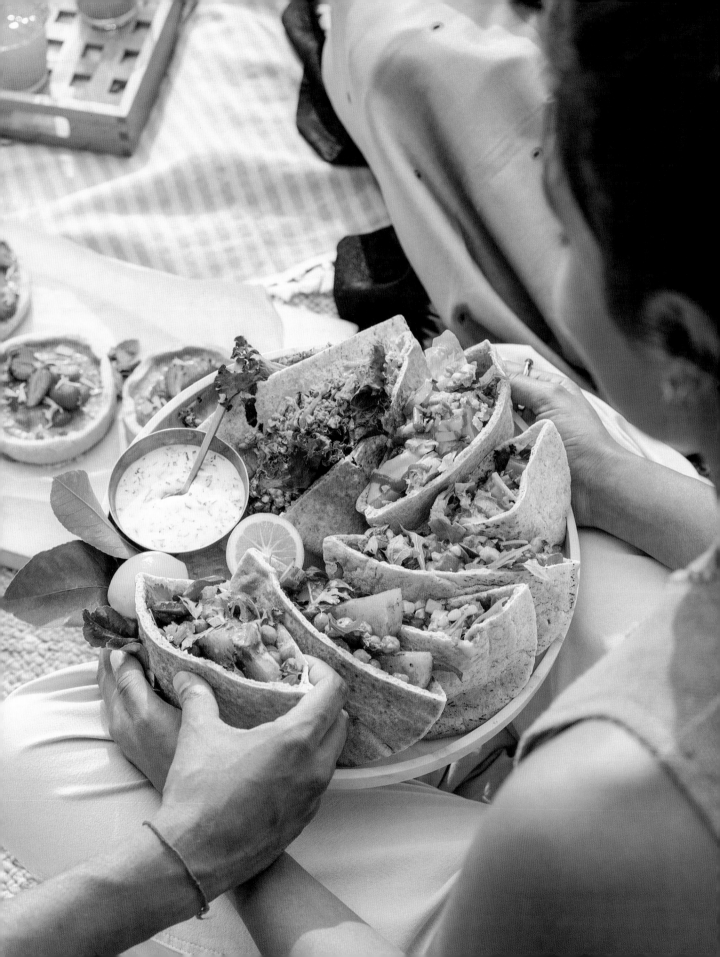

CHEESY SWEET CORN

MAKES *4 sandwiches*
TOTAL TIME: *15 minutes*

- 1 tablespoon extra-virgin olive oil
- 1 tablespoon tomato paste
- ¼ teaspoon asafoetida
- 1 cup finely chopped vegetables (I love a mix of zucchini and red bell pepper, but use whatever you have in the crisper!)
- 1 cup fresh sweet corn kernels (from about 2 ears) or thawed frozen
- 5 slices pickled jalapeño peppers, chopped
- 1 tablespoon nutritional yeast
- 1 tablespoon ketchup (optional)
- 1 tablespoon chopped fresh or dried herbs of your choice (I like parsley)
- 1 teaspoon spicy English or Dijon mustard
- 1 teaspoon Italian seasoning
- ½ teaspoon sea salt
- ⅓ cup shredded vegan cheese
- 4 pitas, sliced widthwise into pockets
- 4 tablespoons hummus
- 1 cup arugula

In a medium skillet, heat the oil over medium heat. Add the tomato paste and asafoetida and cook, stirring, until fragrant, just 1 minute or so. Add the chopped vegetables and cook, stirring, until soft, about 5 minutes. Add the corn, jalapeño, yeast, ketchup (if using), fresh or dried herbs, mustard, Italian seasoning, and salt. Stir to combine and cook until everything is smelling delicious and warmed through, about 2 minutes. Stir in the cheese and remove the pan from the heat.

For each sandwich, spread 1 tablespoon of the hummus inside a pita, scoop in one-quarter of the vegetable filling, and top with ¼ cup of the arugula.

If you aren't making all 4 sandwiches, leftover filling can be stored in a sealed container in the refrigerator for up to 3 days.

TOFU TIKKA STUFFED PITAS

MAKES *4 sandwiches*
TOTAL TIME: *25 minutes*

- 1 tablespoon tomato paste
- 1 tablespoon plain vegan yogurt
- 1 teaspoon smoked paprika
- ½ teaspoon garam masala or Ground CCF Masala (page 49)
- ½ teaspoon asafoetida
- ⅛ teaspoon ground turmeric
- 1 tablespoon sunflower or avocado oil
- 1 tablespoon liquid aminos
- 1 teaspoon dried fenugreek leaves (optional)
- ½ teaspoon finely chopped hot Indian or Thai green chile or ½ tablespoon sambal oelek
- 2 tablespoons finely chopped fresh cilantro leaves
- ½ small head cabbage, grated (about 3 cups)
- ½ teaspoon sea salt
- 2 cups pressed and grated firm tofu (see page 139)
- 4 pitas, sliced widthwise into pockets
- 1 cup shredded romaine lettuce
- Yogurt Mint Sauce (page 245), for serving

In a small bowl, stir together the tomato paste, yogurt, paprika, garam masala, asafoetida, and turmeric.

In a large skillet, heat the oil over medium-low heat. Stir in the liquid aminos, fenugreek (if using), green chile, cilantro, plus the tomato paste–yogurt mixture. Cook, stirring, for 2 minutes to let the spices warm through and release their oils and fragrance.

Add the cabbage and salt and cook, stirring, until softened, 3 to 4 minutes. Add the tofu and cook, stirring, until the cabbage almost melts and the flavors come together, about 7 minutes more.

Divide the mixture among the pitas and top with the shredded lettuce and yogurt mint sauce.

If you are not making all 4 sandwiches, leftover filling can be stored in a sealed container in the refrigerator for up to 3 days.

ROASTED BUTTERNUT AND CHICKPEA SHAWARMA

SERVES *4*

TOTAL TIME: *40 minutes*

ROASTED BUTTERNUT AND CHICKPEA SHAWARMA

- Sunflower or avocado oil for the baking sheet
- ½ medium butternut squash (halved lengthwise), peeled and seeded
- 1 cup cooked or canned chickpeas (rinsed and drained if canned)
- ½ cup chopped red bell pepper (about ½ large pepper)
- 3 tablespoons tahini
- 1 tablespoon fresh lemon juice
- 1 tablespoon sunflower or avocado oil
- 1 teaspoon ground cumin
- 1 teaspoon ground coriander
- ½ teaspoon ground ginger
- ½ teaspoon paprika
- ½ teaspoon sea salt
- ¼ teaspoon freshly ground black pepper
- ¼ teaspoon ground cinnamon
- ¼ teaspoon ground turmeric
- ⅛ teaspoon asafoetida
- 2 tablespoons finely chopped fresh cilantro leaves

SANDWICHES

- 4 pitas, toasted
- 4 tablespoons hummus (homemade, page 239, or store-bought), tahini, vegan mayonnaise, or So Much More Than a Burger Sauce (page 235)
- Arugula, for serving (optional)

Preheat the oven to 400°F. Line a baking sheet with parchment paper and lightly oil the parchment.

Slice the squash into 10 slices, each about ¼ inch thick (a mandoline works well here). Cut those slices in half and transfer the slices to a bowl. Add the chickpeas and red bell pepper. Set aside.

In a small bowl, whisk together the tahini, lemon juice, oil, cumin, coriander, ginger, paprika, salt, pepper, cinnamon, turmeric, and asafoetida. Add the spice mixture to the vegetables and toss to coat.

Spread the vegetables over the prepared baking sheet, cover with foil, and cook until the squash is tender, 20 to 25 minutes.

Remove the foil and set the oven to broil. Broil the vegetables until lightly charred, about 5 minutes. Sprinkle the cilantro over the roasted vegetables and set aside.

SPREAD THE INSIDE OF EACH PITA WITH YOUR SPREAD OF CHOICE: hummus, tahini, mayo, or tangy vegan sauce. Add a scoop of the butternut-chickpea mixture, top with some arugula, if you like, and serve immediately.

If you are not making all 4 sandwiches, leftover filling can be stored in a sealed container in the refrigerator for up to 3 days.

NOTE You can use tofu in place of the squash, which will only make the dish slightly less sweet. Use 8 ounces extra-firm tofu, press it as directed in Pressing Tofu (page 139). Cut it into 1-inch cubes and proceed with the recipe as written.

MAKE-AHEAD The filling mixture for each of these four sandwiches keeps well in the fridge, which means you can prep it ahead of time and have lunch, dinner, or a snack right when you need it.

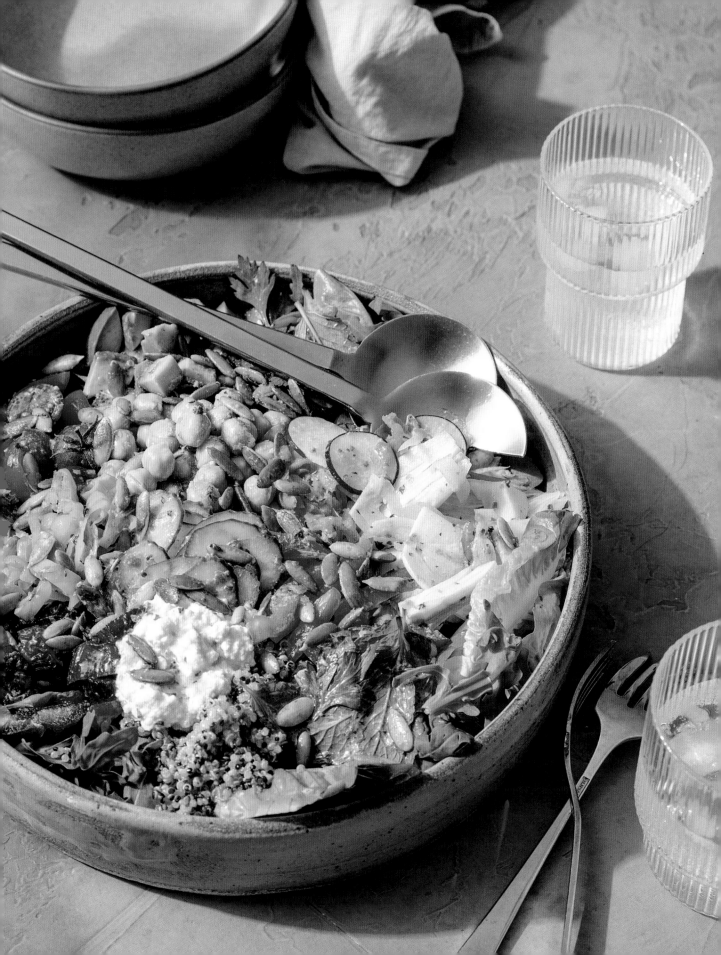

SALADS

The recipes in this chapter have layer upon layer of crunchy, creamy, salty, sweet, bright, and savory flavor and texture, plus all the sauces, dressings, and drizzles you could possibly want. In other words, these are not a few wimpy leaves with dressing that you suffer through to be plant-based or "healthy." There's a lot of love here!

While salad is usually thought of as a "light" meal, raw foods can be more difficult to digest than cooked. They take longer to break down thanks to all that belly-loving raw fiber. That said, even though lunchtime is the perfect time to eat a salad because your digestive fire is at its peak, it can be a lovely, nourishing way to end the day as well. The spiced dressings and healthy fats will aid with digestion, but you should still be sure to give your body at least a few hours to process your meal before it's time to power down for the night.

MY EVERYTHING PACKED SALAD

This salad is perfectly named because it has everything you want and everything you need, all heaped in a bowl. I like to tell people that this is the salad that you'll not only crave every single day—seriously, I sometimes eat it on repeat for months and months—but it's actually a great thing for you to have in your usual rotation because of the well-rounded nutrition it delivers. You'll find all the macro- and micronutrients you need to feel nourished in this crunchy, creamy, leafy, zippy, fresh, bright mishmash masterpiece.

SERVES *2 or 3*
TOTAL TIME: *25 minutes*

- 2 heads Little Gem lettuce or other tender lettuce, trimmed and chopped
- 1½ cups diced cucumber (about 1 medium cucumber)
- 1 cup cooked grain or legume of your choice (see Note)
- 1 cup arugula
- 1 medium carrot, peeled and grated
- 1 small head fennel, trimmed and thinly sliced
- 8 cherry tomatoes, quartered
- ½ cup chopped red bell pepper (about ½ large)
- ½ avocado, diced
- 5 Medjool dates, pitted and chopped
- 3 medium radishes, ends trimmed and thinly sliced
- ¼ cup chopped fresh mint leaves
- ¼ cup fresh parsley leaves
- ¼ cup vegan parmesan or vegan ricotta cheese
- 2 tablespoons chopped pepperoncini or pickled jalapeño peppers
- Herby Vinaigrette (recipe follows)
- "Popcorn" Pumpkin Seeds (page 255), for serving

In a large bowl, gently toss together the lettuce, cucumber, grain or legume, arugula, carrot, fennel, tomatoes, bell pepper, avocado, dates, radishes, mint, parsley, parmesan, and pepperoncini. Drizzle as much or as little dressing as you like over the salad and toss to coat. Top with the toasted pumpkin seeds and serve.

Herby Vinaigrette
MAKES *about 1 cup*
TOTAL TIME: *10 minutes*

- ½ cup fresh lemon juice (from 4 lemons)
- ½ cup extra-virgin olive oil
- 1½ tablespoons agave nectar
- 1½ teaspoons Dijon mustard
- ¾ teaspoon sea salt
- ½ teaspoon dried basil
- ½ teaspoon dried oregano
- ½ teaspoon freshly ground black pepper

In a medium bowl, whisk together the lemon juice, olive oil, agave, mustard, salt, basil, oregano, and pepper until well combined.

NOTE I like tossing cooked grains or beans (I love quinoa or chickpeas here) into this salad to make it extra filling. It's a great way to use up leftovers, but you could also cook a batch of your favorite grain, bean, or lentil and store it in the fridge for up to 3 days. That way any time can be salad time. Or in a pinch, go with rinsed and drained canned beans and call it a day!

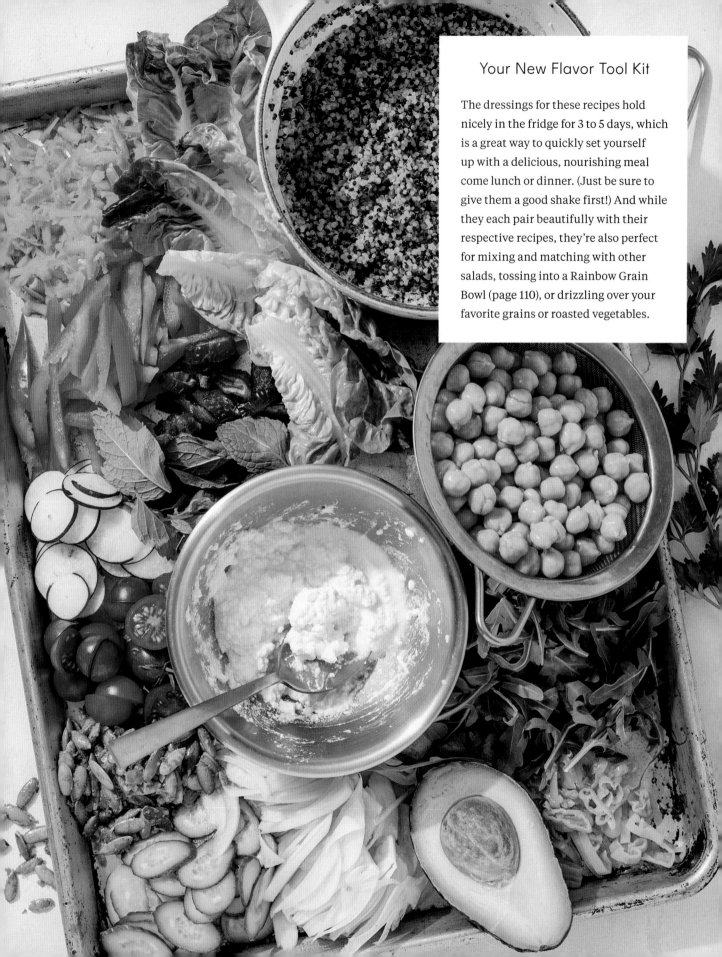

Your New Flavor Tool Kit

The dressings for these recipes hold nicely in the fridge for 3 to 5 days, which is a great way to quickly set yourself up with a delicious, nourishing meal come lunch or dinner. (Just be sure to give them a good shake first!) And while they each pair beautifully with their respective recipes, they're also perfect for mixing and matching with other salads, tossing into a Rainbow Grain Bowl (page 110), or drizzling over your favorite grains or roasted vegetables.

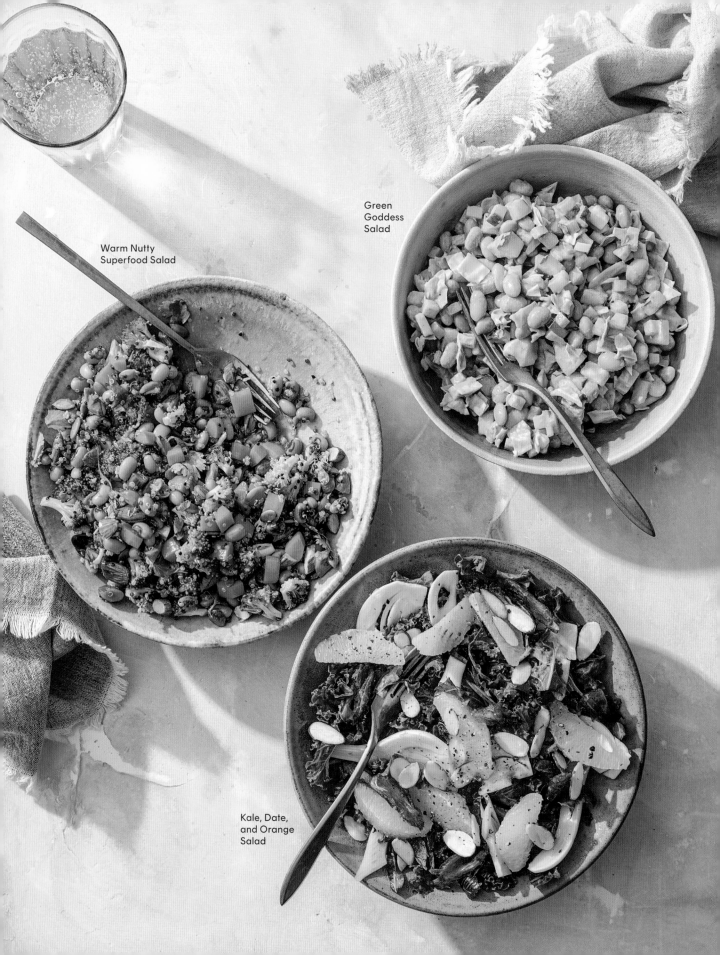

Green
Goddess
Salad

Warm Nutty
Superfood Salad

Kale, Date,
and Orange
Salad

KALE, DATE, AND ORANGE SALAD
with Citrus Vinaigrette

I always think of kale as a bougie sort of leaf—she needs to be pampered and massaged in order to bring out her optimal texture and flavor. But can you really blame her for needing a little extra love? After these tender, sweet-bitter greens have had their spa moment with a little olive oil and freshly squeezed orange juice, they become the perfect backdrop for fresh fennel, jammy dates, and a peppery orange dressing.

SERVES *2*
TOTAL TIME: *15 minutes*

- 2 bunches curly or Tuscan kale, leaves stripped of midribs and chopped, or 4 loosely packed cups baby kale
- 2 tablespoons extra-virgin olive oil
- 2 tablespoons freshly squeezed orange juice
- 1 large navel orange, peeled and cut into 8 wedges or slices
- 2 small heads fennel, trimmed and very thinly sliced
- 10 pitted Deglet Noor dates, roughly torn
- ¼ cup sliced almonds
- Citrus Vinaigrette (recipe follows)

In a large bowl, combine the kale, olive oil, and orange juice. Using your hands, firmly massage the kale to work in the juice and oil. When the kale has begun releasing its green chlorophyll and is tender, you're done, 3 to 5 minutes.

Arrange the massaged kale over a serving platter and top with the orange pieces, fennel, dates, and almonds. Drizzle the dressing over the top, toss well to coat, and serve.

Leftovers can be stored in a sealed container in the refrigerator for up to 2 days.

Citrus Vinaigrette
MAKES *a generous ¾ cup*
TOTAL TIME: *10 minutes*

- ½ cup freshly squeezed orange juice (1 to 2 large navel oranges)
- ⅓ cup extra-virgin olive oil
- 1 teaspoon agave nectar
- ¾ teaspoon sea salt
- ½ teaspoon freshly ground black pepper
- ½ teaspoon Dijon mustard

In a jar with a tight-fitting lid, combine the orange juice, olive oil, agave, salt, pepper, and mustard. Cover and shake vigorously to combine.

WARM NUTTY SUPERFOOD SALAD

Quinoa is like salad's secret weapon for filling you up without weighing you down. I especially love mixing white and red quinoa because the red has a nutty flavor and firmer texture, while the white is milder and creamier. Quinoa is also packed with protein, and here I complement it with other powerhouse ingredients like black-eyed peas, broccoli, and almonds. It all comes together with an Asian-inspired gingery dressing and is served warm, and is generally just an all-around feel-good salad.

SERVES *1*
TOTAL TIME: *25 minutes*

- 1 teaspoon extra-virgin olive oil
- 1 cup chopped broccoli (about ½ small head)
- ¾ cup cooked or canned black-eyed peas (rinsed and drained if canned)
- ½ cup cooked quinoa (I like a mix of red and white)
- ½ cup thin rounds or ¼-inch dice peeled carrots
- ⅓ cup pistachios, toasted in a dry pan until fragrant
- ¼ cup fresh, canned and drained, or frozen and thawed green peas
- ¼ cup pumpkin seeds
- 2 tablespoons chopped fresh cilantro leaves
- ¼ teaspoon sea salt
- ⅓ cup raw almonds, toasted until fragrant in a dry pan and roughly chopped
- Soy-Ginger Dressing (recipe follows)

In a large skillet, heat the oil over medium-high heat. Add the broccoli and cook, stirring, until tender but still firm, 3 to 4 minutes. Add the black-eyed peas, quinoa, carrots, pistachios, green peas, pumpkin seeds, cilantro, and salt and stir to combine. Reduce the heat to low, cover, and cook until the mixture is softened, 10 to 12 minutes.

Remove the pan from the heat and let the mixture cool, uncovered, for 5 minutes. Transfer to a medium bowl or serving plate. Pour the dressing over the warm salad mixture and toss well to coat. Top with the toasted almonds and serve.

MAKE-AHEAD You can make the quinoa ahead and store it in the fridge for up to 3 days, making it easy to throw this salad together on the fly.

Soy-Ginger Dressing
MAKES *about ½ cup*
TOTAL TIME: *10 minutes*

- 2 tablespoons extra-virgin olive oil
- 1½ tablespoons soy sauce
- 1 tablespoon rice vinegar
- 1 tablespoon pomegranate molasses (optional)
- 2 teaspoons light brown sugar
- ½ teaspoon grated fresh ginger
- ¼ teaspoon sea salt

In a jar with a tight-fitting lid, combine the olive oil, soy sauce, vinegar, molasses (if using), brown sugar, ginger, and salt. Shake vigorously to combine.

GREEN GODDESS SALAD

There is something special about the color green in nature. It's the shade of vitality, of vibrancy, of *life*. It also so happens that some of the tastiest ingredients are green, ranging from cool and crunchy to bright and briny to fresh and herbaceous. When combined in a big heap of a chopped salad drizzled with a creamy, fresh, zesty dressing, it's nothing short of ethereal.

SERVES *2*

TOTAL TIME: *15 minutes*

- 2 cups finely chopped green cabbage (about ⅓ small head)
- 1 cup finely diced seedless cucumber (about 1 medium)
- 1 cup peeled and finely chopped jicama (about ⅓ medium)
- 1 cup (8 ounces) shelled edamame, fresh or thawed frozen
- Green Goddess Dressing (recipe follows)

In a large bowl, toss together the cabbage, cucumber, jicama, and edamame. Drizzle as much or as little dressing as you like over the salad and toss to coat. Add more dressing as desired, toss again, and serve.

Green Goddess Dressing

MAKES *about 2 cups*

TOTAL TIME: *10 minutes*

- 1 cup roughly chopped fresh dill
- 1 cup fresh parsley leaves
- 1 cup fresh basil leaves
- 1 cup fresh mint leaves
- ½ cup plain vegan yogurt
- ¼ cup vegan mayonnaise
- 2 tablespoons capers in brine, drained
- 2 tablespoons extra-virgin olive oil
- 2 tablespoons fresh lemon juice
- ½ teaspoon sea salt, plus more to taste
- ⅛ teaspoon asafoetida

In a high-powered blender, combine the dill, parsley, basil, mint, yogurt, mayonnaise, capers, oil, lemon juice, salt, and asafoetida and blend until completely smooth, scraping down the sides of the blender as needed. Season with more salt, if desired. Store the dressing in a sealed container in the fridge for up to 4 days.

SPINACH, CHICKPEA, AND RAISINS

with Curried Cashew Dressing

You know I love my sauces and dressings, so to say that the curried-cashew number on this salad is one of my favorites is some seriously high praise. Between its gorgeous golden color; bold, spiced flavor; and rich, creamy texture, the rest of the salad is *almost* beside the point. And yet, this dish manages to get even more perfect with the Indian-inspired combo of chickpeas and spinach dotted with sweet moments of raisins.

SERVES *2*

TOTAL TIME: *30 minutes*

- 2 cups chopped fresh baby spinach (about 2 ounces)
- 3 red radishes, trimmed and thinly sliced
- ⅓ cup canned chickpeas, rinsed and drained
- ⅓ cup peeled and grated carrot (about 1 small carrot)
- 2 tablespoons raisins
- 2 tablespoons sliced toasted almonds
- Curried Cashew Dressing (recipe follows)

In a large bowl, toss together the spinach, radishes, chickpeas, carrot, and raisins. Drizzle as much or as little dressing as you like over the salad and toss to coat. Top with the sliced almonds and serve.

Curried Cashew Dressing

MAKES *about 2 cups*

TOTAL TIME: *10 minutes, plus soaking time*

- ½ cup sunflower seeds
- ½ cup cashews
- 3 tablespoons fresh lemon juice
- 2 tablespoons extra-virgin olive oil
- 1 tablespoon nutritional yeast
- 2 teaspoons curry powder
- 1 teaspoon sea salt
- ¼ teaspoon asafoetida

In a medium bowl, combine the sunflower seeds and cashews with hot water to cover and soak for at least 20 minutes or up to overnight. Drain well and discard the soaking water.

In a high-powered blender, combine the soaked cashews and sunflower seeds, ¾ cup water, the lemon juice, olive oil, nutritional yeast, curry powder, salt, and asafoetida and blend until completely smooth.

Store in a sealed container in the refrigerator for up to 5 days.

NOTE You can use all sunflower seeds or all cashews for the dressing if you have only one of them.

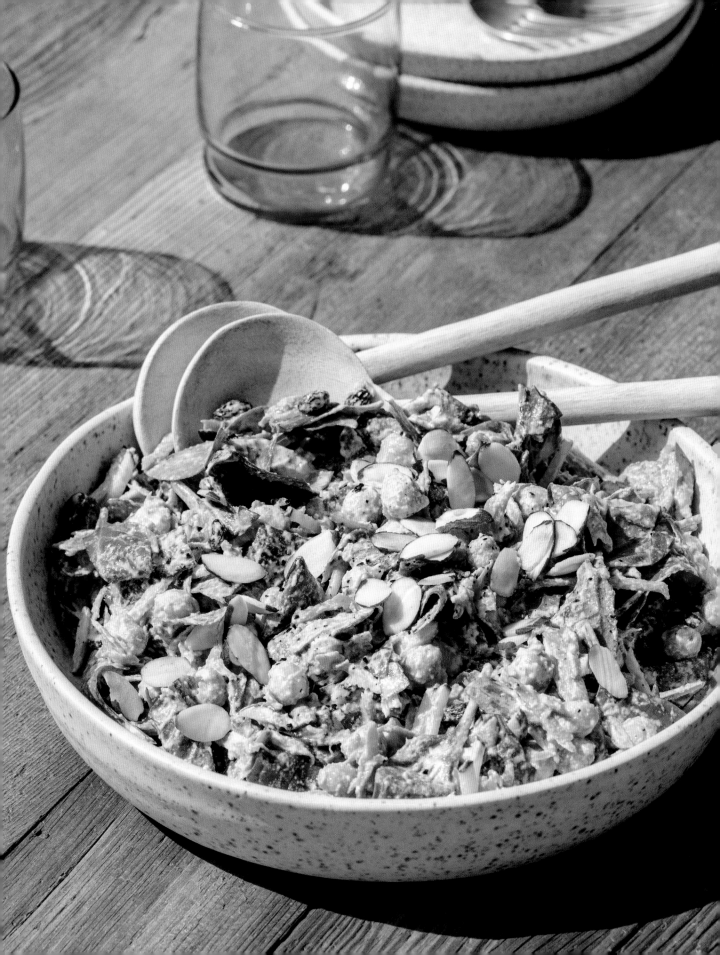

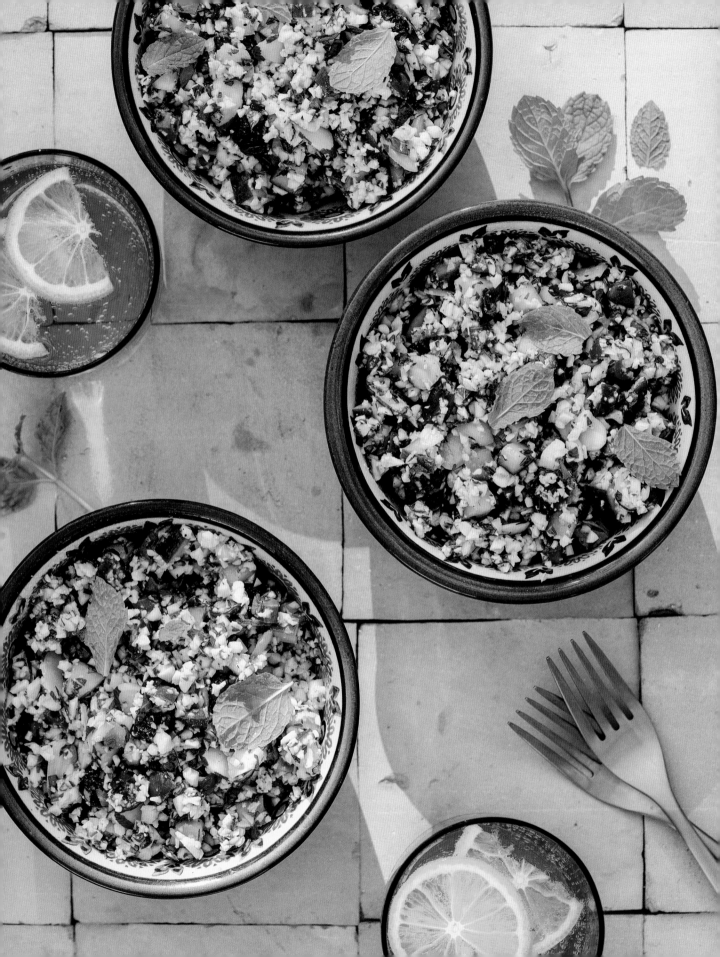

CAULIFLOWER TABBOULEH

Tabbouleh is a Middle Eastern dish that's traditionally made with bulgur, a little pearl of a grain, plus heaps of fresh parsley and mint. Instead of bulgur, I love using crumbled and quickly sautéed cauliflower because of its naturally sweet flavor, lightness, plus all of its disease-fighting antioxidants and phytonutrients. With some sweet-tart dried cranberries, salty olives, and a simple Dijon vinaigrette, it's a light, vibrant salad that you can enjoy on its own as a meal, as a side, or tossed with some greens for a little extra oomph.

SERVES *4*
TOTAL TIME: *15 minutes*

- ½ large head cauliflower, roughly chopped (about 3 cups)
- 1 tablespoon extra-virgin olive oil
- 1 cup finely chopped seedless cucumber (about 1 medium cucumber)
- ½ cup dried cranberries (unsweetened, if you can find them), optional
- ½ cup chopped fresh parsley leaves
- ½ cup chopped fresh mint leaves
- ⅓ cup chopped pitted olives, such as Niçoise
- 2 tablespoons skin-on sliced almonds
- 2 to 3 tablespoons Dijon Vinaigrette (recipe follows)

In a food processor, pulse the cauliflower until it resembles couscous or small grains of rice.

In a large skillet, heat the oil over medium heat. Add the cauliflower and cook until just tender but not mushy, about 5 minutes. Set aside to cool slightly.

Transfer the cauliflower to a large bowl and add the cucumber, cranberries, parsley, mint, olives, and almonds. Toss to combine. Drizzle on the dressing and mix well.

Leftover salad can be stored in a sealed container in the refrigerator for up to 2 days.

Dijon Vinaigrette

MAKES *½ cup*
TOTAL TIME: *10 minutes*

- ¼ cup extra-virgin olive oil
- ¼ cup fresh lemon juice (from 2 lemons)
- 1 tablespoon agave nectar
- 2 teaspoons Dijon mustard
- ½ teaspoon sea salt
- ¼ freshly ground black pepper

In a jar with a tight-fitting lid, combine the olive oil, lemon juice, agave, mustard, salt, and pepper. Seal the jar and shake well to combine. Store in the refrigerator for up to 5 days.

NOTE I hear all the time how cauliflower gives people gas. But when you cook it down—same with beans and legumes—and eat it with healthy fats and spices, it's easier to digest.

BUTTER BEAN AND TOMATO SALAD

Butter beans, or lima beans, are creamy and substantial, which makes them the perfect (and unusual) base for a salad. In the summer, I layer them up with big wedges of heirloom tomatoes, handfuls of fresh basil and parsley, and a sprinkling of salty capers. With a zesty lemony dressing, this dish is effortlessly simple and versatile—enjoy it on its own, as a side, or as an addition to pretty much any meal.

SERVES *2*
TOTAL TIME: *10 minutes*

- ¼ cup fresh lemon juice (from 2 lemons)
- 3 tablespoons extra-virgin olive oil
- 1 teaspoon sea salt
- 1 teaspoon agave nectar
- ¼ teaspoon freshly ground black pepper
- 1 cup cooked or canned butter beans (rinsed and drained if canned)
- 1 cup chopped heirloom tomato (about 1 large tomato)
- ½ cup roughly chopped fresh basil leaves
- ½ cup roughly chopped fresh parsley leaves
- ¼ cup halved and pitted green olives
- 2 tablespoons brined capers, drained
- 3 tablespoons vegan ricotta cheese
- Caraway or Chili Croutons (page 253), for serving (optional)

In a medium bowl, whisk together the lemon juice, olive oil, salt, agave, and black pepper. Add the butter beans, tomato, basil, parsley, olives, and capers and toss gently to coat. Serve topped with the ricotta and croutons (if using).

NOTE Because there are so few ingredients in this dish, the quality of each of them is key. Try to find the best tomatoes you can, ideally from the farmers' market, or at the very least when they're in season. If you don't have or can't find butter beans, you could also use cannellini.

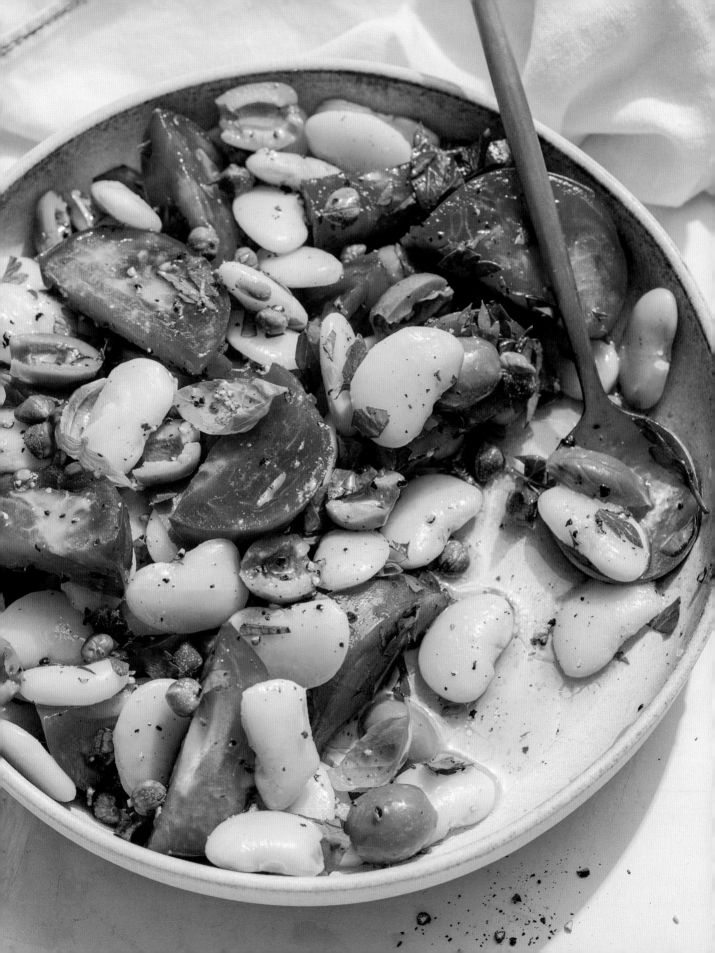

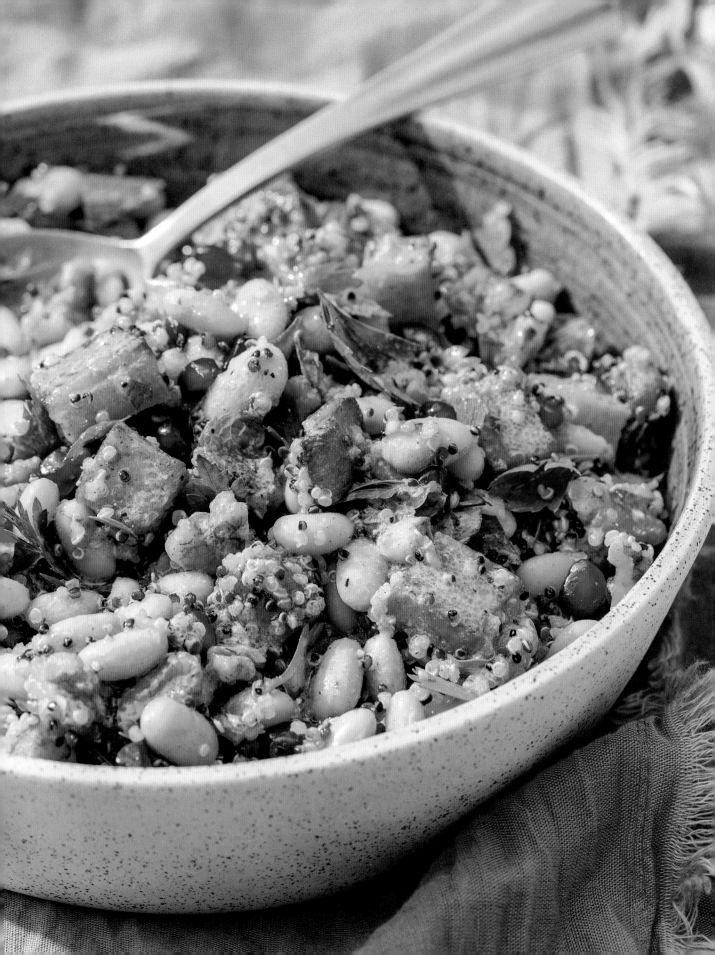

AUTUMN BUTTERNUT SQUASH SALAD

I like to think of this warming salad as the equivalent of wrapping yourself in a cozy sweater on the first chilly day of fall. It embodies moody seasonal flavors—caramelized butternut squash, toasty walnuts, and a kiss of cinnamon—balanced with bright bursts of fresh mint, parsley, and pomegranate seeds and finished off with a paprika vinaigrette. It's a delicious and intuitive way to embrace the transition to cooler months.

SERVES *6 to 8*
TOTAL TIME: *35 minutes*

- 1 medium butternut squash, peeled and cut into 1-inch cubes (about 3 cups)
- 3 tablespoons extra-virgin olive oil
- 1 teaspoon sea salt
- 1 teaspoon ground cumin
- ½ teaspoon ground cinnamon
- ½ teaspoon paprika
- 1 cup cooked white quinoa
- 1 cup cooked or canned cannellini beans (rinsed and drained if canned)
- Seeds of 1 pomegranate (about 2 cups)
- ½ cup walnuts, toasted until fragrant in a dry pan and chopped
- ½ cup fresh mint leaves, chopped
- ½ cup fresh parsley leaves, chopped
- Paprika Vinaigrette (recipe follows)

Preheat the oven to 425°F. Line a baking sheet with parchment paper.

In a large bowl, combine the squash, olive oil, salt, cumin, cinnamon, and paprika and toss well to coat. Spread the squash over the prepared baking sheet in a single layer and bake until the squash is tender and cooked through, 15 to 20 minutes. Set aside to cool slightly.

In a large bowl, combine the roasted squash, quinoa, cannellini beans, pomegranate seeds, walnuts, mint, and parsley. Drizzle as much or as little of the vinaigrette over the salad as you like and toss to coat.

Paprika Vinaigrette

MAKES *about ¾ cup*
TOTAL TIME: *10 minutes*

- ⅓ cup extra-virgin olive oil
- ⅓ cup fresh lemon juice (from 2 to 3 lemons)
- 2 tablespoons agave nectar
- 1 tablespoon Dijon mustard
- 1 teaspoon sea salt
- 1 teaspoon freshly ground black pepper
- ¼ teaspoon paprika
- ⅛ teaspoon asafoetida

In a jar with a tight-fitting lid, combine the olive oil, lemon juice, agave, mustard, salt, pepper, paprika, and asafoetida. Seal the jar and shake well to combine. Store in the refrigerator for up to 5 days.

CHILLED SOBA NOODLE SALAD *with Creamy Sambal Dressing*

Every salad rotation needs a solid cold-noodle dish. A big bowl of chilled buckwheat noodles tossed with raw veggies, toasted nuts, and cilantro, then draped in a creamy, spicy Southeast Asian–inspired dressing is so fresh and satisfying. It's the perfect salad for making in the evening and packing up for lunch the next day.

SERVES *2*
TOTAL TIME: *35 minutes*

- 3½ ounces soba noodles
- 1 cup thinly sliced red bell pepper (about 1 large pepper)
- 1 cup peeled and julienned carrots (about 2 medium carrots)
- 1 cup finely shredded red cabbage (about ½ small head)
- ¼ cup Creamy Sambal Dressing (recipe follows)
- 2 tablespoons crushed peanuts or almonds, toasted in a dry pan until fragrant
- 2 tablespoons finely chopped fresh cilantro leaves
- 1 teaspoon black sesame seeds

Cook the soba noodles according to package directions. Drain and rinse with cold water.

In a large bowl, toss the noodles with the bell pepper, carrot, and cabbage. Drizzle the dressing over the salad and toss again to coat.

Serve sprinkled with the peanuts, cilantro, and sesame seeds.

Creamy Sambal Dressing

MAKES *about 1 cup*
TOTAL TIME: *10 minutes*

- ½ cup unsweetened almond butter
- ¼ cup soy sauce
- ¼ cup fresh lime juice (2 to 3 limes)
- 1 tablespoon toasted sesame oil
- 1 tablespoon agave nectar
- 1 teaspoon sambal oelek

In a blender, combine the almond butter, ¼ cup water, the soy sauce, lime juice, sesame oil, agave, and sambal and blend until smooth. Store in a sealed container in the refrigerator for up to 3 days.

NOTE You could sauté the vegetables and make this a warm noodle dish instead.

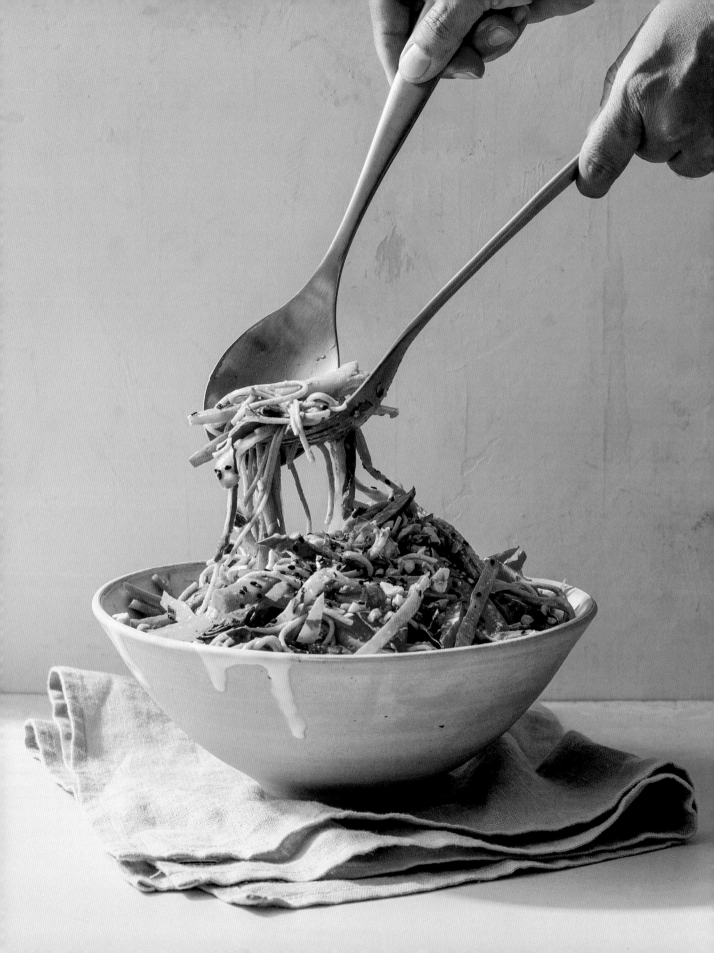

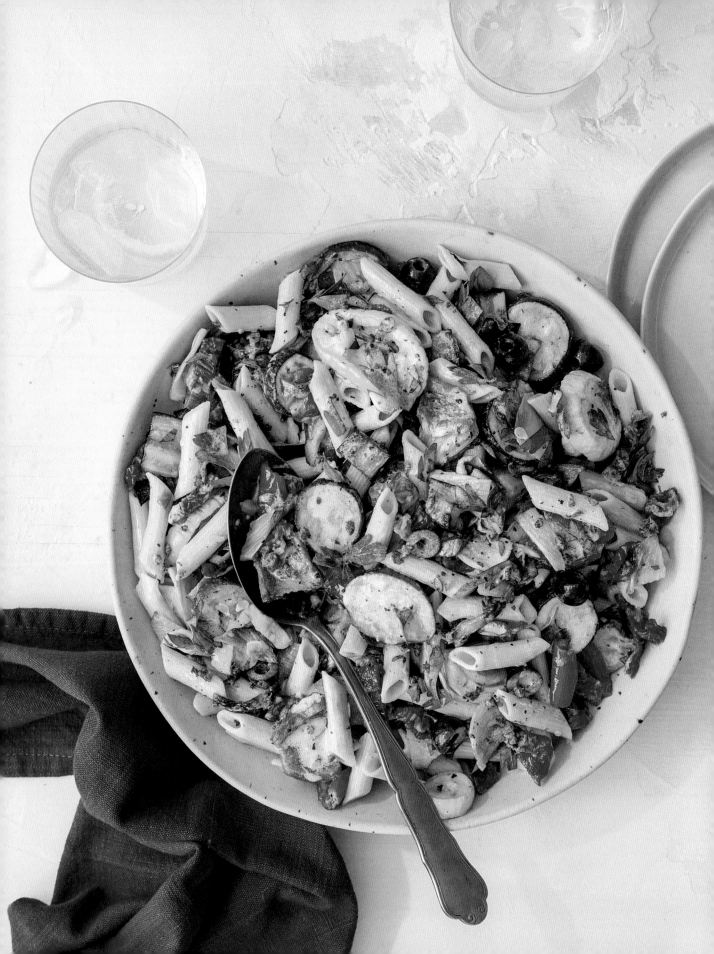

CLASSIC PASTA SALAD

Sometimes an occasion calls for a hearty but fresh pasta salad—BBQs, picnics, Tuesdays . . . Whenever the mood strikes, I whip up a bowl of this recipe, which is chock-full of veggies (zucchini, eggplant, fennel, peppers), fresh herbs, and zippy sun-dried tomatoes and olives. It's also my go-to dish to bring with me whenever I travel because it only gets more delicious as all the ingredients love up on one another, and I know I'll have something tasty to eat on the plane while feeling like I'm getting some of the good stuff in, too.

SERVES *4*

TOTAL TIME: *30 minutes*

ROASTED VEGETABLES

- 1 medium eggplant, trimmed and chopped (about 2 cups)
- 1 medium zucchini, chopped (about 1¼ cups)
- 1 medium yellow squash, chopped (about 1¼ cups)
- 1 medium head fennel, trimmed and chopped (about 1¼ cups)
- 2 large red bell peppers, chopped (about 2 cups)
- 3 tablespoons extra-virgin olive oil
- 1 tablespoon Italian seasoning
- 1 teaspoon paprika
- ½ teaspoon sea salt

DRESSING

- ¼ cup extra-virgin olive oil
- ¼ cup fresh lemon juice (from 2 lemons)
- 2 tablespoons vegan mayonnaise
- 1 tablespoon agave nectar
- ½ tablespoon yellow English or Dijon mustard
- ½ tablespoon dried basil
- ½ teaspoon dried oregano
- ½ tablespoon dried parsley
- ½ teaspoon sea salt
- ¼ teaspoon freshly ground black pepper

PASTA SALAD

- 1 cup brown rice penne pasta
- Extra-virgin olive oil
- ¼ cup finely chopped oil-packed sun-dried tomatoes
- ¼ cup finely chopped pitted black olives
- ¼ cup chopped fresh parsley leaves

ROAST THE VEGETABLES: Preheat the oven to 425°F. Line two baking sheets with parchment paper.

In a large bowl, toss together the eggplant, zucchini, squash, fennel, bell pepper, olive oil, Italian seasoning, paprika, and salt and toss to coat. Spread the vegetables over the prepared baking sheets in an even layer and bake until soft and just beginning to caramelize, about 15 minutes. Set aside.

MEANWHILE, MAKE THE DRESSING: In a jar with a tight-fitting lid, combine the olive oil, lemon juice, mayonnaise, agave, mustard, basil, oregano, parsley, salt, and pepper. Seal the jar and shake well to combine.

ASSEMBLE THE PASTA SALAD: In a medium saucepan, cook the pasta according to package directions. Do not rinse the cooked pasta with cold water, just toss it with a little olive oil to prevent sticking and set aside to cool slightly.

In a large serving bowl, toss together the roasted vegetables, cooked pasta, sun-dried tomatoes, olives, and parsley. Add the dressing and toss once more to coat. Serve immediately or refrigerate for 40 minutes before serving.

Leftover salad can be stored in a sealed container in the refrigerator for up to 3 days.

NOTE   Feel free to toss in any combination of vegetables that you like or that you need to clean out of the veggie drawer!

Tuning In with Your Breath

Breath is the bridge between your mind and your body, so it makes sense that whenever you want to feel more focused, more present, more connected with your body, or just want to experience a different frequency, you go back to where it all begins. Doing just a few minutes of these breathwork exercises throughout the day can pull you back into the moment and return you to the rhythm of the day.

THE RISE AND SHINE: SURYA NAMASKAR

There's a reason this stretch-breathwork combo is called "sun salutations"—it's meant to greet the rising sun (and shake the desire to hit the snooze button again). These ten simple yoga postures prepare your body for whatever is to come that day. There are tall, proud stances, surrendering stances, challenging stances—it's almost like they are a dress rehearsal for the feelings and moods that may arise during the day. Do just one round, and do it deeply, and it will be a very powerful practice.

THE GLOW UP: FULL YOGIC BREATH

Full Yogic Breath revitalizes the entire body with prana (essential life force). It literally breathes new life into our vital organs, which can become stagnant and constricted with emotional and physical tension. (Yes, organs get stressed, too!) Full Yogic Breath relieves stress and unwinds tension, mainly by soothing the parasympathetic nervous system, which is a network of nerves responsible for recalibrating your body after periods of stress or danger, helping you return to a calm, relaxed state. So when you support this vital—and frequently used—function, you'll feel refreshed, clear-minded, and balanced. You can reach for this breath any time, but it's especially beneficial early in the morning, preferably on an empty stomach.

Start by inhaling slowly into your lower abdomen. Then bring your breath into the midsection of your torso, followed by the diaphragm and ribs, and finally, into the upper chest and shoulders. To exhale, release your breath just as slowly and in the reverse order—chest, diaphragm, midtorso, lower belly. A full round is both the inhale and exhale. Aim for at least 5 minutes every day and work your way up to 15, imagining you are filling your entire body with sunshine as you breathe.

THE PUMP-UP: BREATH OF FIRE

This quick, dynamic breath delivers a hit of oxygen to your brain (its name, kapalabhati, literally translates to "shining skull breath"), which is perfect for feeling focused and energized.

Sit comfortably, then begin taking in short, quick breaths through the nose and exhaling deeply from your stomach through your mouth (making a "ha" sound). Start with 1 minute, which is plenty to wake up your body.

THE EQUALIZER: ANULOM VILOM

Anulom vilom, or alternate nostril breathing, is perfect for when you're transitioning from the high-intensity midday pitta energy to slower, gentler end-of-day vata energy, maybe getting a little sluggish, and want calm focus without feeling like you've just had a shot of espresso (which also happens to be the effect of my Iced Matcha Tahini Latte, page 50).

Anulom vilom brings alertness and balance to the left and right hemispheres of your brain. Begin by folding down your ring and pinky fingers on one hand and place your middle and pointer finger on your third eye (the spot on your forehead between your eyebrows). Use the knuckle of your ring finger to gently close one nostril and take a deep inhale. Hold for a few seconds, then release that nostril and plug the other nostril with your thumb. Exhale deeply through the second nostril. Breathe in through that same nostril and reverse the process, alternating nostrils and breathing like this for 1 to 2 minutes. You may notice that one nostril brings in air more effortlessly; that corresponds to the opposite hemisphere of your brain, which is likely your dominant side (i.e., left brain or right brain). When you're finished, you'll feel calm, awake, and refreshed.

THE NIGHTCAP: DEEP BELLY BREATHING

When it's time to wind down and prepare your body for sleep, it's the perfect moment to focus on deep breathing. You can do this lying or sitting in bed.

Take a deep inhale through your nose and feel the breath flowing down your throat, to your chest, and finally, filling up your belly. Then release it from your belly, feeling the breath come back through your chest, neck, and out of your mouth. Breathe deeply and slowly, focusing on the *completion* of the inhalation and exhalation. At the bottom of each breath, you should have no breath left to inhale or exhale, which will help release any stagnant air sitting in your belly. Notice your thoughts, sit with them, and observe them like clouds, then let them pass by. You can also focus on a different body part with each breath—I like to work from my feet up to my head. Think about completely relaxing that part of your body with each exhale. I recommend 5 minutes of this to give yourself time to unwind from the events of the day.

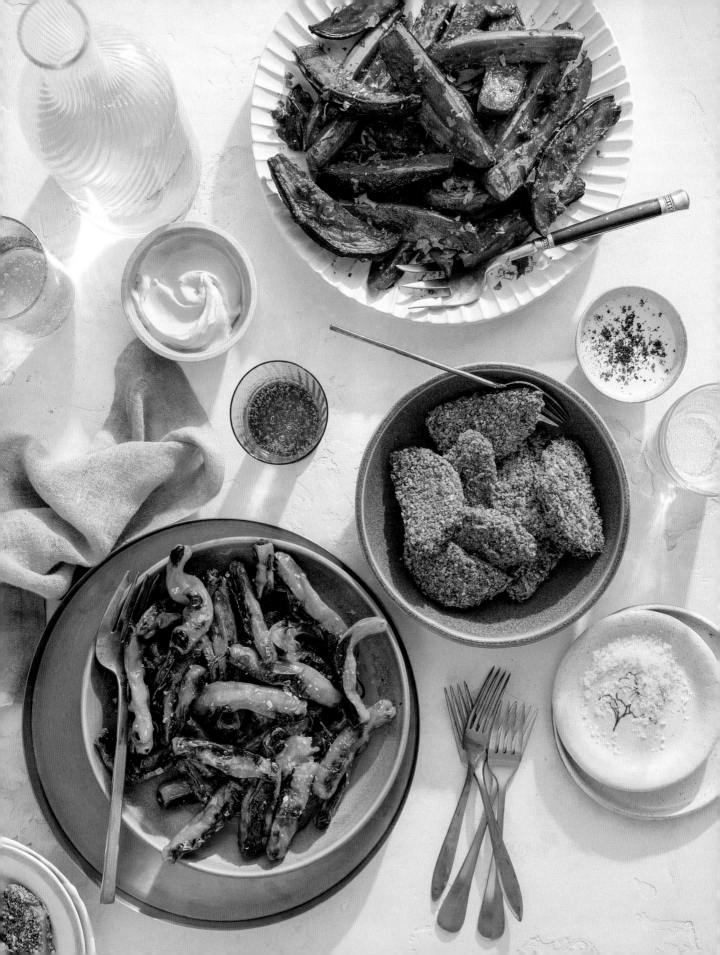

HERO VEG

When I first heard someone unapologetically call veg-forward dishes "hero vegetables," I fell in love with the idea that instead of being the sidekick in a dish or hidden in the background, vegetables could hold the spotlight. Each of the dishes in this chapter is like a love letter to some of my favorite vegetables; they're my way of saying "thank you" for sharing their beautiful natural, nourishing gifts. Feel free to enjoy them as main dishes, as sides, or mixed and matched to create a bountiful spread.

GOLDEN CARAMELIZED FENNEL *with Creamy Cilantro Sauce*

I try so hard not to play favorites when it comes to vegetables, but with fennel it's impossible not to. It has such a unique flavor, whether it's raw, crisp, and anise-y or cooked down and deeply sweet. And then there are all of its superpowers, like helping to cool an overworked liver, where much of our bodies' detoxification happens, taming inflammation, and keeping your organs supple and hydrated. For this dish, we're going with succulent caramelized fennel that's been turned sunny yellow with turmeric and paired with a creamy, refreshing cilantro yogurt sauce. Don't tell the other veg, but you're about to fall in love.

SERVES *2 to 4*

TOTAL TIME: *20 minutes*

FENNEL

- 1 large or 2 small heads fennel, stalks removed
- 2 tablespoons vegan butter
- 1½ teaspoons cumin seeds
- ½ teaspoon sea salt
- ¼ teaspoon ground turmeric
- ⅛ teaspoon asafoetida

SAUCE

- 1 cup plain Greek-style vegan yogurt
- 1 cup chopped fresh cilantro leaves
- 1 teaspoon fresh lemon juice
- Pinch of sea salt

If using small fennel bulbs, cut each bulb into 4 wedges. If using a large bulb, cut into 8 wedges. In both cases, keep the core of the fennel intact so the wedges will hold together better as they cook.

In a medium skillet, heat the butter over high heat. Add the cumin seeds and cook, stirring occasionally, until they pop, about 2 minutes. Reduce the heat to medium-low and add the salt, turmeric, and asafoetida. Cook, stirring, until fragrant, about 30 seconds.

Add the fennel, cover the pan, and cook until the fennel is just tender but still crisp, about 10 minutes. Uncover, increase the heat to medium-high, and cook, turning the fennel occasionally, until it is deeply golden brown, 2 to 3 more minutes. Remove the pan from the heat and set aside.

MAKE THE SAUCE: In a blender, combine the yogurt, cilantro, lemon juice, and salt and blend until smooth.

Create a bed of the sauce on a serving plate and arrange the fennel wedges on top, or simply dollop the top of the fennel with the sauce. Serve warm.

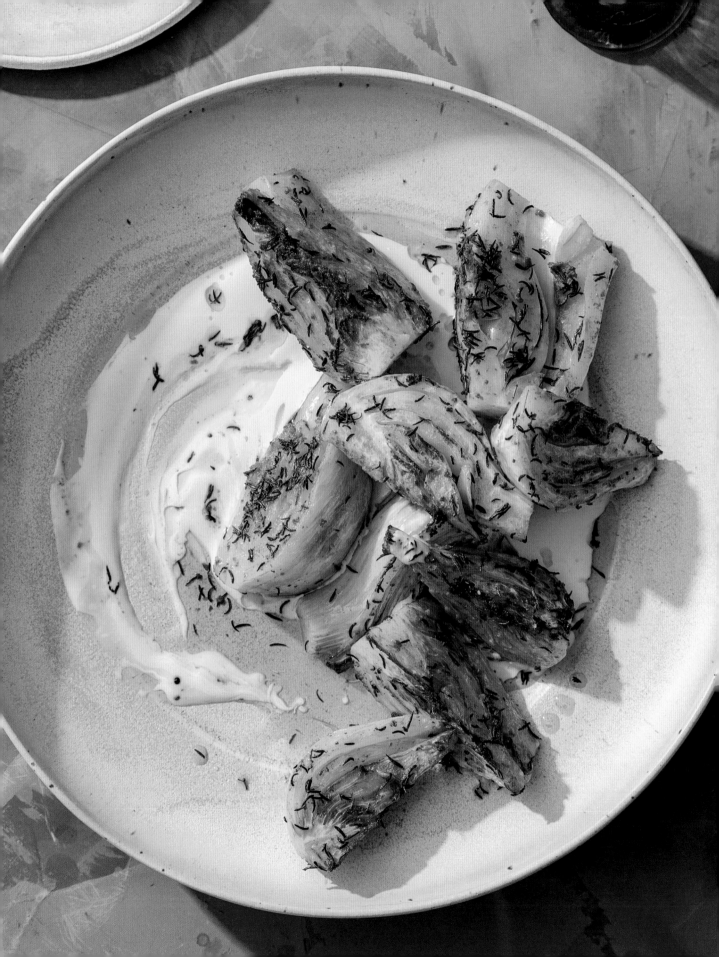

MIDDLE EASTERN CHARRED CAULIFLOWER

This dish was made for eating with your senses. There's the aromatic blend of hot paprika and earthy za'atar, the crunchy roasted pistachios, and the vibrant rainbow cauliflower that looks beautiful on the plate (while also delivering inflammation-fighting antioxidants). It all gets served on a bed of rich tahini sauce with a drizzle of date syrup, which is like the most luxurious sweet-savory combination you could dream of. Enjoy this dish on its own or bundle it up in a Proper Good Naan (page 156) wrap.

SERVES *4*

TOTAL TIME: *35 minutes*

- 2 tablespoons extra-virgin olive oil
- 1 tablespoon paprika
- 1 tablespoon za'atar
- 1 teaspoon ground coriander or cumin
- 1 teaspoon ground cinnamon
- 1 teaspoon sea salt
- ½ teaspoon ground sumac
- ½ teaspoon ground turmeric
- ¼ teaspoon asafoetida
- 4 cups cauliflower florets (about 1 medium head)
- Tahini Drizzle (page 241)
- Date syrup, for drizzling
- Fresh micro cilantro or cilantro leaves, for garnish
- Unsalted roasted pistachios, for garnish

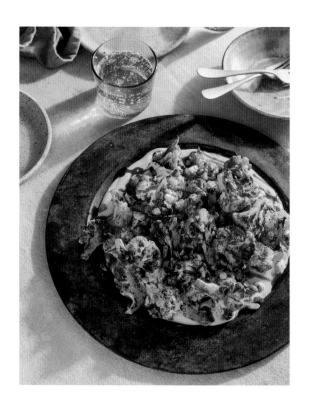

Preheat the oven to 400°F.

In a large bowl, whisk together the olive oil, paprika, za'atar, coriander, cinnamon, salt, sumac, turmeric, and asafoetida. Add the cauliflower and toss to coat well.

Spread the cauliflower over a baking sheet and bake until soft and golden brown, 20 to 25 minutes.

Spread the tahini drizzle over a serving plate. Pile the roasted cauliflower on top and drizzle with the date syrup. Sprinkle with the cilantro and pistachios and serve.

CORNMEAL AND CUMIN-CRISPED OKRA

Okra has a reputation for being a little tricky (and sticky) to prepare well, but it's actually not difficult to bake into a light, spiced, perfectly crispy number that reminds me of popcorn bites. Okra is also incredibly nourishing. It is considered ojas-building, meaning its life force–promoting nutrients are beneficial to almost every element of your health from immunity to strength to mood.

SERVES *4*

TOTAL TIME: *35 minutes*

- 1½ tablespoons extra-virgin olive oil
- 1 teaspoon cumin seeds
- 1 teaspoon curry powder
- 1 teaspoon sea salt
- ⅛ teaspoon asafoetida
- 1 pound okra (30 to 40 pods), trimmed and sliced into rounds ¼ inch thick
- 1 tablespoon cornmeal
- 1 tablespoon white sesame seeds

Preheat the oven to 450°F. Line a baking sheet with parchment paper.

In a large bowl, whisk together the oil, cumin seeds, curry powder, salt, and asafoetida. Add the okra and toss well to coat. Sprinkle the cornmeal and sesame seeds over the okra and toss again to coat.

Spread the okra over the prepared baking sheet in a single layer. Bake until the okra is cooked through, browned, and crispy, about 30 minutes, flipping it halfway through. Enjoy fresh out of the oven.

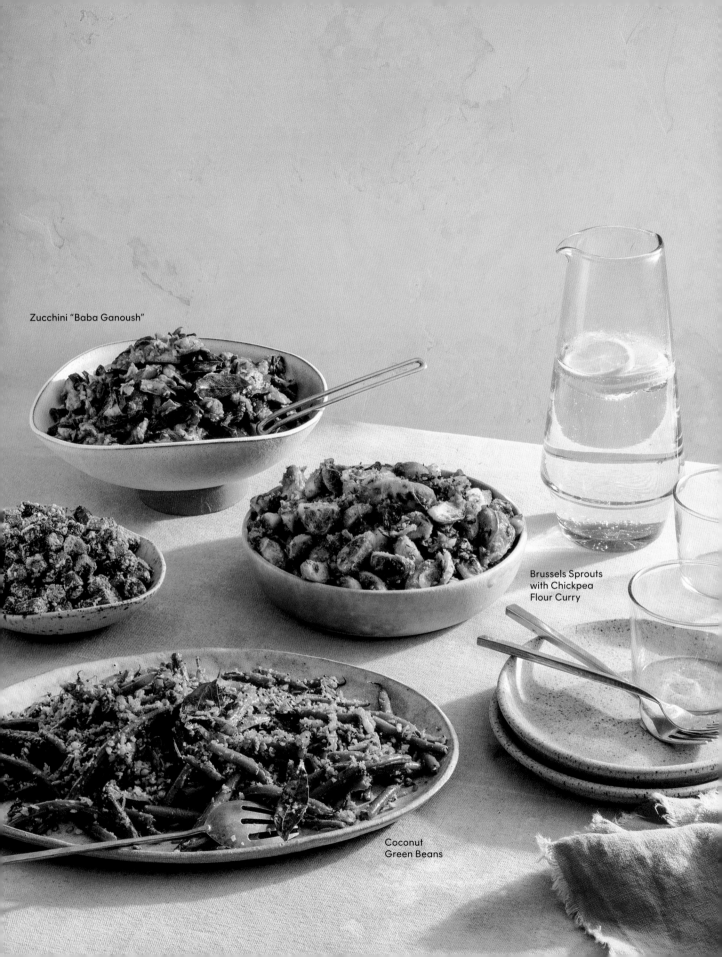

Zucchini "Baba Ganoush"

Brussels Sprouts
with Chickpea
Flour Curry

Coconut
Green Beans

COCONUT GREEN BEANS

Green beans are high in B vitamins, which are associated with elevating your mood—which completely tracks, because this dish makes you feel so good. The South Indian–inspired flavors and textures of rich, creamy coconut, mustard seeds, and crunchy sautéed lentils bring out the natural butteriness of the green beans.

SERVES *4 to 6*
TOTAL TIME: *25 minutes*

- 1½ tablespoons vegan butter or coconut oil
- 10 fresh or dried curry leaves
- 1 teaspoon mustard seeds
- 1½ tablespoons dried urud lentils
- 1 tablespoon sesame seeds (optional)
- ½ teaspoon ground turmeric
- ½ teaspoon garam masala
- ½ teaspoon ground cumin
- ½ teaspoon ground coriander
- ⅛ teaspoon asafoetida
- 1 pound green beans, trimmed
- 1 teaspoon sea salt
- ¼ cup grated frozen or fresh coconut
- Chopped fresh cilantro leaves, for serving

Melt the butter in a large skillet over medium heat. Add the curry leaves and mustard seeds and heat until the seeds begin to pop, about 1 minute. Add the lentils and reduce the heat to medium-low. Cook, stirring frequently, until the lentils are golden brown, about 1 minute. Stir in the sesame seeds (if using), turmeric, garam masala, cumin, coriander, and asafoetida and cook, stirring, until the spices have released their fragrance and oils, about 2 minutes.

Add the green beans, salt, and ¼ cup water to the pan. Stir to combine, then cook, covered, until the green beans are bright green and still slightly crisp, 8 to 10 minutes.

Remove the lid and continue cooking, tossing frequently, as the water evaporates and the green beans crisp slightly, about 2 minutes more. Stir in the coconut and cook until the coconut has softened and the flavors have melded, about 5 minutes.

Sprinkle with cilantro and serve.

ZUCCHINI "BABA GHANOUSH"

In the Gujarat region of India, where my grandparents are from, we have a dish called ringna no oro, which is eggplant charred over a fire and then cooked in tomatoes and aromatic spices. It's essentially like a delicious thick, earthy, smoky stew, sort of an Indian baba ghanoush. But because eggplants are nightshades and are best eaten in moderation, my mum created this zucchini-based version—which also calls for using the oven and not a fire so it's a little easier to make regularly—and it's almost impossible to tell the difference, especially scooped up with Proper Good Naan (page 156), spooned onto a bowl of grains, or spread over roasted or grilled vegetables, then drizzled with Raita (page 246).

SERVES *4*

TOTAL TIME: *35 minutes*

- 5 small to medium zucchini (about 6 ounces each), trimmed and halved lengthwise
- 1 tablespoon sunflower or avocado oil, plus more for drizzling
- 1 teaspoon cumin seeds
- 10 to 15 fresh or dried curry leaves
- 1 teaspoon minced fresh ginger
- 1 teaspoon garam masala or Ground CCF Masala (page 49)
- 1 teaspoon ground coriander
- 1 teaspoon sea salt
- ½ teaspoon minced hot Indian or Thai green chile
- ¼ teaspoon asafoetida
- ¼ teaspoon ground turmeric
- 1 tablespoon chopped fresh cilantro leaves
- 1 teaspoon white sesame seeds

Preheat the oven to 425°F. Line a baking sheet with parchment paper.

Place the zucchini on the prepared baking sheet and drizzle with the oil. Rub them all over to coat and then arrange the halves so they're all cut-side down. Roast until completely softened and browned, about 30 minutes, turning them halfway through.

In a large nonstick skillet, heat the oil over medium-low heat. Add the cumin seeds and let them toast, stirring frequently, until they pop, about 1 minute. Add the curry leaves, ginger, garam masala, coriander, salt, green chile, asafoetida, and turmeric and cook, stirring, until fragrant, about 2 minutes. Remove the pan from the heat.

Use two forks to shred and tear the roasted zucchini, then add it to the pan with the spices and mix thoroughly. Return the pan to medium-low heat and cook for another 10 minutes to cook off any extra liquid from the zucchini and to completely marry the flavors.

Serve topped with the cilantro and sesame seeds.

Leftovers can be stored in a sealed container in the refrigerator for up to 3 days.

BROCCOLI OR BRUSSELS SPROUTS *with Chickpea Flour Curry*

Many of my cooking skills have come from watching my mum make magic in the kitchen. One of my favorite and most frequently used tricks is to toss vegetables in chickpea flour mixed with spices like garam masala, coriander, and turmeric. You get a crisp, hearty coating that makes the veggies even more substantial-feeling and flavorful, which is what makes this recipe such a keeper. You could make this with just about any vegetable you'd add to a stir-fry—green beans, broccoli, carrots—but I'm partial to Brussels sprouts for their blood-nourishing vitamin K and vitamin C, and to broccoli for its disease-preventing antioxidants and fiber. I love enjoying these as part of a traditional Indian meal with daal and roti or rice.

SERVES *2 to 4*
TOTAL TIME: *25 minutes*

- ½ cup chickpea flour (chana lot)
- 1 tablespoon ground coriander
- ½ tablespoon garam masala or Ground CCF Masala (page 49)
- ½ teaspoon ground turmeric
- ¼ teaspoon asafoetida
- 2 tablespoons sunflower or avocado oil
- 1 teaspoon cumin seeds
- 2 tablespoons white sesame seeds
- 1 teaspoon grated or finely minced fresh ginger
- 4 heaping cups small broccoli florets or quartered or shaved Brussels sprouts
- ½ teaspoon sea salt
- 1 teaspoon fresh lemon juice

In a small bowl, whisk together the chickpea flour, coriander, garam masala, turmeric, and asafoetida until well combined. Set aside.

In a large skillet, heat 1½ tablespoons of the oil over medium heat. Add the cumin seeds and cook, stirring, until they start to pop, about 1½ minutes. Stir in the sesame seeds and ginger and cook, stirring, for 1 minute.

Add the broccoli or Brussels sprouts, salt, and 1 tablespoon water. Cover and cook for 5 minutes to partially cook the vegetables. Uncover and sprinkle the chickpea flour mixture evenly over the top, along with the remaining ½ tablespoon oil. Mix well.

Cover, reduce the heat to low, and cook until the vegetables are tender, 10 to 12 minutes, checking about halfway through to stir and add a splash of water if the pan is dry.

Uncover, increase the heat to medium, and cook, stirring, until the vegetables are cooked through to your preference, 3 to 5 minutes. Squeeze the lemon juice over the dish and serve warm.

SWEET AND SALTY BROCCOLINI

I don't know anyone who can resist the combination of salty and sweet, and I've turned it up to a 10 for this dish. The pairing of savory, umami miso with jaggery (cane sugar in its rawest form that has a deep molasses-like flavor) creates an almost naughty-feeling saucy, sticky broccolini dish that is perfect as a side or tossed with noodles. While you could use coconut sugar instead of jaggery, I highly recommend seeking it out. It tastes just like brown sugar, and yet because it hasn't been processed, it is still rich in important minerals such as calcium, magnesium, and potassium, as well as digestive enzymes and iron. It's the perfect main dish with your favorite grains, bread, and/or daal, or can be enjoyed as a side.

SERVES *2 to 4*
TOTAL TIME: *15 minutes*

- 2 tablespoons boiling water
- 1 tablespoon yellow miso
- 1 tablespoon jaggery or coconut sugar
- 1 tablespoon sambal oelek
- 1 tablespoon rice vinegar
- ⅛ teaspoon sea salt
- 1 tablespoon toasted sesame oil
- 10 broccolini stalks (about 6 ounces)
- 1 teaspoon white sesame seeds

In a small bowl, whisk together the boiling water, miso, jaggery, sambal, vinegar, and salt and set aside.

In a wok or large nonstick skillet, heat the sesame oil over medium-high heat. Add the broccolini and 2 tablespoons water, cover, and steam the broccolini until just tender, about 5 minutes.

Uncover and let any excess water evaporate from the pan as it simmers. Reduce the heat to medium-low, stir in the reserved sauce, and cook, turning the broccolini occasionally, until the sauce becomes sticky and thick and coats the vegetables, 3 to 5 minutes. Remove the pan from the heat.

Serve warm topped with the sesame seeds.

Leftovers can be stored in a sealed container in the refrigerator for up to 2 days.

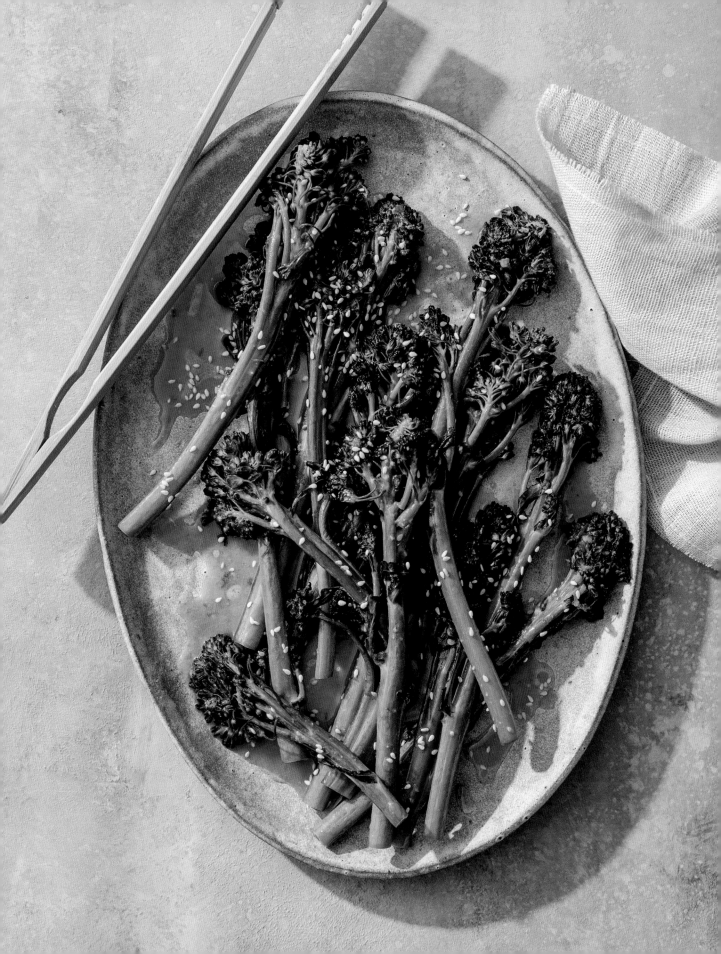

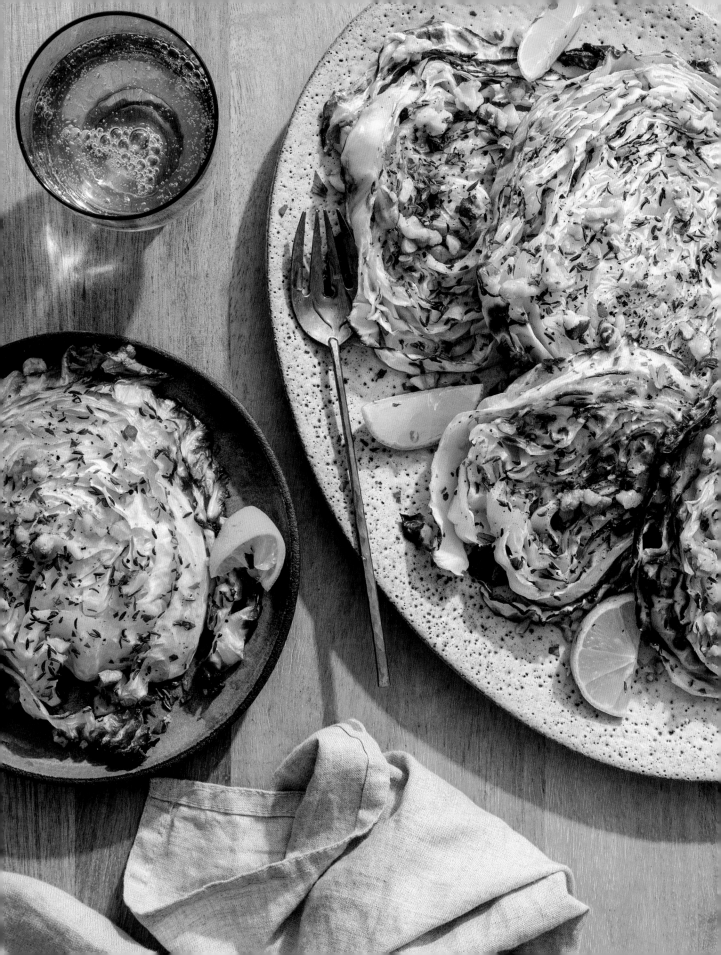

BUTTERY CARAWAY CABBAGE

Cabbage comes into season just as the weather is getting colder and you find yourself wanting to reach for dishes that feel comforting and nourishing. That's when I love cooking down finely shredded cabbage in an almost inappropriate amount (but not quite) of vegan butter plus caraway seeds, which bring a nutty, anise-y fragrance to the tender vegetable. There's really nothing like a bowlful of this on a chilly day, which also delivers a high concentration of vitamin C just in time for those winter coughs and colds to start making the rounds. Enjoy it on its own, maybe drizzled with tahini sauce, as a side veggie to a carb-heavy meal, or as part of a big tapas-y spread for a dinner party.

SERVES *2*
TOTAL TIME: *10 minutes*

- 1½ tablespoons unsalted vegan butter
- 1 tablespoon caraway seeds
- 4 cups shredded cabbage (about ½ medium head)
- ¼ teaspoon sea salt
- ⅛ teaspoon asafoetida

In a large skillet, heat the butter over low heat. Add the caraway seeds and cook, stirring, until fragrant, about 30 seconds. Increase the heat to medium and add the cabbage, salt, and asafoetida. Cook, stirring frequently, until the cabbage begins to soften and sweat, about 5 minutes. Depending on your cabbage and your tastes, you can take it off the heat at this point to retain some bite, or cook it down a bit more until completely soft, usually about 5 minutes more. Serve warm.

Leftovers can be stored in a sealed container in the refrigerator for up to 2 days.

SWEET POTATOES *with Cavolo Nero Pesto*

I don't think any vegetable tastes quite as decadent as creamy, caramelized, antioxidant- and vitamin-packed, blood sugar–stabilizing cubes of roasted sweet potato. And it's truly irresistible when you toss them with a lemony cavolo nero (Tuscan kale) pesto, which makes for a side dish that will always hit that sweet-salty spot. Or you could enjoy this combination over greens, wrapped up in naan or a taco, or even piled on top of a pizza.

SERVES *4*
TOTAL TIME: *35 minutes*

- 4 cups chopped sweet potatoes (about 4 medium), unpeeled (see Note)
- 2 teaspoons extra-virgin olive oil
- 3 tablespoons Cavolo Nero Pesto (recipe follows), plus more to taste
- Vegan parmesan, for serving (optional)

Position an oven rack in the top third of the oven and preheat the oven to 400°F. Line a baking sheet with parchment paper.

In a medium bowl, toss the sweet potatoes with the olive oil. Spread out on the prepared baking sheet and bake until tender and cooked through, 20 to 25 minutes. Switch the broiler on and broil the sweet potatoes until just crisp on top, a minute or so. Set aside.

Toss the sweet potatoes with about 3 tablespoons of the pesto, until coated. Top with the vegan parmesan and serve.

NOTE You should leave the peel on if possible, as it is packed with fiber and nutrients!

Cavolo Nero Pesto

MAKES *about 2½ cups*
TOTAL TIME: *10 minutes*

- 3 cups chopped Tuscan kale (cavolo nero) leaves (about 1 bunch)
- 1 cup chopped fresh parsley leaves
- ¼ cup sunflower seeds
- ¼ cup pine nuts
- 3 tablespoons extra-virgin olive oil
- 1 teaspoon grated lemon zest
- 2 tablespoons fresh lemon juice
- 2 tablespoons nutritional yeast
- 1 tablespoon brined capers, drained
- ¼ teaspoon sea salt
- ⅛ teaspoon asafoetida

In a food processor, combine the kale, parsley, sunflower seeds, pine nuts, olive oil, lemon zest, lemon juice, yeast, capers, salt, and asafoetida and pulse to blend. I like keeping the pesto a little chunky rather than fully blended because those bigger bits deliver more flavor. Store the pesto in a sealed container in the refrigerator for up to 4 days.

NOTE I like my pesto a little bit chunkier, but for a creamier blended pesto, you can blanch the kale for 3 minutes in salted water, rinse under cold running water for a bright green color, and proceed with the pesto recipe as written.

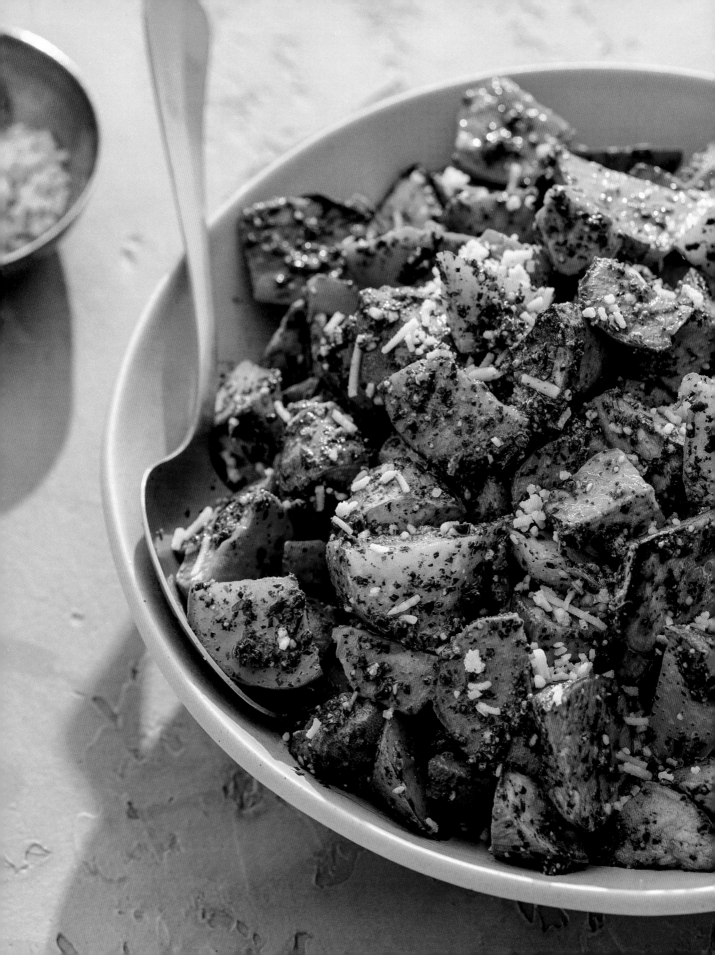

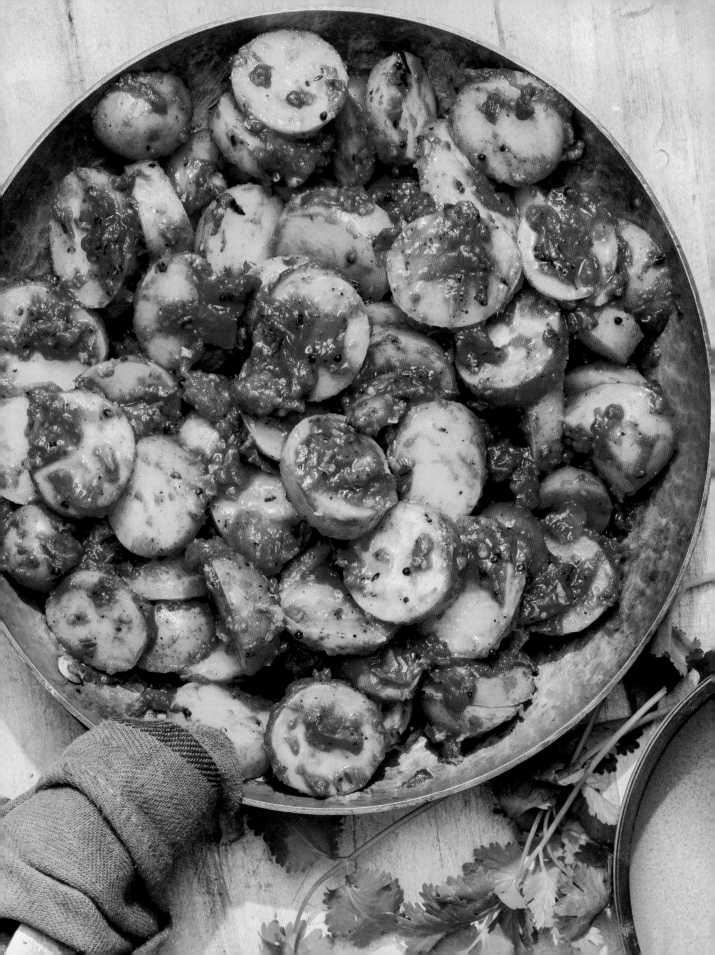

CHUNKY BOMBAY MASALA POTATOES

I do love a good ol' simple roasted potato, but here's how we Indians do it! It's all about bold, fresh spices like garam masala, coriander, and cumin, plus bright, green heat from fresh chiles. And yet this comes together just as easily as the simplest potato dish. It's a comforting, satisfying, and nourishing dish that doesn't require more than a drizzle of raita or yogurt and some naan or rice to make it a cozy, carb-y meal.

SERVES 6
TOTAL TIME: *30 minutes*

- 2 pounds baby potatoes, cut into ½-inch slices (about 5 cups)
- 1 tablespoon extra-virgin olive oil
- 1 teaspoon cumin seeds
- 1 teaspoon brown or black mustard seeds
- ½ tablespoon grated fresh ginger
- ½ to 1 teaspoon chopped hot Indian or Thai green chile
- ½ teaspoon ground turmeric
- 1 teaspoon garam masala or Ground CCF Masala (page 49)
- 1 teaspoon ground coriander
- 1 teaspoon ground cumin
- 1 cup canned crushed tomatoes
- ¼ cup chopped fresh cilantro leaves

Bring a large pot of water to boil over medium-high heat. Add the potatoes and cook until just fork-tender, 8 to 10 minutes. Drain the potatoes and let them steam dry in a colander.

Meanwhile, in a large skillet, heat the oil over medium heat. Add the cumin seeds and mustard seeds and cook until they pop, about 1 minute. Add the ginger and green chile and cook, stirring, until fragrant, 1 minute or so. Stir in the turmeric, garam masala, coriander, and ground cumin and cook, stirring, until the spices release their oils and aromas, 1 to 2 minutes. Add the crushed tomatoes, reduce the heat to low, and simmer until the sauce thickens slightly, 3 to 4 minutes. You want it to be able to hug the potatoes.

Add the potatoes to the spiced tomato sauce and continue simmering until the potatoes are warmed through, about 5 minutes.

Serve hot topped with the cilantro.

Leftovers can be stored in a sealed container in the refrigerator for up to 2 days.

CRISPY SUNCHOKES *with Golden Aioli*

Growing up, I'd never tried a Jerusalem artichoke (aka sunchoke), but when I started coming across them after I moved to LA and heard that they had the texture of a potato and the flavor of an artichoke heart—both of which I love—I knew I needed this vegetable in my life. Sure enough, when you thinly slice the sunchokes, crisp 'em up in a bit of oil or vegan butter, and dunk 'em in a creamy aioli, it's a really elevated fries and dip situation. Show me any other French fry that also has prebiotic properties (meaning it feeds the beneficial bacteria in your gut), heaps of potassium (the mineral your brain needs for optimal function), iron, amino acids, and liver-detoxifying properties.

SERVES *4*
TOTAL TIME: *30 minutes*

SUNCHOKES

Olive oil cooking spray or avocado oil

1 pound sunchokes (about 7 medium), cleaned, dried, and very thinly sliced (I like using a mandoline for this)

1½ tablespoons extra-virgin olive oil or unsalted vegan butter

½ teaspoon fine sea salt

2 teaspoons fresh thyme leaves, chopped

½ teaspoon flaky salt, such as Maldon

GOLDEN AIOLI

¼ cup vegan mayonnaise

¼ cup plain vegan yogurt

½ teaspoon Dijon mustard

½ teaspoon fresh lemon juice

¼ teaspoon ground turmeric

⅛ teaspoon sea salt

ROAST THE SUNCHOKES: Preheat the oven to 425°F. Line a baking sheet with parchment paper and lightly coat with cooking spray or brush with avocado oil.

In a large bowl, toss the sunchokes with the olive oil and fine sea salt. Spread the sunchokes over the prepared baking sheet in a single layer and roast until crisp and golden, 15 to 20 minutes. While still hot, toss the sunchokes with the thyme and flaky salt.

MEANWHILE, MAKE THE AIOLI: In a medium bowl, whisk together the mayonnaise, yogurt, mustard, lemon juice, turmeric, and salt.

Set the bowl of aioli in the center of a plate and surround it with the crispy sunchokes. You can also drizzle the aioli over the sunchokes, if you like.

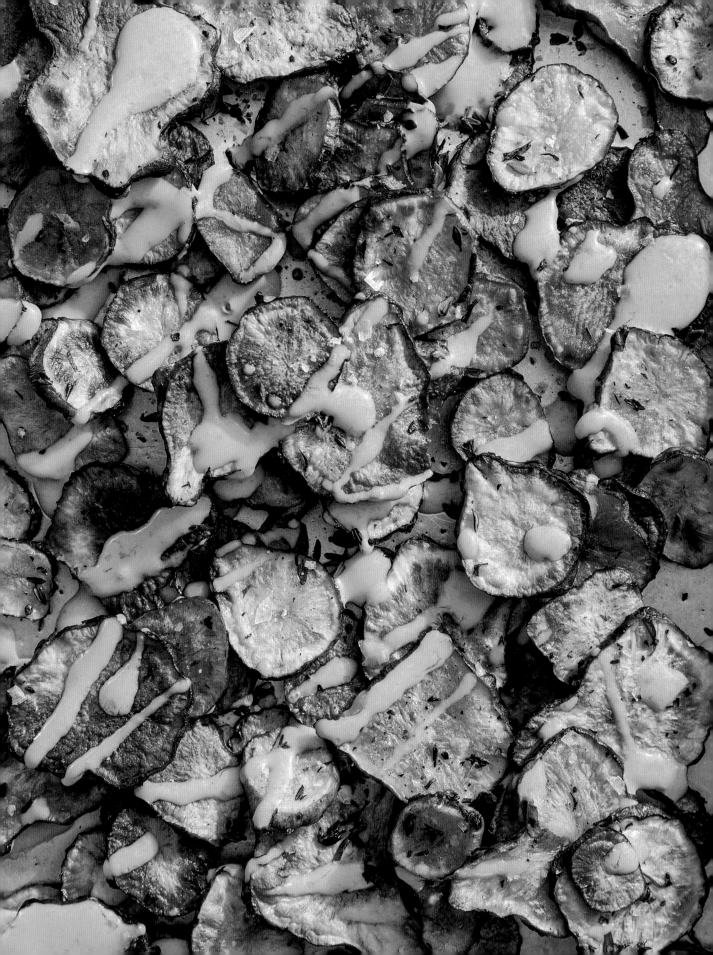

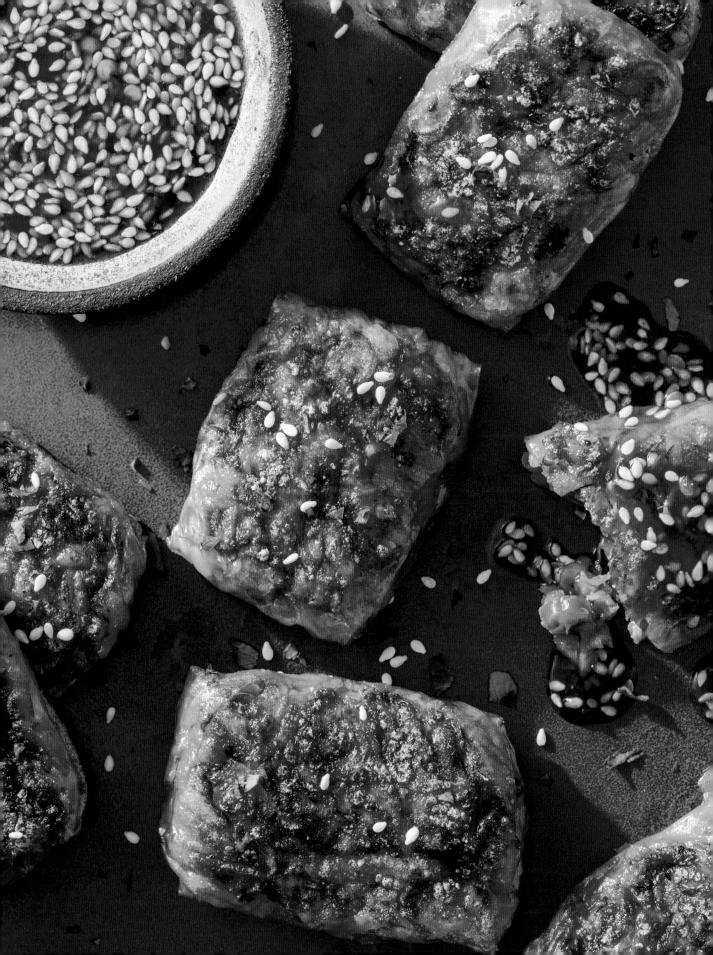

VEGGIE RICE PAPER DUMPLINGS

Pretty much anything wrapped in rice paper, pan fried, and dunked in salty, spicy sauce is going to hit the spot. I stuff these with cabbage, carrots, and green beans, but you can use any combination of your favorite vegetables.

MAKES *8 to 10 dumplings*
TOTAL TIME: *25 minutes*

FOR THE DIPPING SAUCE

- ¼ cup soy sauce
- 2 tablespoons sriracha or sambal oelek
- 2 tablespoons agave nectar
- 1 teaspoon white sesame seeds

FOR THE DUMPLINGS

- 1 tablespoon toasted sesame oil
- 1½ cups grated or finely chopped Chinese cabbage
- ½ cup chopped bean sprouts
- ½ cup grated carrots
- ½ cup finely chopped green beans
- 2 tablespoons liquid aminos
- ¼ teaspoon minced fresh ginger
- 8 to 10 3-inch round rice paper wrappers (see Note)
- 2 tablespoons sunflower or extra-virgin olive oil, for frying

MAKE THE DIPPING SAUCE: In a small bowl, whisk together the soy sauce, sriracha, agave nectar, and sesame seeds. Set aside.

MAKE THE DUMPLINGS: Heat the sesame oil in a medium skillet over medium-high heat. Add the cabbage, bean sprouts, carrots, green beans, aminos, and ginger and cook, stirring, until the vegetables are tender but still crisp, about 5 minutes. Remove the pan from the heat and let cool for 5 minutes.

Fill a wide, shallow bowl with an inch or so of lukewarm water. Working with one sheet of rice paper at a time, submerge the rice paper until it begins to soften, 5 to 10 seconds. Transfer to a nonstick surface, such as a silicone mat or plastic wrap, and place 2 tablespoons of the filling in the center of the wrapper. Fold in the two sides, followed by the top and bottom, and gently but firmly pinch the edges to seal. Set the dumpling on a large plate and repeat with the remaining wrappers and filling.

Heat the 2 tablespoons of oil in a large skillet over medium-low heat. Working in batches if needed so as not to crowd the pan, add the dumplings to the hot oil and cook until golden and crispy on each side, 3 to 5 minutes total. Repeat with any remaining dumplings and serve immediately with the dipping sauce.

NOTE: You can add an extra wrapper to your dumplings if you want a thicker dumpling or insurance against tearing.

HEART CAKES

I love finding ways to use plants to replicate the flavors people enjoy from animal products. In this case, I've called on the unique meaty texture of hearts of palm and artichoke to stand in for crab in these "crab cakes." With their crispy breaded coating, I've tricked many an unsuspecting guest into thinking these cakes are the real deal. They're always a popular addition to a spread, especially when served over a salad, on a bun with a slather sauce, or as a side.

MAKES *10 to 12 cakes*
TOTAL TIME: *25 minutes*

HEART CAKES

- 2 14-ounce cans artichoke heart quarters, drained
- 2 14-ounce cans hearts of palm, drained
- ⅓ cup vegan mayonnaise
- 1 tablespoon liquid aminos
- 2 teaspoons Old Bay seasoning or 1½ teaspoons paprika
- 1 teaspoon dried parsley
- 1 teaspoon celery salt
- 1 teaspoon yellow mustard
- ½ teaspoon freshly ground black pepper
- ½ cup chopped fresh parsley leaves, for serving

SAUCE

- 1 small cooked red beet (see Note on page 224)
- ½ cup plain vegan yogurt
- ½ cup vegan mayonnaise
- 1½ tablespoons prepared horseradish or yellow mustard
- 2 teaspoons apple cider vinegar
- ½ teaspoon sea salt

ASSEMBLY

- ¼ cup all-purpose flour
- ¼ cup plain unsweetened vegan milk
- ½ teaspoon sea salt
- 1 cup panko bread crumbs
- ¼ cup cornstarch
- Extra-virgin olive oil, for cooking

MAKE THE HEART CAKES: Line a baking sheet with parchment paper and set aside.

Squeeze the water out of the artichokes, thinly slice or shred them, and add them to a large bowl.

Use your hands to pull apart the hearts of palm into stringy pieces and add them to the same bowl. If they have a thick outer husk, you can either discard it or finely chop it with a knife. Add the mayonnaise, liquid aminos, Old Bay, parsley, celery salt, mustard, and pepper to the bowl and mix well to combine.

Using a ¼- or ⅓-cup measure (depending on the size of cakes you'd like), form the mixture into 1½- to 2-inch-wide patties (you will get 10 or 12, depending on what size you've chosen) and place them on the prepared baking sheet. Refrigerate for about 15 minutes to firm up.

MEANWHILE, MAKE THE SAUCE: In a high-powered blender, combine the beet, yogurt, mayonnaise, horseradish, vinegar, and salt and blend until completely smooth. Set aside while you assemble the heart cakes.

TO ASSEMBLE: Set up a dredging station with two medium bowls. In one bowl, whisk together the flour, milk, and salt until smooth and thick. In the second bowl, combine the panko and cornstarch.

Line a plate with paper towels and have at the ready. Pour about 1 inch oil into a large skillet and heat over medium heat. Working in batches of four, use a pastry brush to coat the cakes with the batter, then use your hands to gently coat them in the panko mixture. When the oil shimmers, add the cakes to the hot oil and fry for 5 minutes per side. Increase the heat to high and brown the sides of the cakes, rolling them in the pan. Transfer the cooked cakes to the paper towels to drain.

Serve each cake with a spoonful of the sauce and sprinkle with the parsley.

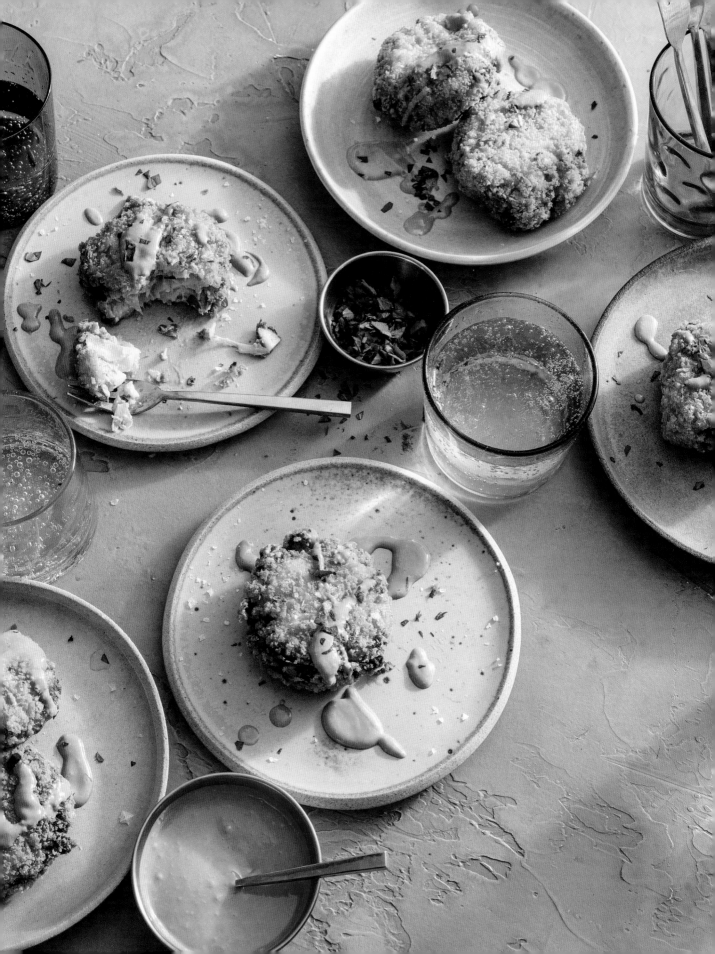

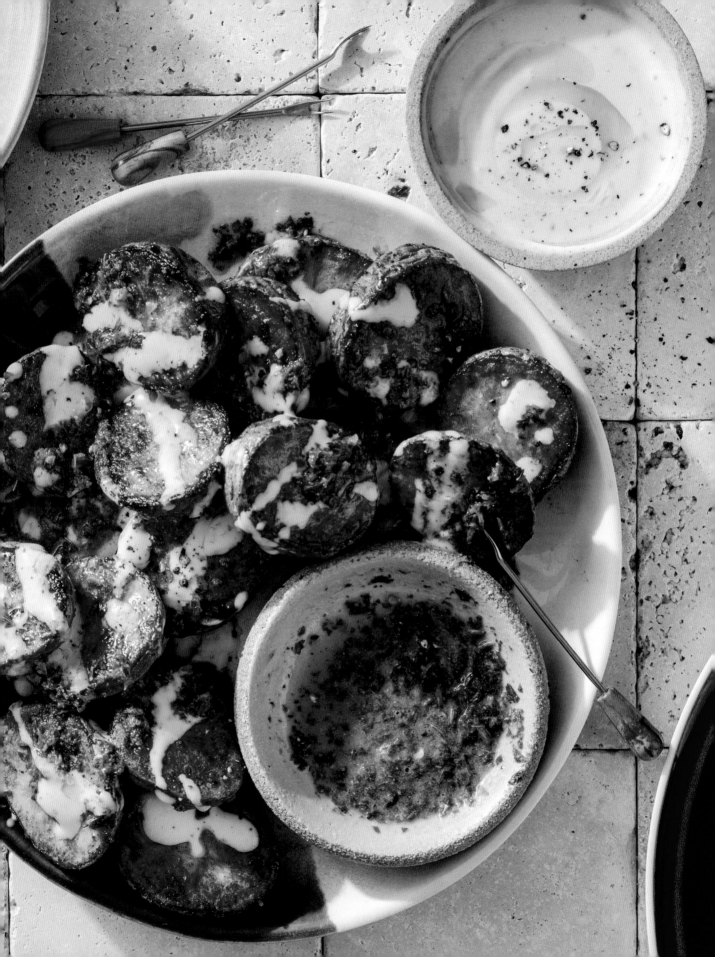

CRISPY ROASTED POTATOES *with Zhoug and Zesty Yogurt*

I've never met a buttery, crispy potato that I didn't devour with pleasure. For this dish, I've paired the potatoes with zhoug, a Yemeni hot sauce that packs serious but fresh green heat from jalapeño. Then a drizzle of lemony yogurt cools it all down. You'll never look at potatoes in quite the same way.

SERVES *6 to 8*
TOTAL TIME: *45 minutes*

CRISPY POTATOES

- 8 medium Yukon Gold potatoes (about 1½ pounds), unpeeled (see Note) and sliced into 1-inch-thick rounds
- 3 tablespoons extra-virgin olive oil
- ½ tablespoon minced fresh parsley leaves
- ½ tablespoon minced fresh cilantro leaves
- 1 teaspoon sea salt
- 1 teaspoon paprika
- ¼ teaspoon freshly ground black pepper

ZESTY YOGURT

- ½ cup plain vegan yogurt
- 1 tablespoon vegan mayonnaise
- 1 teaspoon fresh lemon juice
- ¼ teaspoon sea salt
- ¼ teaspoon freshly ground black pepper

FOR SERVING

Zhoug (recipe follows)

MAKE THE CRISPY POTATOES: Preheat the oven to 450°F. Line a baking sheet with parchment paper.

In a large bowl, toss the potatoes with the olive oil, parsley, cilantro, salt, paprika, and pepper until evenly coated.

Arrange the potato slices on the prepared baking sheet in a single layer. Bake until just starting to brown, about 15 minutes. Turn and cook until crispy, browned, and cooked through, another 10 to 15 minutes.

MEANWHILE, MAKE THE ZESTY YOGURT: In a medium bowl, whisk together the yogurt, mayonnaise, lemon juice, salt, and pepper.

TO SERVE: Arrange the crispy potatoes on a serving plate and dollop the zhoug all around and over the potatoes. Drizzle the yogurt on top and serve warm.

NOTE   You can peel the potatoes if you prefer, but the peels are packed with fiber and nutrients!

Zhoug

MAKES *about 1 cup*
TOTAL TIME: *10 minutes*

- 1 cup fresh cilantro leaves
- ¼ cup fresh parsley leaves
- 3 tablespoons fresh lemon juice
- 2 small hot Indian or Thai green chiles, stemmed but whole
- 1 teaspoon turbinado sugar
- 1 teaspoon ground cumin
- 1 teaspoon caraway seeds (optional)
- ¼ teaspoon sea salt
- ⅛ teaspoon asafoetida
- Pinch of red chile flakes
- 3 tablespoons extra-virgin olive oil

In a food processor or high-powered blender, combine the cilantro, parsley, lemon juice, green chiles, sugar, cumin, caraway (if using), salt, asafoetida, and chile flakes and pulse until coarsely chopped. Add the oil and pulse again to create a chunky paste. Store in a sealed container in the refrigerator for up to 5 days.

NOTE   While you're at it, make a bonus batch to punch up any savory dish.

Eating with Your Senses

Finding sensory pleasure in your food isn't just a feel-good idea that sounds nice for when we have the time; it's an essential part of kick-starting digestion. When you experience the texture of each ingredient in your hands as you take the time to prepare it for a meal, smell the aroma of it cooking, hear it crackling in the pan, and see it beautifully arranged on a plate, maybe vibrant with a spray of fresh herbs, your mouth releases digestive enzymes and your stomach produces acid. These processes are key to breaking down your food and accessing its nutrients.

When you prepare food in a way that stimulates your hearing, sight, smell, taste, and touch and then allow yourself to fully experience those sensations, you're actually enhancing the health benefits of that meal. Your eyes, ears, nose, mouth, and hands feel wholly and agreeably sated. Which means that your body is getting what it needs *and* what it wants.

I also love refining and enhancing the use of our senses because it makes us more aware of all the abundance and bliss in our lives.

It is very simple to cook and eat with your senses. Here are some examples:

TASTE

- Enhance flavor with spices and herbs and round out your plates with a variety of flavors, especially the six tastes (see Build Meals with the Six Tastes in Mind, page 35).

SMELL

- Mix up your cooking preparations, because they each create different aromas: Roast, grill, bake, and sauté.

- Use herbs and spices, especially spices that you toast first, which releases their fragrance.

SIGHT

- Mix up your color palette! For example, use red peppers instead of green if you're already using spinach.

- Use a variety of knife cuts; slice some ingredients, chop others.

- Finish dishes with bright fresh herbs, and look to nature for other edible adornments, such as flowers and fronds.

FEEL

- Layer different textures, such as crunchy, soft, and creamy.

- Combine different temperatures in a dish.

- Best of all, eat with your hands! Traditionally in India—and many other parts of the world, such as the Middle East, Africa, and South America—there was no cutlery; the cutlery was our hands. Westerners thought this was animalistic and uncivilized, so utensils started to appear on tables as part of the pressure to assimilate. But touching your food is more than just the lack of silverware. It signals your body to start producing digestive enzymes, while also allowing a real connection to your food. It's a full sensory experience. Research has even shown that food actually tastes better when you eat with your hands! Yes, it can get messy, but that's what napkins are for.

SOUND

If you tune in, you'll hear the symphony of your dish:

- Cook with various consistencies in mind so you can slurp, crunch, and chew.

- Listen for the popping of spices in the pan as you toast them and grind them.

- Hear the sizzle of an ingredient hitting a hot pan.

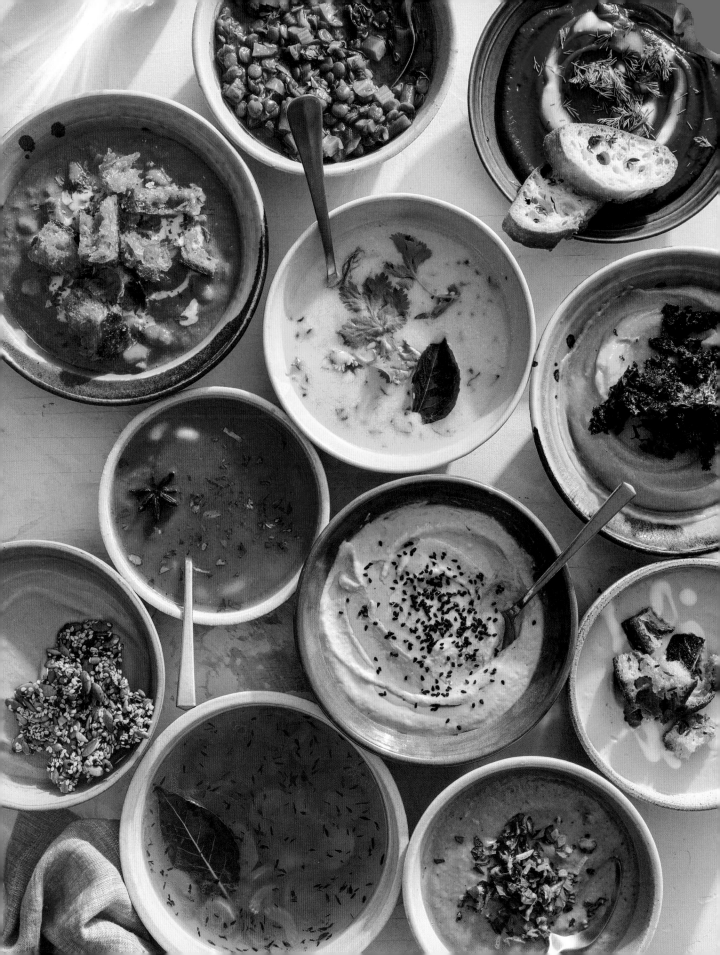

SOUPS

When the sun descends at the end of the day and the temperature falls along with it, our digestive energies also start to wane. It's time to shift from the go go go fiery energy of the sun and let the moon's cozy blanket of calm take over. That's why when I think about the perfect dinner, my mind immediately goes to soups. They're already cooked down and blended, so they're easier to digest. Plus, there's nothing like a warm, soothing bowlful to get you into the (sleepy) mood. But don't be fooled—these recipes are still filling and would be satisfying any time of day.

BAA'S WEDDING DAAL

SPLIT YELLOW PIGEON PEAS IN SWEET-SOUR BROTH

For as long as I can remember, my grandma has made this Gujarati yellow split pigeon pea daal that's traditionally served at weddings and also every Monday at her house. My mum has continued the tradition, and she's passed the recipe down to my sister and me—and now my niece and nephew regularly request "Baa's Daal," which to them is "Nani's [my mum's] Daal." Everyone knows it's the best! It has a soupier consistency than other daals, and its complex broth is scented with cinnamon, ginger, and star anise, plus a combination of jaggery (or coconut sugar) and kokum (see Note), which make it sweet and sour. The warm broth and strong flavors also make this a powerful home remedy, like the kind of soup you reach for when you need to clear your sinuses or generate a healing heat in your body. I make it in my own kitchen weekly, and I feel so connected to all the women in my family when I do. The only update I've made is occasionally using a pressure cooker to prepare the toor daal when I want to save a little time (see Variation).

SERVES *4 to 6*

TOTAL TIME: *50 minutes, plus soaking time*

1 cup toor daal (split yellow pigeon peas)

¼ cup peanuts

4 dried kokum or 3 tablespoons fresh lemon juice

1 tablespoon sunflower or avocado oil

1 teaspoon cumin seeds

½ teaspoon brown mustard seeds

2 whole star anise

1 small cinnamon stick

5 fresh or dried curry leaves (optional)

1 tablespoon garam masala or Ground CCF Masala (page 49)

2 teaspoons sea salt

2 teaspoons red chile powder

1 teaspoon ground coriander

½ teaspoon ground turmeric

1 teaspoon minced hot Indian or Thai green chile

½ cup canned crushed tomatoes

1 tablespoon jaggery or coconut sugar

Warm cooked basmati rice, for serving

Chopped fresh cilantro leaves, for serving

In a bowl, soak the toor daal in water for at least 30 minutes or up to 2 hours. (Or skip completely, if you're really in a rush!) Rinse and drain.

In a large pot, combine the pigeon peas, peanuts, kokum (if you're using lemon juice, you'll add it after the pigeon peas are cooked), and 6 cups water. Bring to a boil over high heat, reduce the heat to a simmer, and cook, stirring occasionally, until the pigeon peas are completely tender, about 25 minutes. Remove the pot from the heat. If using lemon juice, stir it in now.

In a medium skillet, heat the oil over medium heat. Add the cumin and mustard seeds and cook, covered, until they pop, 30 seconds to 1 minute. Reduce the heat to medium-low and add the star anise, cinnamon stick, curry leaves, garam masala, salt, chile powder, coriander, and turmeric and cook, stirring, just until fragrant, about 15 seconds. Add the green chile and cook briefly, stirring, for 15 seconds. Add the crushed tomatoes and jaggery and cook, stirring, until the flavors have come together, 2 to 3 minutes.

Add the spiced tomato mixture to the pigeon pea mixture and stir well to combine. If you'd like a thicker consistency, return the pot to low heat and cook until the mixture has thickened up to your liking, another 8 to 10 minutes.

Serve over rice and top with chopped cilantro.

Leftovers can be stored in a sealed container in the refrigerator for up to 3 days.

NOTE This recipe calls for kokum, which is a type of dried fruit that has a slightly sour taste and medicinal qualities that can calm the mind and uplift the mood. (It promotes the production of serotonin, which is the feel-good hormone.) You can find packages of it online, but you could also substitute lemon juice, if you prefer.

VARIATION *Pressure Cooker Wedding Daal:* To make this in an electric pressure cooker, follow the directions for cooking the pigeon peas on the stove, but reduce the water to 4 cups and cook on high pressure for 7 minutes. If you have time, you can let the pressure release naturally, or you can just do it manually.

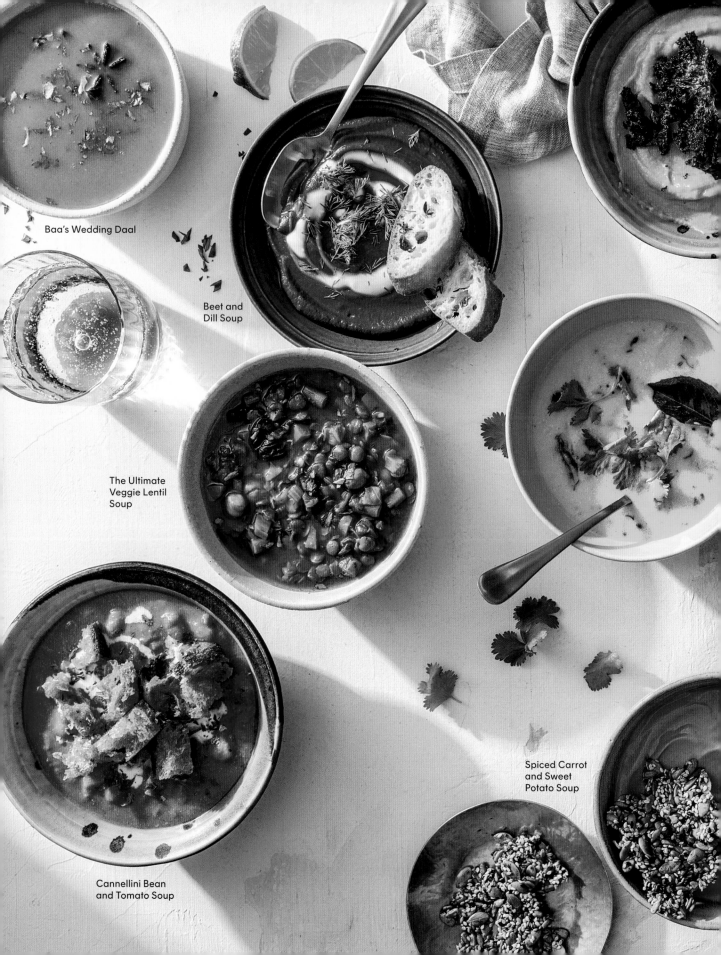

Baa's Wedding Daal

Beet and Dill Soup

The Ultimate Veggie Lentil Soup

Cannellini Bean and Tomato Soup

Spiced Carrot and Sweet Potato Soup

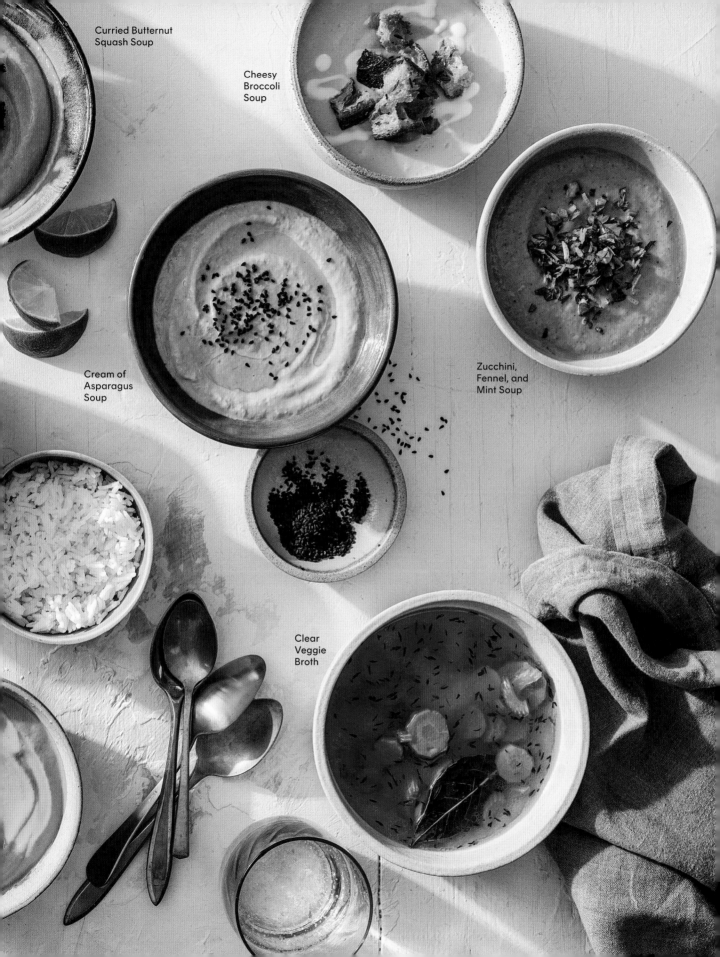

Curried Butternut
Squash Soup

Cheesy
Broccoli
Soup

Cream of
Asparagus
Soup

Zucchini,
Fennel, and
Mint Soup

Clear
Veggie
Broth

CREAM OF ASPARAGUS SOUP

with Crisped Kalonji Seeds

According to Ayurveda, asparagus purifies the blood and cleanses excess fluid from the lymphatic system (which is why you may pee a little more after eating it). I created this heavenly soup when my teacher, His Holiness Radhanath Swami, visited. He always takes soup as his evening meal, and I felt inspired to treat him to the perfect bowlful after a day spent in meditation, reflection, and conversation. Since he loves asparagus, I challenged myself to come up with a recipe that celebrated the vegetable's unique woody, earthy taste. The result is a refreshingly simple soup with a clean, pure flavor, and I've been making it in service and gratitude ever since.

SERVES *2 or 3*
TOTAL TIME: *20 minutes*

- 1 tablespoon unsalted vegan butter or coconut oil
- 1 cup chopped celery (about 2 stalks)
- 2 cups chopped asparagus (about ½ pound)
- ⅓ cup cashews
- ⅛ teaspoon asafoetida
- Canned full-fat coconut milk or plain vegan cream, for drizzling
- Extra-virgin olive oil, for drizzling
- Kalonji (nigella) seeds, for garnish

In a heavy medium pot, melt the butter or coconut oil over medium heat. Add the celery, asparagus, cashews, and asafoetida and cook, stirring, until fragrant, about 2 minutes. Add 1½ cups water, cover, and cook until the vegetables are super soft and mushy, about 15 minutes.

Using an immersion blender, puree the soup until creamy and smooth. (Alternatively, carefully transfer the soup to a stand blender and blend until smooth.)

Divide the soup among bowls and drizzle with coconut milk and/or olive oil and sprinkle with nigella seeds.

Leftovers can be stored in a sealed container in the refrigerator for up to 3 days.

THE ULTIMATE VEGGIE LENTIL SOUP

The name says it all, people! You've got loads of vegetables, loads of spices, loads of fresh herbs, plus lentils in this extremely hearty and filling soup. If you've ever been skeptical that a bowl of soup could actually fill you up, doubt no more!

SERVES *4 to 6*
TOTAL TIME: *45 minutes*

- ½ tablespoon extra-virgin olive oil
- ½ tablespoon sea salt
- 1 teaspoon ground cinnamon
- 1 teaspoon ground coriander
- 1 teaspoon sweet paprika
- ½ teaspoon smoked paprika
- ¼ teaspoon asafoetida
- ¼ teaspoon ground turmeric
- 2 bay leaves
- 1 cup green or brown lentils, rinsed and drained
- 1 cup canned crushed tomatoes
- 1 cup peeled and finely chopped carrots
- ½ cup finely chopped celery
- ½ cup finely chopped cabbage
- ½ cup finely chopped green beans
- ½ cup spinach leaves
- ¼ cup cooked or canned chickpeas (optional), rinsed and drained if canned
- 1 tablespoon cornstarch, tapioca starch, or potato starch
- ¼ cup chopped fresh cilantro leaves
- ¼ cup chopped fresh parsley leaves

In a large pot, heat the oil over medium heat. Add the salt, cinnamon, coriander, sweet paprika, smoked paprika, asafoetida, turmeric, and bay leaves and cook, stirring, until the spices release their oils and aromas, about 1 minute. Reduce the heat to medium-low and add 2 cups water, the lentils, crushed tomatoes, carrots, celery, cabbage, green beans, spinach, and chickpeas (if using). Cover and cook, stirring occasionally, until the vegetables and lentils are tender and the mixture is perfumed with the spices, about 30 minutes.

In a medium bowl, whisk the cornstarch with 1 cup water until smooth. Stir the slurry into the soup and cook until thickened, about 5 minutes. Add up to ½ cup water if needed to loosen the consistency to your liking. Remove the pot from the heat and stir in half of the cilantro and parsley.

Divide the soup among bowls and garnish with the remaining herbs.

Leftovers can be stored in a sealed container in the refrigerator for up to 3 days.

SPICED CARROT AND SWEET POTATO SOUP

with Super-Seed Brittle

It probably comes as no surprise that in Ayurveda, the sweet flavor is one of the most sattvic. It is thought to offer feelings of calmness, happiness, and mental clarity, and has a cooling effect on the body. I couldn't think of a more perfect wavelength for ending the day and sending yourself off to bed! Creamy sweet potato and carrot are balanced with rich tahini and deep, warm spice from paprika and cumin. It's like the soup equivalent of pulling on the most buttery-soft pair of sweatpants.

While the savory-sweet-smoky seed brittle offers beautiful texture to this otherwise silky soup and makes this a bit more filling as a meal, it is certainly not required.

SERVES *4 to 6*

TOTAL TIME: *40 minutes*

1 tablespoon extra-virgin olive oil

¼ cup chopped celery

½ teaspoon ground cumin

½ teaspoon ground coriander

¼ teaspoon asafoetida

¼ teaspoon freshly ground black pepper

4 cups peeled and chopped carrots (about 2 pounds)

2 cups chopped peeled sweet potato (about 2 medium)

1 fresh mild red chile, such as Anaheim, stemmed and chopped, or 1 teaspoon paprika

1½ teaspoons sea salt

⅓ cup tahini, stirred well

Super-Seed Brittle (page 255)

In a large pot, heat the oil over medium heat. Add the celery, cumin, coriander, asafoetida, and black pepper and cook, stirring, for 1 minute. Add the carrots, sweet potato, chile, and salt and cook, stirring to coat the vegetables. Add 4 cups water, reduce the heat to a simmer, cover, and cook until the carrots and sweet potatoes are soft and mashable and have been infused with the spices, about 20 minutes.

Add the tahini and use an immersion blender to blend the soup until completely smooth. (Alternatively, carefully transfer the soup to a stand blender and blend until smooth.)

Divide the soup among bowls, top with the seeded brittle, and serve.

Leftovers can be stored in a sealed container in the refrigerator for up to 3 days.

ZUCCHINI, FENNEL, AND MINT SOUP

with Pistachio Gremolata

Soup can also be, somewhat surprisingly, a way to cool and energize your body in warmer months. The combination of hydrating zucchini and invigorating mint feels fresh and light yet substantial thanks to a pistachio gremolata. It's the recipe I want whenever I'm feeling a little overheated—in body or spirit—or when I've had a few days of heavier meals and desire something that feels cleansing.

SERVES *4*

TOTAL TIME: *30 minutes*

- 2 tablespoons extra-virgin olive oil
- 2 large or 3 medium zucchini, cut into ½-inch cubes (about 3 heaping cups)
- 1 medium head fennel, stalks trimmed, cut into ½-inch cubes (about 2 cups)
- 1 cup chopped celery (about 2 stalks)
- 2 teaspoons sea salt
- ¼ teaspoon asafoetida
- 2 cups packed spinach leaves (optional; for a hit of extra greens)
- ¼ cup chopped fresh mint leaves
- 1 tablespoon fresh lemon juice
- Pistachio Gremolata (page 253)

In a large heavy-bottomed pot, heat the oil over medium heat. Add the zucchini, fennel, celery, salt, and asafoetida and cook, stirring, until the vegetables are fully coated in the oil, about 2 minutes. Stir in 1 cup water. Cover, reduce the heat to a simmer, and cook, stirring occasionally, until the vegetables are soft, about 15 minutes. Fold in the spinach (if using), mint, and lemon juice and remove the pot from the heat.

Carefully transfer the hot soup mixture to a high-powered blender and blend until completely smooth.

Divide the soup among bowls and top with the pistachio gremolata.

Leftovers can be stored in a sealed container in the refrigerator for up to 3 days.

NOTE   The gremolata is a versatile condiment that has the ability to complement and enhance the flavor of almost any dish, so I always find that any leftovers are quickly put to good use. But this soup would still be delicious without it.

BEET AND DILL SOUP

with Thyme Crostini

This hot pink soup is gorgeous, a reminder that food is a powerful way to experience nature's vibrant beauty. But yes, it's also very delicious thanks to the classic combination of slightly sweet beets and fresh dill, plus coconut milk for richness, a pop of lime for lift, and thyme-scented crostini for crunch factor. The beet doubters in your life have only to take one look at this bowl to know there's good things to come.

Any time I have something crunchy and herby to dip into a soup like these thyme crostini, I know I'm in for a special treat!

SERVES *2*
TOTAL TIME: *40 minutes*

- 3 cooked medium beets (see Note), peeled and chopped
- 1 cup canned full-fat coconut milk
- ¼ cup plain unsweetened almond milk (or more coconut milk)
- 1 teaspoon sea salt
- 1 bay leaf
- ¾ cup chopped fresh dill, plus more for serving
- 1 medium lime, quartered
- Vegan cream, for drizzling
- 6 to 8 Thyme Crostini (page 254)

In a large pot, combine the beets, coconut milk, almond milk, 1½ cups water, the salt, and bay leaf and bring to a boil over medium-high heat. Cover, reduce the heat to medium-low, and simmer until you can easily pierce the beets with a paring knife, about 30 minutes. Remove the pot from the heat.

Discard the bay leaf. Carefully transfer the soup mixture to a high-powered blender. Add the dill and the juice of 1 lime quarter (about ½ tablespoon) and blend until completely smooth.

Divide the soup among bowls and drizzle with cream. Top with more dill and serve with the remaining lime quarters and crostini.

NOTE To save yourself quite a bit of time and effort, I suggest using store-bought cooked and peeled beets, which is typically what I do when making beet soups and dips. Otherwise, you can wrap each beet in foil and roast at 400°F until you can pierce them easily with a knife, 50 to 60 minutes. Wait for them to cool slightly, then slip off their skins.

CANNELLINI BEAN AND TOMATO SOUP
with Torn Chili Croutons

This is pretty much the creamy tomato soup of your dreams. The secret is using beans for extra thickness and body, plus a dab of miso for that can't-quite-place-it layer of deep, savory umami flavor. It would be perfect on its own, but why deprive yourself of simple chili croutons and a drizzle of coconut milk?

SERVES *4*
TOTAL TIME: *35 minutes*

- 2 tablespoons extra-virgin olive oil or unsalted vegan butter
- 1 heaping cup chopped celery (about 2 stalks)
- 2 tablespoons chopped fresh basil leaves
- 2 bay leaves
- ⅛ teaspoon asafoetida
- 2 cups canned crushed tomatoes
- 1 15-ounce can cannellini beans, rinsed and drained
- ¾ cup canned full-fat coconut milk
- 3 tablespoons nutritional yeast
- 1 teaspoon yellow miso
- ½ teaspoon sea salt, plus more to taste
- Vegan cream or more coconut milk, for serving
- Fresh or dried parsley, for serving
- Chili Croutons (page 253), for serving

In a heavy-bottomed pot, heat the oil or butter over medium-high heat. Add the celery, basil, bay leaves, and asafoetida and cook, stirring, until the celery starts to sweat and soften, about 3 minutes. Add the tomatoes, beans, coconut milk, ½ cup water, the nutritional yeast, miso, and salt. Reduce the heat to low and simmer until the flavors have come together, the soup has thickened, and the aromas coming from the pot make it impossible to wait any longer, 15 to 20 minutes. Season with a bit more salt, if needed.

Divide the hot soup among bowls and drizzle with a bit of vegan cream or coconut milk. Garnish with parsley and a handful of chili croutons.

Leftovers can be stored in a sealed container in the refrigerator for up to 3 days.

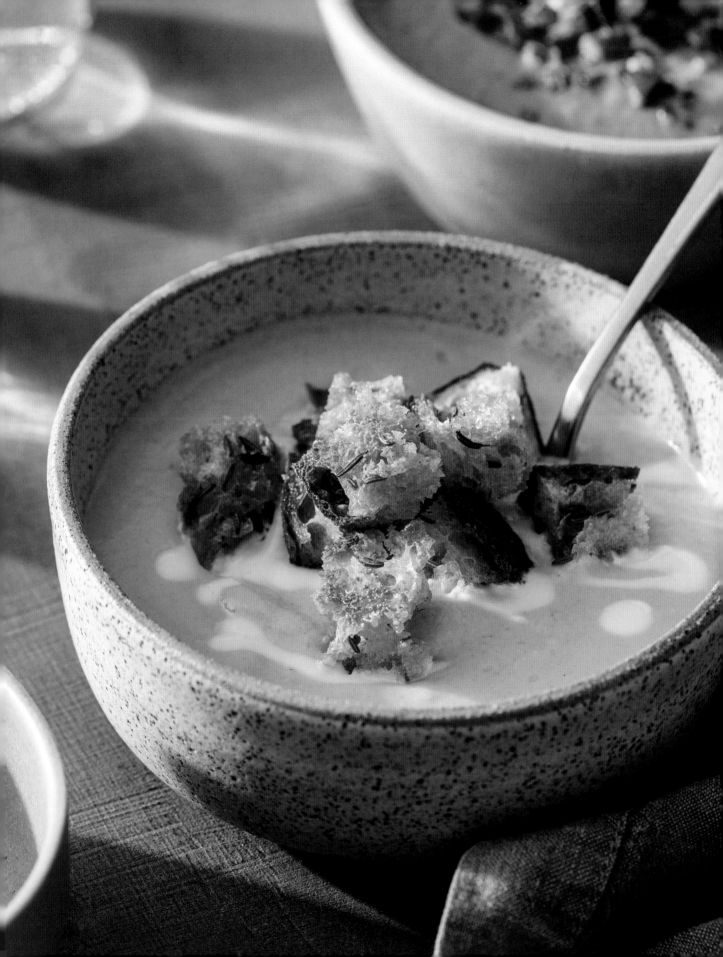

CHEESY BROCCOLI SOUP
with Caraway Croutons

Every time I make this dish, I'm reminded of just how magical it is. It's one of those great throw-everything-in-a-pot recipes that takes barely any time. The heat does all the work for you because it brings out the natural sweetness of the broccoli, which doesn't need much more to be delicious—except maybe nutritional yeast for its savory cheese-like flavor. Then once everything's blended, you have this super-rich yet light cream of broccoli soup. Done and dusted.

    Though I do love serving this with a drizzle of caraway-infused oil and the caraway croutons because the anise-y spice complements the subtly sweet broccoli, this soup would be just as delicious without one or either of these elements.

SERVES *4 to 6*
TOTAL TIME: *50 minutes*

CARAWAY OIL

    2 tablespoons extra-virgin olive oil

    1 teaspoon caraway seeds

SOUP

    2 tablespoons vegan butter

    ¾ cup finely chopped celery

    2½ cups plain unsweetened almond milk

    2 cups chopped broccoli florets

    ½ cup cashews

    3 tablespoons nutritional yeast

    ½ teaspoon sea salt

    ¼ teaspoon asafoetida

    Caraway Croutons (page 253), for serving

    Vegan cream, for serving (optional)

MAKE THE CARAWAY OIL: In a small skillet, heat the oil over medium heat. Add the caraway seeds and heat until fragrant, 30 seconds to 1 minute. Remove the pan from the heat and set aside to cool.

MAKE THE SOUP: In a medium pot, melt the butter over medium-high heat. Add the celery and cook, stirring, until softened, about 3 minutes. Add the almond milk, ½ cup water, the broccoli, cashews, nutritional yeast, salt, and asafoetida. Cover, reduce the heat to a slow simmer, and cook until the vegetables are very soft, 15 to 20 minutes. Remove the pot from the heat.

Carefully transfer the hot soup mixture to a high-powered blender and blend until completely smooth, adding a splash of water if needed to loosen the consistency to your liking.

Divide the soup among bowls and top with the croutons and caraway oil. If desired, add a drizzle of cream.

Leftovers can be stored in a sealed container in the refrigerator for up to 3 days.

CURRIED BUTTERNUT SQUASH SOUP

with Cheesy Curry Crispy Kale

There's a quietness to this soup, making it extra soothing at the end of a long day when your senses don't necessarily want to be engaged. The squash is naturally silky and sweet, and it's balanced by just the right amount of heat from ginger and chiles. I call for using curry powder here, too, which isn't quite as bold as garam masala but has the same warming effect. To make this soup even more special, I add a sprinkling of curried kale chips, but the soup is also delightful on its own.

SERVES *4*

TOTAL TIME: *40 minutes*

- 1 tablespoon extra-virgin olive oil
- 1 cup finely shredded cabbage (about ¼ small head)
- 2 bay leaves
- 1½ teaspoons sea salt
- 1 teaspoon finely grated fresh ginger
- 1 teaspoon minced fresh hot red chile, such as Fresno or Thai red chile
- ¼ teaspoon asafoetida
- 3 cups ½-inch cubes peeled butternut squash (about 1 medium squash)
- 1 teaspoon curry powder
- ½ cup canned full-fat coconut milk
- ½ tablespoon fresh lime juice
- Cheesy Curried Crispy Kale (page 254), for serving

In a large pot, heat the olive oil over medium-low heat. Add the cabbage, bay leaves, salt, curry powder, ginger, red chile, and asafoetida and cook, stirring, until fragrant, about 1 minute.

Add the squash, curry powder, and 1 cup water and simmer for 10 minutes. Stir in the coconut milk and another 1 cup water and cook until the squash is soft and mushy, another 15 to 20 minutes.

Transfer the mixture to a high-powered blender and blend until smooth. Stir in the lime juice.

Divide the soup among bowls and serve topped with the crispy curried kale.

Leftovers can be stored in a sealed container in the refrigerator for up to 3 days.

CLEAR VEGGIE BROTH

Soup is a powerful way to offer your body deep nourishment while requiring very little digestive effort, which is what also makes it such a healing food. This broth offers both of these benefits while also being especially gentle because there's nothing for your digestive system to break down. The vegetables release all their nutrients and flavor, while ginger, thyme, and peppercorns infuse their warm, fragrant, naturally antiviral and anti-inflammatory properties. I make this as a soothing antidote whenever I'm feeling a little run-down, or I'll enjoy it anytime I want a gentle nutrient boost, maybe with some noodles for something a little heartier.

SERVES *2*
TOTAL TIME: *50 minutes*

- 1 tablespoon extra-virgin olive oil
- 2 large carrots, peeled and chopped
- 2 medium celery stalks, chopped
- 2 sticks lemongrass, trimmed and chopped
- ½ cup fresh parsley leaves
- 1 2½-inch piece of fresh ginger, peeled and sliced
- 3 fresh or dried bay leaves
- ¼ teaspoon dried thyme leaves
- 4 black peppercorns
- ⅛ teaspoon asafoetida
- Cooked thin rice or ramen noodles (optional)

Heat the olive oil in a large skillet over medium heat. Add the carrots, celery, lemongrass, parsley, ginger, bay leaves, thyme, peppercorns, and asafoetida and cook, stirring, until fragrant, about 2 minutes.

Add 4 cups of water, reduce the heat to low, and cover. Simmer until the vegetables are completely softened and their flavor has infused into the broth, about 45 minutes.

From here, you can strain out the vegetables and aromatics and drink this as a hot broth, leave the vegetables in and remove only the bay leaves and peppercorns for a vegetable soup, or add cooked noodles for something a little heartier.

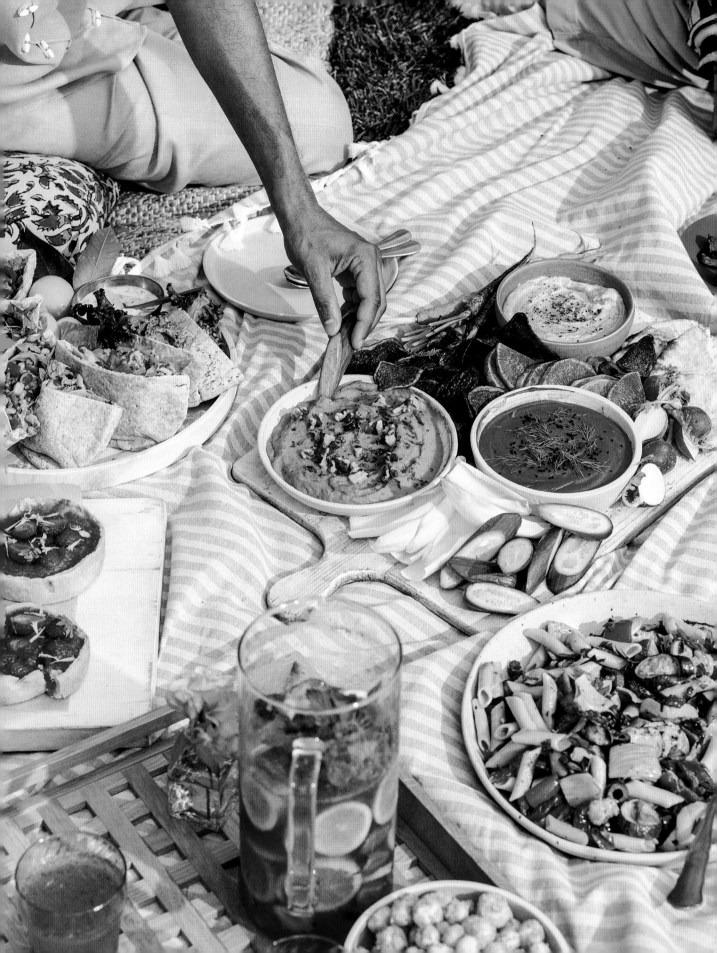

CONDIMENTS, DIPS, AND CRUNCHY BITS

This is where layers of flavor are born. Whether you're into rich and creamy, cool and tangy, bright and fresh, sweet and sour, herbaceous and savory, or all of the above (the correct answer, in my opinion), the recipes in this chapter will take your cooking and eating game to the next level. I highly recommend keeping an assorted stash in the fridge, which means that something tasty to eat is never going to be more than a few minutes away. Unless otherwise noted, all recipes in this chapter will last in the fridge when stored in a sealed container for 3 to 5 days.

Sauces, Condiments, Dips, and Spreads:
Dress for Success

I have never been a sauce or dip traditionalist. I believe in free condiment love—meaning that no matter whether something's called a dip, a dressing, or a drizzle, it can be used all manner of ways in your cooking. Creamy spreads are just as nice smeared on naan or scooped up with raw veggies as they are stirred into bowls; a vinaigrette can dress greens, grains, or mains; a sauce can just as easily be layered in a sandwich as it can be draped over your favorite roasted vegetables. Get the idea? And, as always, the more, the merrier! Now go forth and sauce! (For more dress-spiration, see How to Make a Rainbow Bowl, page 110.)

MUHAMMARA

SYRIAN WALNUT AND RED PEPPER DIP

To me, the perfect spread is lusciously creamy, has several levels of flavor, and is irresistible for dipping and slathering. Lucky for us, muhammara—a traditional Syrian dip made from omega 3-rich walnuts, red bell peppers, pomegranate molasses, and bread crumbs—is *all* of those things. It's smoky, it's sweet, it's tangy, it's nutty, it's spicy—a little bit like me. And it has the most vibrant orange hue.

SERVES *4*

TOTAL TIME: *5 minutes*

FOR THE DIP

    2 cups chopped roasted red peppers (about 2 jarred roasted peppers)

    ½ cup walnuts, toasted in a dry pan until fragrant (see Note)

    ¼ cup extra-virgin olive oil

    ¼ cup plain bread crumbs

    1 tablespoon pomegranate molasses

    1 tablespoon fresh lemon juice

    1 teaspoon paprika

    ½ teaspoon sea salt

    ½ teaspoon ground sumac

    ⅛ teaspoon asafoetida

FOR SERVING

    Chili oil, to taste

    Pomegranate molasses, to taste

    2 tablespoons chopped toasted walnuts

    2 tablespoons chopped fresh parsley

MAKE THE DIP: In a high-powered blender, combine the roasted peppers, walnuts, olive oil, bread crumbs, pomegranate molasses, lemon juice, paprika, salt, sumac, and asafoetida and blend until completely smooth.

TO SERVE: Transfer the dip to a serving bowl. Drizzle with the chili oil and pomegranate molasses and finish with a sprinkle of the walnuts and parsley.

NOTE I've also made this recipe with tahini instead of walnuts, and it's just as delicious!

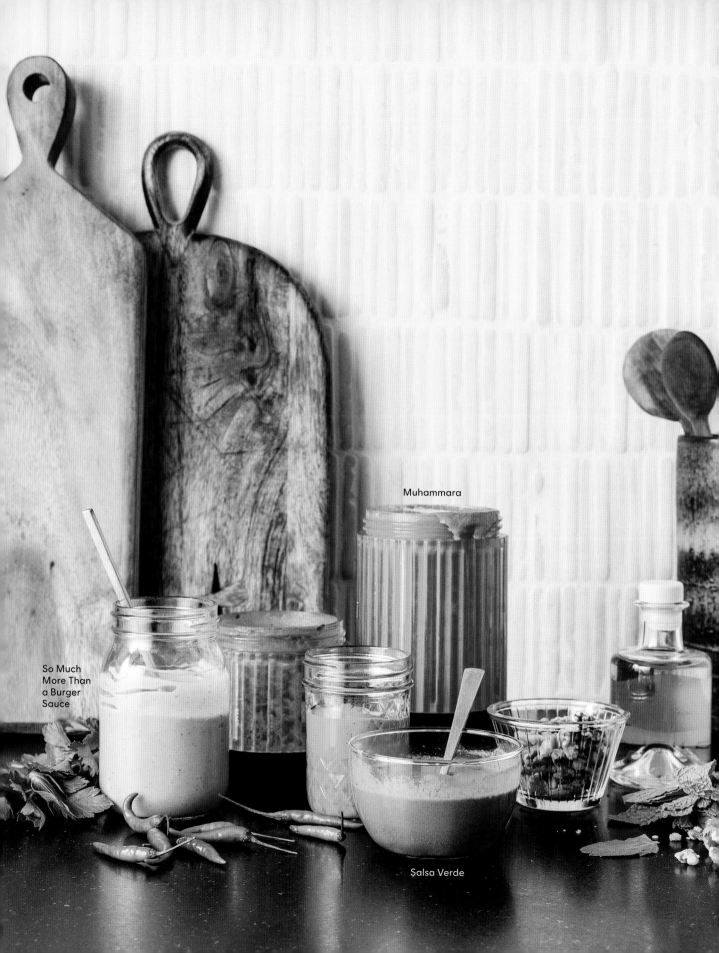

Muhammara

So Much
More Than
a Burger
Sauce

Salsa Verde

SO MUCH MORE THAN A BURGER SAUCE

Since I moved to LA, I've heard so much about In-N-Out Burger, especially their incredible tangy, creamy sauce that's made from a whole mess of condiments—which is my love language. I wanted to create a vegan version, and it's become a staple during burger nights or a dip with chips when friends are coming over. You can smother it all over a Spicy Bean Burger (page 147), a fully loaded Everything Sandwich (page 146), or anywhere else you want that deluxe saucy experience.

MAKES *about 1¼ cups*
TOTAL TIME: *5 minutes*

- ½ cup ketchup
- ½ cup vegan mayonnaise
- 1 tablespoon pickle juice or pickled jalapeño juice
- ½ tablespoon yellow mustard
- ½ teaspoon apple cider vinegar
- ¼ cup finely chopped dill pickles (optional)

In a medium bowl, whisk together the ketchup, mayonnaise, pickle juice, mustard, vinegar, and pickles (if using). Store in a sealed container in the refrigerator for up to 2 weeks.

SALSA VERDE

A version of salsa verde is a staple in some of the best cuisines in the world—Spanish, Italian, Mexican—and for good reason. It's a bright, fresh condiment packed with herbs in addition to capers and chiles, plus it gets a few good glugs of olive oil to ensure that all that green goodness can be effortlessly drizzled over pretty much anything. There is not a roasted or grilled veggie in the world that wouldn't be most grateful for a spoonful of this.

MAKES *about 1½ cups*
TOTAL TIME: *5 minutes*

- ¾ cup fresh cilantro leaves
- ¾ cup fresh parsley leaves
- ½ cup fresh mint leaves
- ¼ cup extra-virgin olive oil
- 1 hot Indian or Thai green chile, halved
- 2 tablespoons brined capers, drained
- 1 tablespoon fresh lemon juice

In a high-powered blender, combine the cilantro, parsley, mint, oil, green chile, capers, lemon juice, and 1 tablespoon water and blend until completely smooth.

BEET, PINE NUT, AND FETA DIP

Give me a hot-pink dip and I am one happy lady. Especially when that vibrancy is from fiber- and glutamine-rich beets, which help detoxify the body and reduce inflammation. This is a spread that's just as happy dressed up for a party as it is at home in its comfies spread on toast.

MAKES *about 2½ cups*
TOTAL TIME: *5 minutes*

- 1½ cups vegan feta cut into ½-inch cubes, plus crumbled feta for garnish
- 1 cup sliced cooked beets (see Note on page 224)
- ½ cup pine nuts, plus more for garnish (optional)
- 3 tablespoons thick unsweetened vegan yogurt
- 1 tablespoon dried dill or 3 tablespoons chopped fresh dill (optional)
- ½ tablespoon fresh lemon juice
- ½ teaspoon sea salt
- ½ teaspoon ground cumin

In a high-powered blender, combine the feta, beets, pine nuts (if using), yogurt, dill (if using), lemon juice, salt, and cumin. Blend until silky smooth. Serve garnished with crumbled feta and pine nuts (if using).

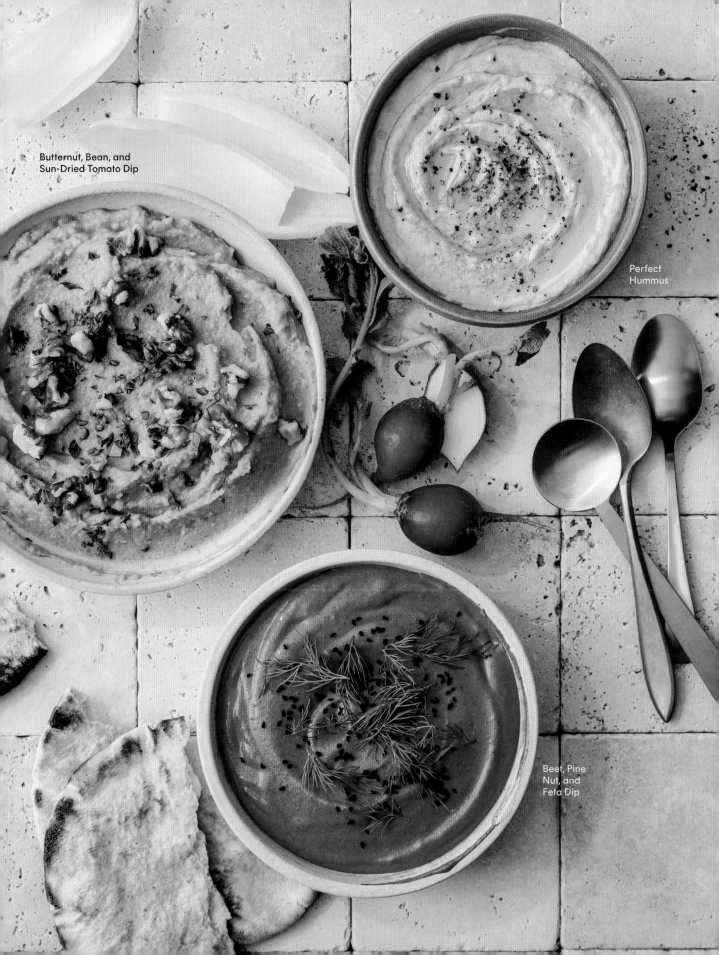

Butternut, Bean, and
Sun-Dried Tomato Dip

Perfect
Hummus

Beet, Pine
Nut, and
Feta Dip

BUTTERNUT, BEAN, AND SUN-DRIED TOMATO DIP

Roasted butternut squash is already perfectly creamy, but I wanted to see what would happen if I gave it even more body with pureed butter beans, cheesy richness from nutritional yeast, plus the salty kick of sun-dried tomatoes. The result is a spread that lives somewhere between sweet and savory and is perfectly suitable for dolloping over a variety of dishes, especially those with subtly sweet ingredients like my Everything Sandwich (page 146) and Chopped Salad Stuffed Pita (page 160).

MAKES *about 3 cups*
TOTAL TIME: *5 minutes*

1 medium butternut squash, halved and seeds scooped out

1½ cups cooked or canned butter beans (rinsed and drained if canned)

10 oil-packed sun-dried tomatoes

1 tablespoon nutritional yeast

1 tablespoon extra-virgin olive oil, plus more for roasting the squash

1 tablespoon chili oil (or more olive oil)

1 teaspoon English or Dijon mustard

1 teaspoon sea salt, plus more to taste

⅛ teaspoon asafoetida

Chili oil, chopped fresh parsley, chopped toasted walnuts, for garnish (optional)

Preheat the oven to 400°F. Line a baking sheet with parchment paper. Lay the squash cut side up on the baking sheet, lightly brush the tops with olive oil, and season with salt. Roast until very tender, 45 to 55 minutes. Allow the squash to cool slightly, then scoop out 1 cup of the flesh. The remainder can be saved for another use.

In a high-powered blender, combine the cooked squash, butter beans, ¼ cup water, the sun-dried tomatoes, nutritional yeast, olive oil, chili oil, mustard, salt, and asafoetida and blend until smooth.

If serving as a dip, transfer the puree to a serving bowl and garnish as desired with chili oil, parsley, and walnuts. Otherwise, spread, smear, and spoon as you please.

NOTE   You can use the extra roasted squash for the Roasted Butternut and Chickpea Shawarma (page 163) or the Curried Butternut Squash Soup (page 228).

PERFECT HUMMUS

Hummus is my all-time love. I went through a phase of eating it with everything—and when I say everything, I mean it got to the point where I was even adding a spoonful to my curries. (Which, by the way, is insanely delicious and absolutely correct.) But one thing I kept running into was not being able to make the silky-smooth hummus of my dreams at home. With a little research and experimenting, I finally discovered the secrets: boiling canned chickpeas with baking soda, removing the skins, using ice water when blending, and swirling in more tahini than you think you need. Brace yourself, because you are about to add a whole lot of hummus to your life.

Scoop this on Hummus Bruschetta (page 71), Baked Falafel Pita Sandwiches (page 126), The Everything Sandwich (page 146), Cheesy Sweet Corn Stuffed Pita (page 162), Roasted Butternut and Chickpea Shawarma Stuffed Pita (page 163), or Chopped Salad Stuffed Pita (page 160). Or use anytime you're in the mood for a rich, creamy condiment or dip.

MAKES *1½ cups*
TOTAL TIME: *35 minutes*

- 1 15-ounce can chickpeas, drained and rinsed
- ½ teaspoon baking soda
- 3 tablespoons tahini
- 2 tablespoons fresh lemon juice
- ½ teaspoon sea salt
- ¼ teaspoon asafoetida
- 2 to 3 tablespoons ice water
- 2 tablespoons extra-virgin olive oil, plus more for drizzling

In a medium saucepan, bring 2 cups water to a boil over medium-high heat. Add the drained chickpeas and baking soda, reduce the heat to medium, and cook until the chickpeas are soft, bloated, and the skins have started wilting off, about 20 minutes. (You can skip this step if you're in a hurry, but it's worth it.)

Remove the pan from the heat and transfer the chickpeas to a fine-mesh sieve. Rinse the chickpeas under cold water and rub them lightly with your fingers to further loosen the skins.

Return the chickpeas to the saucepan and cover with 2 to 3 inches cold water. Stir the chickpeas a couple times, then let the skins float to the top of the water. Use a spider or small sieve to skim them off and discard. Repeat the process until there are very few, if any, chickpea skins left. Drain the chickpeas and set aside.

In a high-powered blender, combine the chickpeas, tahini, lemon juice, salt, and asafoetida and blend until the mixture is thick and creamy. With the machine running, slowly stream in 2 tablespoons of the ice water, scraping down the sides of the blender as needed. If the hummus is still very thick and chunky, add the third tablespoon. Stream in the olive oil and continue blending for another minute or two.

Transfer the hummus to a serving bowl or platter. Drizzle generously with olive oil and serve.

MANGO SALSA

This fresher than fresh chunky salsa is like a little vacation in a bowl. It layers the traditional flavors of pico de gallo (tomato, jalapeño, cilantro) with the unexpected burst of sweet, juicy mango and bits of creamy avocado. It's perfect with chips as a dip or scooped onto salads and Tandoori Tacos (page 159) for a pop of bright flavor.

MAKES *about 2 cups*
TOTAL TIME: *10 minutes*

- ½ cup finely diced mango or pineapple (about ⅓ medium mango or ⅛ medium pineapple)
- ¼ cup finely chopped Roma tomato
- 2 tablespoons finely chopped fresh jalapeño pepper (about 1 medium pepper)
- 2 tablespoons chopped fresh cilantro leaves
- Juice of 1 medium lime

In a medium bowl, toss together the mango or pineapple, tomato, jalapeño, cilantro, and lime juice. Serve fresh as it's best enjoyed the day it's made.

CORN SALSA *with a Kick*

There's no quicker way to round out the flavor of a dish than to add a big scoop of salsa that brings acidity from lime juice, fresh green heat from jalapeño, and sweet, juicy pops of corn. Serve this with Mango Salsa (above) as part of a proper chip 'n' dip, sprinkle it over salads, or—my personal favorite—add it to your Spicy Bean Burgers (page 147).

MAKES *about 3 cups*
TOTAL TIME: *10 minutes*

- 1 cup fresh sweet corn kernels (from about 2 ears) or thawed frozen
- 1 cup diced avocado (about 1 medium avocado)
- ½ cup chopped cherry tomatoes (about 7 small) or Roma tomatoes (about 1 medium)
- ¼ cup chopped pickled jalapeño peppers
- ¼ cup chopped fresh cilantro leaves
- 1 tablespoon fresh lime juice
- ¼ teaspoon sea salt

In a medium bowl, gently toss together the corn, avocado, tomatoes, pickled jalapeños, cilantro, lime juice, and salt. Serve fresh as it's best enjoyed the day it's made.

TAHINI DRIZZLE

I seriously love tahini, a creamy paste made from toasted sesame seeds. Its subtle nuttiness gives unmistakable depth and richness to pretty much anything—sauces, dips, marinades, even a latte! I include it in my cooking for extra calcium or when I want to bring some creaminess to a dish. In particular, I love this simple preparation, which blends tahini paste with lemon juice and asafoetida to make an all-purpose drizzling sauce. It's especially perfect with Baked Falafel Pita Sandwiches (page 126) and Middle Eastern Charred Cauliflower (page 190).

MAKES *about 1¼ cups*
TOTAL TIME: *5 minutes*

- ½ cup tahini
- ½ cup cold water, plus more as needed
- 2½ tablespoons fresh lemon juice
- ½ teaspoon sea salt
- ⅛ teaspoon asafoetida

In a high-powered blender, combine the tahini, cold water, lemon juice, salt, and asafoetida and blend until completely smooth. For a runnier consistency, add more cold water 1 tablespoon at a time with the blender running to help loosen the sauce.

NOTE   To make this more like a dip, start with 2 tablespoons of cold water and add more until you get to your desired consistency.

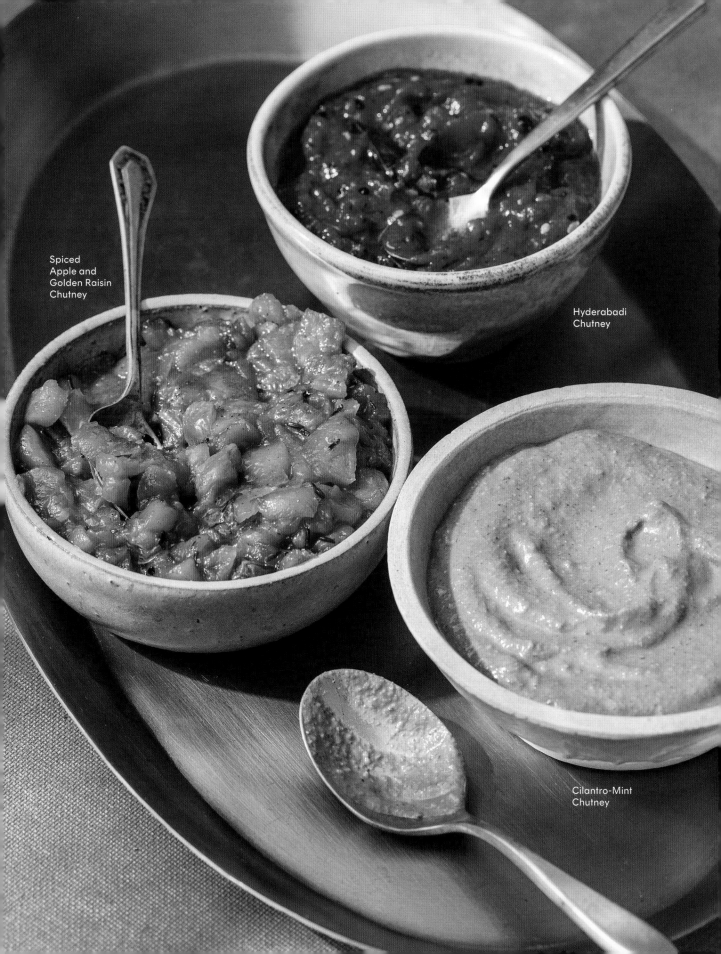

Spiced
Apple and
Golden Raisin
Chutney

Hyderabadi
Chutney

Cilantro-Mint
Chutney

CHUTNEY THREE WAYS

"Chutney" is just another name for dip, and when it comes to dipping, we Indians know a thing or two about how to accentuate *all* the flavors of a dish by offering chutneys alongside most of our meals. Traditional chutneys range from sweet and sour to bright and herbaceous, and almost like magic, they manage to completely balance a dish and bring all the different elements into sharper focus. They also contain botanicals, such as fresh herbs and spiced fruit, which help you digest, too. Much respect, chutney!

HYDERABADI CHUTNEY

MAKES *2 cups*
TOTAL TIME: *10 minutes*

- 2 tablespoons sunflower or avocado oil
- 1 teaspoon kalonji (nigella seeds)
- 1 teaspoon cumin seeds
- 10 fresh or dried curry leaves
- ½ teaspoon minced hot Indian or Thai green chile or 2 dried red chiles, such as Sichuan, left whole
- ½ tablespoon white sesame seeds
- 2 cups canned crushed tomatoes
- 1 teaspoon sea salt
- 1 tablespoon chopped fresh cilantro leaves, for garnish

In a medium skillet, heat the oil over medium heat. Add the nigella seeds and cumin seeds and cook, stirring, for just a few seconds for them to release their oils and fragrance. Add the curry leaves, chile, and sesame seeds and cook, stirring, for a few seconds for the seeds to just begin smelling nutty. Add the tomatoes and salt, reduce the heat to low, and cook, stirring, until the flavors have combined, 3 to 4 minutes. If you used dried chiles, remove and discard.

Transfer the chutney to a bowl, let cool, and garnish with the cilantro.

CILANTRO-MINT CHUTNEY

MAKES *1½ cups*
TOTAL TIME: *5 minutes*

- 2 cups tightly packed roughly chopped fresh cilantro leaves and stems
- ½ cup cashews, sunflower seeds, or peanuts (or a combination)
- ½ hot Indian or Thai green chile
- 4 fresh or dried curry leaves (optional)
- 2 teaspoons English mint sauce or 1 additional teaspoon lemon juice
- 1 teaspoon fresh lemon juice
- 1 teaspoon jaggery or coconut sugar or 1 pitted Medjool date
- ½ teaspoon sea salt

In a high-powered blender, combine the cilantro, cashews (or nut/seed combination), green chile, curry leaves (if using), mint sauce or lemon juice, jaggery, salt, and ¼ cup water. Process until completely smooth.

Recipes Continue

SPICED APPLE AND GOLDEN RAISIN CHUTNEY

This can be a condiment like the other chutneys, but I also love it with crackers and vegan cheese.

MAKES *about 1¾ cups*
TOTAL TIME: *45 minutes*

½ tablespoon unsalted vegan butter or extra-virgin olive oil

1 teaspoon cumin seeds

1 teaspoon Ground CCF Masala (page 49) or ½ teaspoon ground coriander

¼ teaspoon freshly ground black pepper

¼ teaspoon kalonji (nigella seeds)

⅛ teaspoon ground cardamom

⅛ teaspoon asafoetida

4 Braeburn apples, peeled, cored, and diced

½ cup golden raisins

1 tablespoon jaggery, coconut sugar, or light brown sugar, plus more as needed

1 small hot Indian or Thai green chile, minced, or 2 dried red chiles, such as Sichuan, left whole

8 fresh or dried curry leaves

½ teaspoon grated fresh ginger

½ teaspoon sea salt

In a large saucepan, heat the butter or oil over medium heat. Add the cumin, CCF masala, pepper, nigella seeds, cardamom, and asafoetida and cook, stirring until fragrant, about 1 minute. Add the apples, raisins, jaggery, chile, curry leaves, ginger, salt, and ½ cup water and stir to combine. Cover, reduce the heat to a simmer, and cook, stirring occasionally, until most of the liquid has evaporated, about 40 minutes. Remove the pan from the heat. If you used whole dried chiles, remove and discard.

Let the chutney cool to room temperature. For a smooth sauce, you can blend this chutney, or leave it chunky (which is what I like). Transfer it to a sealed container and store it in the refrigerator for up to 1 month.

YOGURT THREE WAYS

You'll frequently find yogurt served with Indian meals because it counterbalances the spices with a bright tanginess and creaminess and provides a nice, cooling effect on the palate—especially cucumber-flecked Raita (page 246). It's also no coincidence that yogurt (including vegan versions) supports digestion thanks to its beneficial bacteria. All of these variations would be at home drizzled over or stirred into just about any recipe in this book, or can be used to pull together a simple meal, such as a bowl of rice and daal.

SPICED YOGURT WITH CHARRED TOMATOES

Serve this on its own as a dip or drizzled over any grain, daal, or veggie dish in this book.

SERVES *4*
TOTAL TIME: *20 minutes*

CHARRED TOMATOES

- 1 small hot Indian or Thai green chile or a jalapeño, chopped
- 1 tablespoon extra-virgin olive oil
- ½ teaspoon cumin seeds
- ¼ teaspoon paprika
- ¼ teaspoon sea salt
- ⅛ teaspoon asafoetida
- 15 cherry tomatoes

YOGURT

- ½ cup plain vegan yogurt
- 4 ounces plain vegan cream cheese or additional yogurt (optional; it'll make the dish even creamier)
- 1 tablespoon fresh lemon juice
- ¼ teaspoon sea salt (omit if using cream cheese)
- Flaky salt, such as Maldon, for serving
- Chopped fresh cilantro leaves, for serving

CHAR THE TOMATOES: Position an oven rack in the top third of the oven and preheat the oven to 400°F. Line a baking sheet with parchment paper.

In a large bowl, combine the chile, olive oil, cumin, paprika, salt, and asafoetida and mix well. Add the cherry tomatoes and toss to combine.

Spread them over the prepared baking sheet and bake until the tomatoes have softened, about 10 minutes. Switch the oven to broil and broil the tomatoes until charred in spots and caramelized all over, checking them frequently and shaking the pan as needed to prevent burning, about 5 minutes. Set aside.

MAKE THE YOGURT: In a medium bowl, whisk together the yogurt, cream cheese (if using), lemon juice, and salt (if using). Transfer the mixture to a plate or a shallow bowl and spoon the tomatoes over the yogurt. Sprinkle with flaky salt and fresh cilantro.

Leftovers can be stored in a sealed container in the refrigerator for up to 3 days.

YOGURT MINT SAUCE

Drizzle this over Shahi Vegetables (page 120), Dum Aloo (page 121), Tandoori Tacos (page 159), Tofu Tikka Stuffed Pitas (page 162), or any grain, daal, or vegetable dish in this book.

SERVES *4*
TOTAL TIME: *5 minutes*

- 1 cup plain vegan yogurt
- 1 tablespoon English mint sauce or 2 tablespoons Cilantro-Mint Chutney (page 243)
- ¼ teaspoon sea salt

In a small bowl, whisk together the yogurt, mint sauce, and salt.

Recipes Continue

RAITA

Drizzle this over Zucchini "Baba Ghanoush" (page 194), any of the pilaus (pages 103–4), or any grain, daal, or veggie dish in this book.

SERVES *4*
TOTAL TIME: *10 minutes*

- 1 teaspoon cumin seeds
- 1 cup plain vegan yogurt
- ¼ cup grated seedless cucumber
- 1 tablespoon fresh lemon juice
- ¼ teaspoon sea salt
- ⅛ teaspoon asafoetida

Heat a small skillet over medium-low heat. Add the cumin seeds and toast until lightly browned and fragrant, about 30 seconds. Coarsely crush the seeds with a mortar and pestle or spice grinder.

In a medium bowl, whisk together the yogurt, crushed toasted cumin seeds, cucumber, lemon juice, salt, and asafoetida.

VARIATION *Tzatziki:* For a Greek-inspired version of traditional Indian raita, omit the cumin seeds and add ¼ cup chopped fresh dill and a few cracks of black pepper.

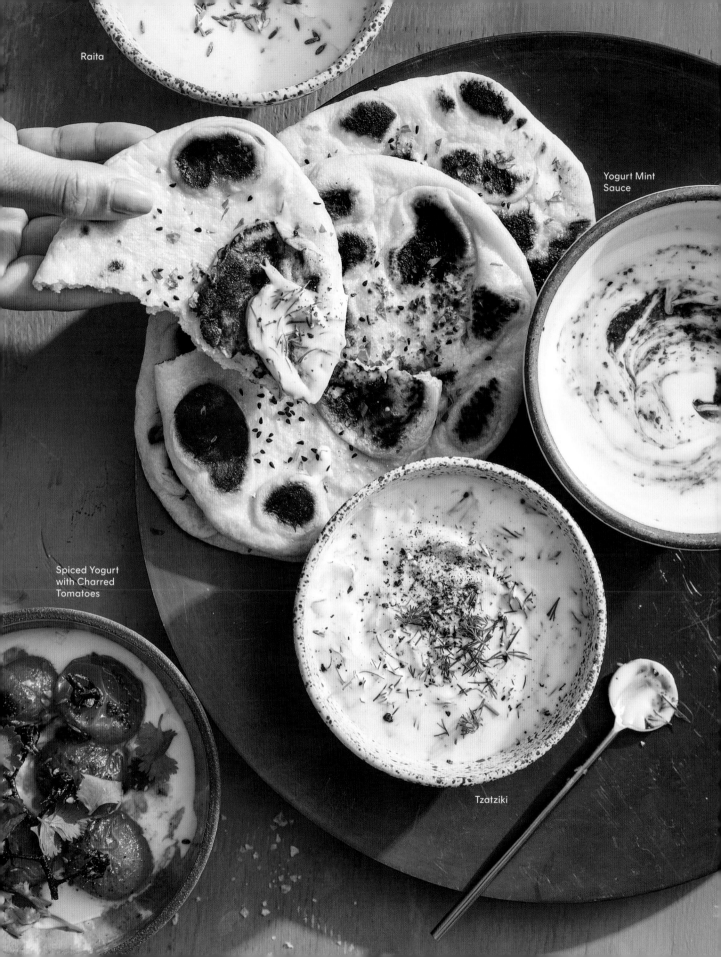

Raita

Yogurt Mint
Sauce

Spiced Yogurt
with Charred
Tomatoes

Tzatziki

NIGHTSHADE-FREE "TOMATO" SAUCE

Ayurveda says that nightshade vegetables, such as tomatoes, can cause inflammation in the body. While I haven't gotten to the point where I can completely let go of my dear nightshades, I have become more mindful of how frequently I eat them, and I choose days to avoid them. To help with that, I developed this sauce, which can be used in any dish that calls for canned tomatoes, tomato puree, or tomato sauce. It has the same deep, savory flavor as the "real" thing thanks to the natural richness that these non-nightshade vegetables develop as they cook down. This is one recipe I always make in a pressure cooker because I can soften the vegetables more quickly, so I've included that option as well.

Try this with Cheesy Bread (page 151), Shahi Vegetables (page 120), Dum Aloo (page 121), Polenta Bake with Creamy Mushrooms and Chili-Spiked Tomato Sauce (page 109), Spicy Pineapple Supreme Naan Pizzas (page 154), or Spicy Indian Pasta (page 90).

MAKES *about 2 cups*
TOTAL TIME: *30 minutes*

3 medium carrots, peeled and roughly chopped (about 1½ cups)

2 celery stalks, trimmed and roughly chopped (about 1 cup)

1 small red beet, trimmed

1 fresh or dried bay leaf

1 teaspoon sea salt

2 tablespoons fresh lemon juice

¼ teaspoon asafoetida (optional)

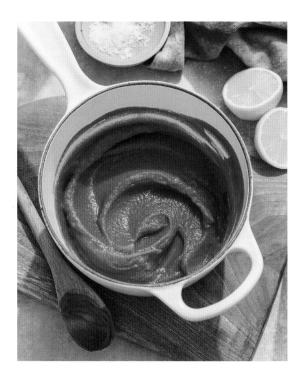

In a medium saucepan, combine the carrots, celery, beet, bay leaf, salt, and 1 cup water. Bring to a boil over high heat and cook until the vegetables are completely soft, about 25 minutes.

Drain the vegetables and discard the cooking liquid and bay leaf. Let the beet cool until it's safe to handle, then slip off the skin and discard.

In a high-powered blender, combine the cooked carrots, celery, peeled beet, lemon juice, asafoetida, and ¼ cup water. Blend until completely smooth, adding more water if needed to thin the sauce to your desired consistency.

VARIATION *Pressure Cooker "Tomato Sauce":* To make this in an electric pressure cooker, combine the carrots, celery, beet, bay leaf, salt, and 1 cup water in the pot. Cook for 15 minutes on high pressure, then release manually. Continue with the recipe as written.

PICKLES THREE WAYS

Give any Indian grandma a selection of ingredients, and she will make you the most delicious pickles. It's just part of their magic. In India pickles are traditionally enjoyed with our meals because they aid digestion, and their salt and tang add balance and brightness to a dish. In Ayurveda, pickles are believed to stoke your digestive fire by activating digestive juices, as well as round out the six tastes on your plate. While Indian pickles are usually made with a lot of oil, my mum started using these lighter vinegar- and lemon juice–based methods, which give everything a brighter punch of flavor. No matter what I'm serving, even if it's just daal and rice, I like having a little bowlful on the table.

PINK PICKLED TURNIPS AND BEETS

These would be delicious with the falafel from Baked Falafel Pita Sandwiches (page 126), any of your favorite dishes, or on their own straight out of the jar.

MAKES *4 to 5 cups*
TOTAL TIME: *5 days*

- 3 cups water (preferably distilled, which will keep the pickles fresher longer)
- ¼ cup kosher salt
- 1 cup distilled white vinegar
- 2 large turnips, peeled and cut into ½-inch-thick batons (about 3 cups)
- 2 medium red beets, peeled and cut into ½-inch-thick batons (about 1½ cups)
- 2 bay leaves

In a large bowl, stir together the water and salt until the salt has dissolved. Stir in the vinegar. In a 2-quart jar or other container with a tight-fitting lid, combine the turnips, beets, and bay leaves. Pour the vinegar mixture over the top and seal the container.

Refrigerate for 5 days before enjoying. They will keep in the refrigerator for up to 1 month.

PICKLED TURMERIC AND GINGER

These are particularly great in the colder months because turmeric has natural antibiotic properties in addition to aiding digestion and maintaining a healthy balance of beneficial gut bacteria, while ginger is also antibiotic, antiviral, anti-inflammatory, and extremely pro-optimal digestion.

MAKES *about 1 cup*
TOTAL TIME: *8 hours*

- ½ cup thinly sliced peeled fresh turmeric (see Note)
- ⅓ cup peeled and thinly sliced fresh ginger
- ½ cup fresh lemon juice (from 4 lemons)
- 1 teaspoon sea salt

In a 12-ounce jar with a tight-fitting lid, combine the turmeric, ginger, lemon, and salt. Cover and marinate overnight in the refrigerator before enjoying them in small amounts with your meals.

These will last in the refrigerator for up to 1 month. Be sure not to introduce any moisture into the jar, such as using a wet spoon to scoop the pickles, which will cause the pickles to spoil.

NOTE: If you don't have access to fresh turmeric, simply omit it from the recipe.

Recipes Continue

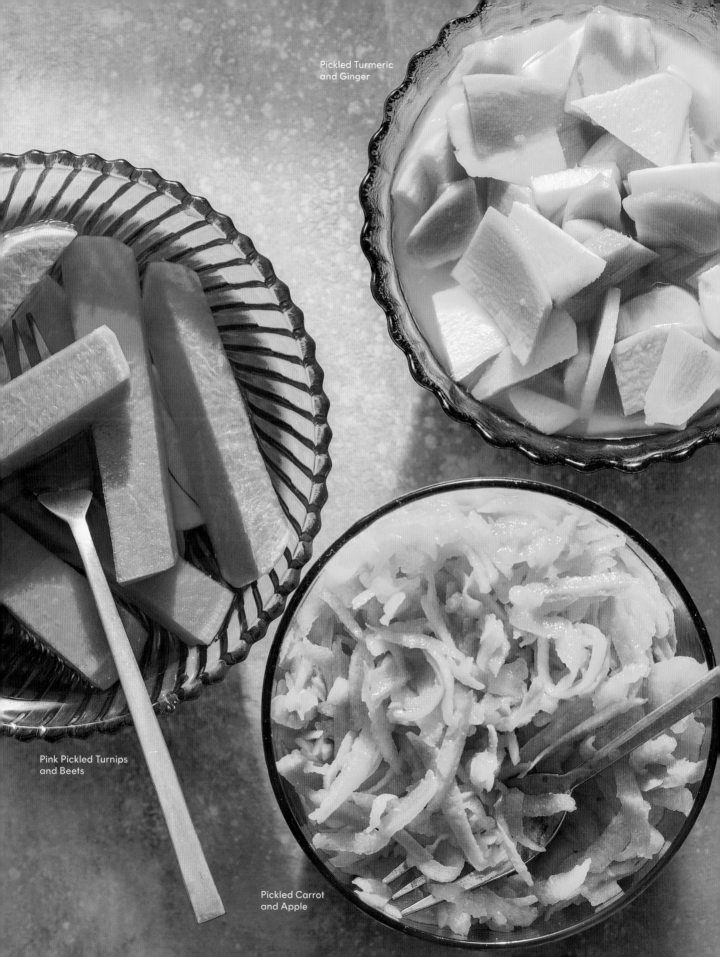

Pickled Turmeric and Ginger

Pink Pickled Turnips and Beets

Pickled Carrot and Apple

PICKLED CARROT AND APPLE

MAKES *about 3 cups*
TOTAL TIME: *11 minutes*

- 2 cups grated peeled sweet-crisp apple, such as Braeburn or Pink Lady (about 2 apples)
- 1 cup peeled and grated carrot (about 2 medium carrots)
- 3 tablespoons fresh lemon juice
- ½ tablespoon sunflower or avocado oil
- 2 teaspoons split mustard seeds or mustard powder, such as Colman's
- 1 teaspoon light brown sugar
- ½ teaspoon ground turmeric
- 1 tablespoon Ground CCF Masala (page 49)
- 1 teaspoon sea salt

In a large bowl, toss together the apples, carrots, and lemon juice. Set aside.

In a large skillet, heat the oil over medium heat. Add the mustard seeds, brown sugar, and turmeric and cook, stirring, until the spices are fragrant and the sugar has dissolved, about 30 seconds.

Add the spice mixture to the bowl with the apples and carrots, along with the CCF masala and salt. Toss well to combine.

Transfer to a 1-quart mason jar or large jar with a tight-fitting lid and refrigerate for at least 3 hours before using. Store refrigerated for up to 2 weeks.

Crunchy Bits

Texture is one of the most important parts of a dish, and the more varied the texture in a dish, the more I feel as though I am eating with the full dimension of my sense of taste. This idea goes back to eating with all your senses and really *feeling* the food in your mouth as part of what makes a dish so satisfying and nourishing. That's why I'm usually looking for a lil' extra crunchy something to finish off a bowl of soup (or salad or veggies or rice or anything, really), whether it's a sprinkling of seeds or nuts that I already have on hand, or a mixture that I make a big batch of to keep for whenever the mood strikes. Here are my favorite bits, which you can reach for however and whenever your heart desires.

PISTACHIO GREMOLATA

Classic Italian gremolata is a bright, freshly chopped condiment made from parsley and lemon zest. I've stayed true to the vibrant flavor profile but added my own twist with the addition of mint plus pistachios, which lend welcome texture wherever you spoon a dollop, especially on top of a bowl of One-Pot Lemony Spaghetti (page 100) or Zucchini, Fennel, and Mint Soup (page 223).

MAKES *about ½ cup*
TOTAL TIME: *10 minutes*

- ⅓ cup unsalted roasted pistachios, finely chopped
- ¼ cup finely chopped flat-leaf parsley leaves
- Grated zest of 2 medium lemons
- 2 tablespoons chopped fresh mint leaves
- ½ teaspoon red chile flakes
- ¼ teaspoon sea salt

In a medium bowl, stir together the pistachios, parsley, lemon zest, mint, chile flakes, and salt.

CROUTONS TWO WAYS: *Caraway and Chili*

These classic olive oily, toasty bits are leveled up with the addition of either nutty, slightly anise-y caraway seeds—which are also beneficial for digestive health—or spicy chili oil. If you'd prefer, you can cut them up into nice little cubes or keep them rustic and torn. Sprinkle these over Cheesy Broccoli Soup (page 227), Cannellini Bean and Tomato Soup with Torn Chili Croutons (page 225), or any other soup, salads, or plate of Hero Veg (page 187–211) for instantly elevated layers of flavor and texture.

MAKES *about 1 cup*
TOTAL TIME: *25 minutes*

- 3 slices sourdough bread, torn into ½-inch pieces or cubed (about 1 cup)
- 2 tablespoons extra-virgin olive oil or 2 tablespoons chili oil (for chili croutons)
- Pinch of sea salt
- 2 teaspoons caraway seeds (for caraway croutons)

Preheat the oven to 325°F. Line a baking sheet with parchment paper.

Add the sourdough pieces to the baking sheet and drizzle them with the olive oil (for the caraway croutons) or chili oil (for the chili croutons). Sprinkle with the salt. If making caraway croutons, also sprinkle with the caraway seeds. Toss with your hands until evenly combined. Spread the bread in an even layer over the baking sheet.

Bake until the croutons are lightly browned, 15 to 20 minutes, checking every few minutes to shake the pan and keep any edges from burning.

Enjoy the croutons now or allow them to cool completely before storing them in an airtight container and storing them at room temperature for up to 1 week.

THYME CROSTINI

As difficult as it is to top good, crusty bread brushed with olive oil and toasted to golden perfection, I've gone and done it by adding thyme. It brings not only its signature earthy, minty flavor but also its naturally antiviral health benefits.

Serve these with Beet and Dill Soup (page 224)—or any other soup—alongside a dip, or topped with your favorite cooked or raw veggies and a saucy drizzle.

MAKES *12 crostini*
TOTAL TIME: *15 minutes*

- 1 narrow, 6-inch-long loaf of crusty bread, such as baguette or ciabatta, cut into ½-inch-thick slices
- 3 tablespoons extra-virgin olive oil
- 1 teaspoon dried thyme leaves
- ½ teaspoon sea salt

Preheat the oven to 400°F. Line a baking sheet with parchment paper.

In a large bowl, combine the bread slices, oil, thyme, and salt and toss well to coat. Spread the slices in an even layer over the prepared baking sheet. Bake until browned and crispy, flipping halfway through, about 10 minutes.

Enjoy the crostini now or allow them to cool completely before storing them in a container at room temperature for up to 5 days.

CHEESY CURRIED CRISPY KALE

There's kale and then there's *kale*. In this case it's smothered in curry and cheesy-tasting nutritional yeast, then baked until delightfully crispy with additional crunch from vitamin E-rich sunflower seeds. These are perfect for sprinkling over Curried Butternut Squash Soup (page 228) and Curried Crispy Kale, Mango Chutney, and Ricotta Naan Pizzas (page 153), in addition to veggies, grains, and salads—or to munch on their own.

MAKES *about 5 cups*
TOTAL TIME: *30 minutes*

- ⅓ cup sunflower seeds
- ¼ cup nutritional yeast
- 1 teaspoon curry powder
- ¼ teaspoon sea salt
- ⅛ teaspoon asafoetida
- 1 bunch curly green or Tuscan kale, leaves stripped of midribs and roughly torn
- 1 tablespoon extra-virgin olive oil

Preheat the oven to 275°F. Line two baking sheets with parchment paper.

In a food processor, combine the sunflower seeds, nutritional yeast, curry powder, salt, and asafoetida and pulse until finely ground.

Add the kale to a large bowl and drizzle with the olive oil. Massage the kale leaves with your hands until softened, about 5 minutes. Add the seed mixture and massage it into the kale until just combined. Spread the kale over the prepared baking sheets in an even layer and bake until the kale is crisp but still green, 18 to 20 minutes.

Set aside to cool slightly before serving. Or allow the kale to cool completely before storing in an airtight container at room temperature for up to 3 days.

SUPER-SEED BRITTLE

Think of this as a sort of savory granola with just a hint of sweet and a kick of paprika. Packed with omega 3-rich seeds and spiced with paprika, it lends the perfect crunch when sprinkled over any dish. I especially encourage you to try this with Spiced Carrot and Sweet Potato Soup (page 222), or to enjoy it on its own as a fortifying protein- and nutrient-rich snack.

MAKES *about 1 cup*
TOTAL TIME: *15 minutes*

- ¼ cup sunflower seeds
- ¼ cup pumpkin seeds
- ¼ cup white sesame seeds
- 1 tablespoon black sesame seeds
- 1 tablespoon unsalted vegan butter or coconut oil, melted
- 1 tablespoon agave nectar
- ½ tablespoon paprika
- ¼ teaspoon sea salt

Preheat the oven to 325°F. Line a baking sheet with parchment paper.

In a medium bowl, combine the sunflower seeds, pumpkin seeds, white sesame seeds, black sesame seeds, melted butter, agave, paprika, and salt and stir well to combine.

Spread the mixture in a thin, even layer on the prepared baking sheet and bake until set but not browned, 8 to 10 minutes. (The brittle may still feel soft but will set into a crunchier texture as it cools.)

Set aside to cool completely and break into bite-size pieces. Store the brittle in an airtight container at room temperature for up to 5 days.

"POPCORN" PUMPKIN SEEDS

Pumpkin seeds are little nutritional powerhouses and are rich in magnesium, which benefits heart health, can lower blood pressure, supports muscle and nerve function, balances hormones, nourishes the skin, and promotes healthy sleep. They're also a great source of heart-healthy fats, are full of antioxidants, and contribute to your protein goals. But I mainly love them because they're supremely crunchy and delicious, especially when toasted up with a sprinkling of sea salt and nutritional yeast, popcorn-style. I can't think of one dish that wouldn't benefit from a sprinkle, and they're a staple on My Everything Packed Salad (page 166).

MAKES *½ cup*
TOTAL TIME: *10 minutes*

- ½ teaspoon extra-virgin olive oil
- ½ cup pumpkin seeds
- ½ teaspoon sea salt
- 1 tablespoon nutritional yeast

In a small skillet, heat the oil over low heat. Add the pumpkin seeds and salt and cook, stirring occasionally, until the seeds brown and begin to pop, 3 to 5 minutes. Add the nutritional yeast and toss to coat.

Remove the pan from the heat and set aside for the seeds to cool completely. Store in a sealed container at room temperature for up to 1 week.

My Mindful and Relaxing *Aaaaaah* Evening Routine

I started a mindful evening routine not to help me fall asleep more easily (although it *does* do that) but because I realized how much it affected my mornings. A structureless evening begat a more haphazard morning. It was harder to get out of bed and harder to prioritize things that I knew would make me feel good, including my morning meditation practice that I was working so hard to cultivate. What really stuck with me was when one of my teachers said, "It's not about the ten minutes or two hours you meditate; it's how you spend the other twenty-two hours."

I also learned that bedtime doesn't just begin the moment you get into bed. Your body is preparing for this winding-down all day long, so as day shifts into evening, it's important to make choices that will help soothe your body. Eventually, I saw how having a sacred evening routine allowed me to have really magical mornings. Of course, I know that not everyone has the luxury of an entire evening to spend winding down, but even I don't do every single step every night. Small changes with deep intentions make all the difference, and consistency is key. Do I have the occasional wild night out until 12 a.m.? Sure I do! But when I saw how much better I felt when I prioritized my routine on a regular basis, it made it easier to say no to things that got in the way. Instead of thinking of it as being selfish, think of it as investing in things that will help make you into a better version of yourself, which means you can show up better for other people, too.

Here are some of my favorite things to do come evening time:

Have a smaller meal at least three to four hours before you plan to get into bed: A light meal that's easy to digest won't put the burden on your body and it allows your body to use the nighttime hours to refuel and replenish, rather than to digest.

Set the mood with essential oils: Aromas can be subtle, but they are incredibly effective in shifting our mood and emotions. They can be energizing and stimulating, or soothing and calming. As the sun sets, I take a moment to change the scent in my diffuser to lavender, rose, jasmine, or sandalwood, which are all sleep-promoting, or any other scent that makes me go *aaaaah*.

Enjoy an Ayurvedic (nonalcoholic) nightcap: Picture this, you're sitting on your sofa, snuggled up with your favorite blanket, reading a really good book, and sipping a mug of Moon Milk (pages 55–56). If that doesn't make you want to curl up right now and take a nap, I'm not sure what else would do the trick.

Avoid stimulating activities: Before bed, you need to be careful about what you allow into your senses. Just as our stomach digests food after we've eaten, our body and our mind digest what we expose our senses to. Watching TV, scrolling on the Internet, playing video games, or even having your lights on too bright can continue to stimulate or even aggravate your mind. And the blue light waves from electronic devices interfere with the production of melatonin, the hormone that encourages sleep and regulates your sleep-wake cycle. Try reading a book, doing a short meditation, journaling, or listening to music. And keep the lights dim in your home, or even better, use candlelight. Whatever you choose, do something sans screen that brings you calm and peace.

Take a hot shower or bath: You know that feeling at the end of a long day when your mind is scrambling all over the place, but then you get into the shower or bath and feel the warm water run over your skin, and your shoulders soften, your mind defogs, and you just feel so cute and cuddly? Major *aaaah* moment. You could also use the same essential oils from your diffuser to help relax the physical body.

Breathe: See Tuning In with Your Breath (page 184) for my favorite evening breathwork practice.

Do an evening abhyanga massage: This is the same as the morning practice, but when practiced in the evening it can feel particularly grounding and soothing, especially if you've warmed up your oils a bit. If you're short on time, just focus on your scalp and your feet—that's where our 70,000 nerves start and finish. Plus, our feet hold a lot of pressure points, so massaging your feet can relieve tension that has built up throughout the body. I often do my scalp massage dry because I don't want oil in my hair every day.

Release your troubles: Sometimes, if you haven't processed everything you're worried about or feeling during the day, your mind continues to chew on it throughout the night. You've probably experienced a disruption in your sleep as a result and have woken up not feeling well rested. By tucking these thoughts and feelings into a journal before bed, you're releasing them—even if for a moment—from your mind. If I've had a really rough day and everything I'm writing is quite negative, I try to end on a good note and write down at least five things I have love and gratitude for in my life. If you can't think of five, try to squeeze out at least one—I promise it will make you feel just a little bit better.

Treat yourself to a skincare routine: In addition to making me look and feel like a glazed doughnut before bed, taking care of my face at night helps me feel like I'm rinsing away the day and heading to bed nice and clean. I try to pamper myself a little bit, too, starting with a face detox massage, spritzing on a spray of jasmine, and finishing with a really nice cleanser and lathering my face in delicious-smelling oils. It's only a few steps and doesn't require investing in a huge number of products (or spending a lot of money), but it's the practice and mindfulness that count.

Finish with an evening meditation or prayer: Just as with my morning routine, this is probably my favorite part of my evening practice. It helps clear my mind, calm my body, and bring a meaningful close to my day. There is no wrong way to pray or meditate; you simply have to tune into your heart, take deep breaths, and invite gratitude.

Sweet dreams!

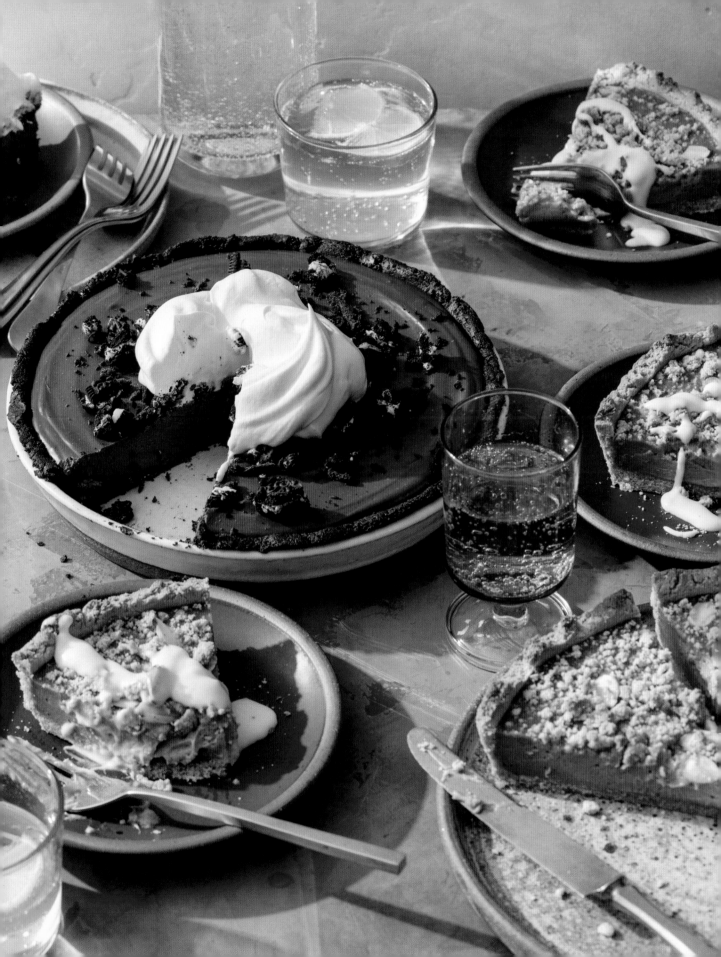

SWEET TREATS

Sweet is one of the essential flavors that helps you taste the sweetness of life and connect you more deeply with the joy and goodness that surrounds you. There's no way I'd take that away from you—or myself! These dishes range from daily delicacies to more indulgent affairs suited for special occasions. But ultimately, it's you and your body who are the judge of what to enjoy when, where, and with whom.

BEET-CARROT HALVA

There is a traditional Gujarati dessert called gajar halva, which is basically carrots that have been simmered in milk, ghee, and sugar until they melt in your mouth. When my family went vegan, my mum figured out how to make the desserts we loved taste just as good using vegan ingredients—which luckily included this dish. Since I, of course, had to add my own twist, I discovered that folding beets into the mix gives the halva a beautiful gem-toned color. And when we accidentally blended the mixture, it created a silky-smooth pudding that is possibly an even better version of the original! But it still makes me think of my mum every time I make it.

SERVES *8*
TOTAL TIME: *40 minutes*

- 2 tablespoons unsalted vegan butter
- 3 cups peeled and grated carrots (about 3 large carrots)
- 2 cups peeled and grated red beets (about 2 medium beets)
- 1 cup plain unsweetened oat milk
- 1 teaspoon ground cardamom
- ¾ cup coconut sugar
- ½ cup canned coconut cream
- 1 tablespoon grated orange zest (optional)
- 1 cup Sweet Cashew Cream (page 263), chilled, or vegan whipped cream or ice cream, for serving
- Chopped roasted pistachios and almonds, for serving

In a heavy-bottomed medium saucepan, heat the butter over medium-low heat. Add the carrots and beets and stir to combine with the butter. Cover and cook for 10 minutes, until the vegetables have softened. Stir in the oat milk and cardamom, cover, and cook until the mixture has thickened and is perfumed with spice, another 10 minutes.

Add the coconut sugar, coconut cream, and orange zest, cover, and cook until the mixture is thick and fudgy, another 10 minutes. For the last 5 minutes, uncover and let the halva simmer to evaporate any excess liquid.

I love enjoying the halva warm with the cold cashew cream generously drizzled on top and a whole lot of pistachios and chopped almonds. It's also delicious chilled and can be stored in a sealed container in the refrigerator for up to 3 days.

NOTE   If you want to turn this dessert into a pudding, simply transfer the mixture, minus the orange zest, to a high-speed blender and blend until silky smooth. Fold in the orange zest, if desired, and serve topped with the cashew cream and nuts.

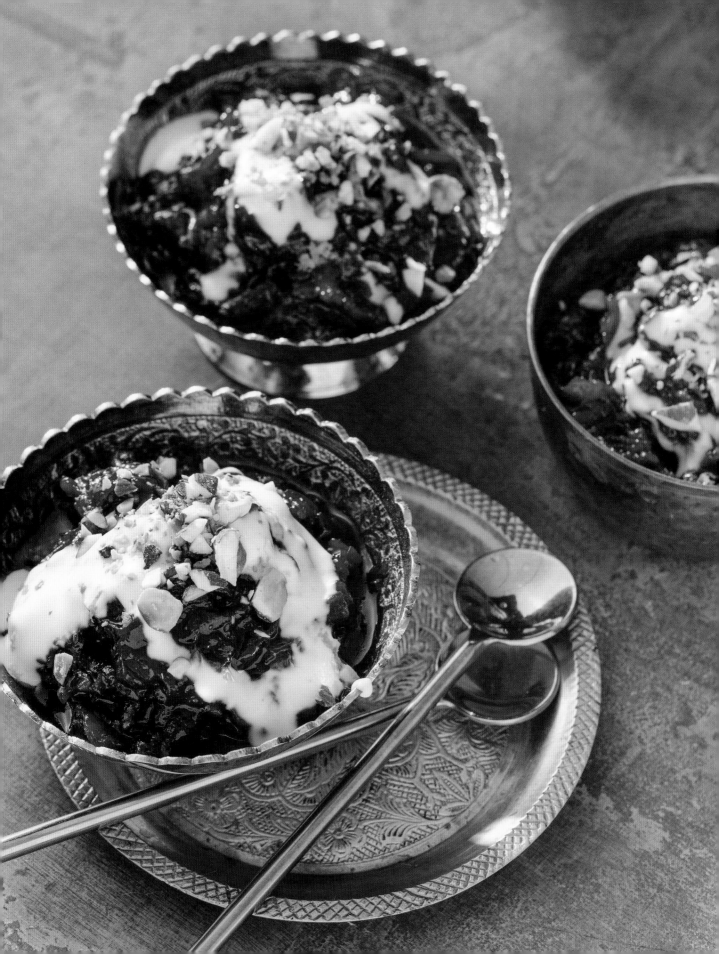

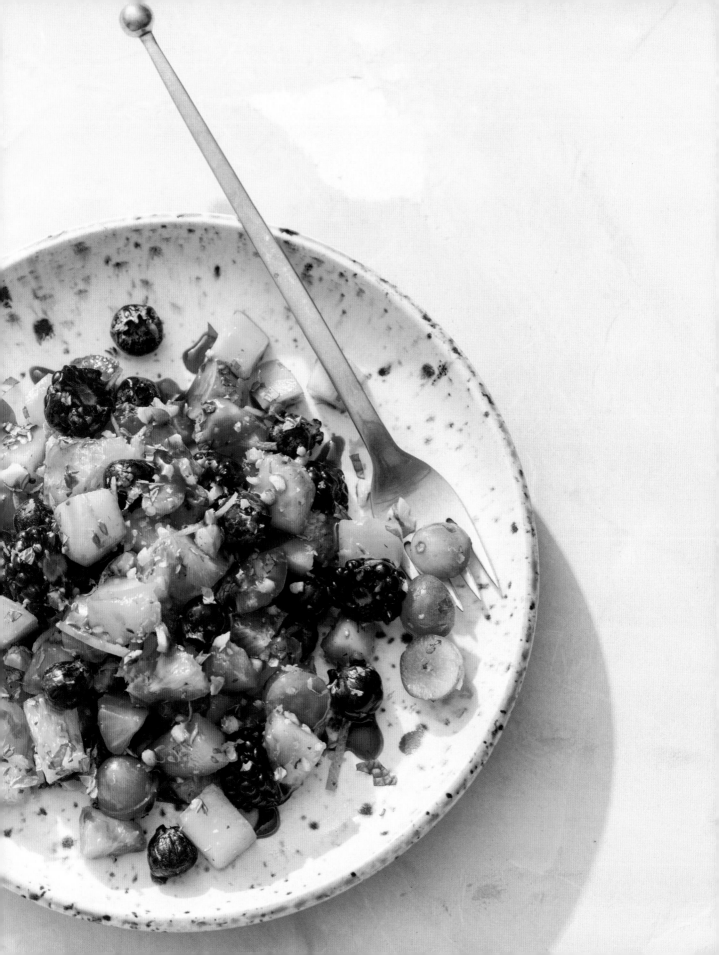

SEASONAL FRUIT SALAD

You don't have to look any further for proof of the miracles of nature than fruit. These jewels of the trees and vines are loaded with vitamins, minerals, antioxidants, phytonutrients, and hydration. Plus, just *look* at them. Whether it's spring's first berries; melons, and stone fruit at the height of summer; figs, quince, apples, and pears in autumn; or citrus in the depths of winter, these fruits are the succulent reminders of life's sweetness. When enjoyed in season, there's not much that good fruit needs in order to be delicious. But for an extra special moment, I like making this salad, which adds even more dimension with nuts and a beautiful mess of fresh herbs.

SERVES *4*
TOTAL TIME: *15 minutes*

- 4 cups diced seasonal fruit
- Grated zest of 1 medium orange
- Grated zest of 1 lemon
- ½ tablespoon fresh lemon juice
- ¼ cup chopped toasted walnuts
- 1 tablespoon minced fresh mint leaves
- ¼ teaspoon minced fresh thyme leaves
- ¼ teaspoon minced fresh rosemary leaves
- Sweet Cashew Cream (recipe follows)
- Spiced Agave (page 73), for drizzling

In a large bowl, toss together the fruit, orange zest, lemon zest, lemon juice, walnuts, mint, thyme, and rosemary.

Divide the salad among bowls. Top each with a dollop of the cashew cream and a drizzle of spiced agave and serve.

Sweet Cashew Cream

Use this as a replacement for heavy cream—for coffees, for desserts, or to just take a nip when you need something sweet. Use it to top pancakes and waffles, in the French Toast Casserole (page 84), Chocolate Mud Pie (page 273), or Didi's Pear and Chocolate Crumble (page 269).

MAKES *about 2 cups*
TOTAL TIME: *5 minutes, plus soaking time*

- 1 cup cashews
- ⅔ cup plain unsweetened almond milk, plus more if needed
- 2 teaspoons maple syrup
- 1 teaspoon vanilla extract
- 1 teaspoon fresh lemon juice

In a bowl, combine the cashews with hot water to cover and let soak for 30 minutes (or plan ahead and soak the cashews overnight). Drain and rinse.

In a high-powered blender, combine the soaked cashews, almond milk, maple syrup, vanilla, and lemon juice and blend until smooth. Add more almond milk if you'd prefer a thinner consistency.

Store in a sealed container in the refrigerator for up to 4 days.

EVERYDAY DATE TARTS

These lil' cuties are perfect if you're someone who likes a daily sweet treat because they're easy to make and have no refined sugars. In addition to being naturally jammy and caramel-like, antioxidant-rich dates are an ojas food, meaning they're balancing and soothing for body and spirit. So these mini confections are providing some nourishing goodness, too!

This recipe calls for two types of gluten-free flour, oat and almond. The oat flour gives baked goods a light, airy crumb, while almond flour is denser, which ensures the tart crusts hold their shape, so the two together is a winning combination.

MAKES *4 small tarts*
TOTAL TIME: *40 minutes*

FILLING

15 Medjool dates, pitted

1 13.5-ounce can full-fat coconut milk

2 tablespoons cornstarch

1 teaspoon vanilla extract

1 teaspoon almond extract

CRUST

1½ cups almond flour

1½ cups oat flour (or another 1½ cups almond flour)

1 tablespoon unsalted vegan butter or coconut oil

2 tablespoons maple syrup

4 tablespoons sliced almonds

Vegan cream, for drizzling

Preheat the oven to 375°F.

MAKE THE FILLING: In a high-powered blender, combine the dates, coconut milk, cornstarch, vanilla, and almond extract and blend until completely smooth. Set aside.

MAKE THE CRUST: In a large bowl, combine the almond flour, oat flour, and butter or oil and use your fingertips to rub it into the flour until the mixture feels like wet sand.

Add the maple syrup and 1 tablespoon water and mix with a silicone spatula until the mixture forms a dough, adding more water as needed, 1 tablespoon at a time. Measure out 2 to 3 tablespoons of dough and set aside for sprinkling.

Divide the remaining dough among four 4-inch tart pans with removable bottoms and press it into the bottoms and up the sides. Divide the filling among the tart pans, leaving a ¼-inch gap at the top of each pan. Top each tart with 1 tablespoon sliced almonds and dots of the reserved dough.

Arrange the tarts on a baking sheet and bake until they're set in the middle, about 25 minutes. Let the tarts cool to room temperature, then refrigerate for at least 1 hour.

Serve the tarts with a generous drizzle of cream on top.

Leftovers can be stored in a sealed container in the refrigerator for up to 3 days.

COOKIES THREE WAYS

I mean, a fresh-baked cookie with a cuppa tea or a lil' warm milk? It doesn't get more heavenly than that. From perfectly chewy, gooey Biscoff cookies (or dough, if you choose to eat them raw, as I often do) to supersized chunky oatmeal raisin cookies inspired by Levain Bakery in New York City to thumbprint cookies dolloped with your favorite jam—these are your afternoon tea nibbles, your Sunday garden-picnic treats, and your reminder to channel your inner child.

THUMBPRINT COOKIES

Buckwheat, despite its name, is not a grain. I love it for its earthy, nutty flavor, which I balance with almond flour. The two together yield a moist, tender cookie.

MAKES *about 8 cookies*
TOTAL TIME: *35 minutes*

- 1 cup light buckwheat flour
- 1 cup almond flour
- ¼ teaspoon baking soda
- ¼ teaspoon baking powder
- 1 flax egg (1 tablespoon flaxmeal mixed with 3 tablespoons water)
- ⅓ cup plus 2 tablespoons maple syrup
- ⅓ cup coconut oil, melted
- 1 teaspoon vanilla extract
- ½ teaspoon apple cider vinegar
- ¼ cup your favorite jam (I love St. Dalfour, or look for one without added sugar)

Position a rack in the middle of the oven and preheat the oven to 350°F. Line a baking sheet with parchment paper.

In a large bowl, whisk together the buckwheat flour, almond flour, baking soda, and baking powder. Set aside.

In a medium bowl, whisk the flax egg. Whisk in the maple syrup, coconut oil, vanilla, and vinegar to combine.

Make a well in the center of the dry mixture and pour in the wet mixture. Use a silicone spatula to mix until just smooth.

Use a spoon or your hands to portion the dough into 1½-tablespoon balls and arrange them on the prepared baking sheet about 2 inches apart. Make an indentation with your thumb in the center of each cookie and fill it with jam (full but not overflowing).

Bake the cookies until slightly golden around the edges, 15 to 20 minutes. Let them cool on the baking sheet for 10 minutes, then transfer to a wire rack to cool completely.

Store in a sealed container at room temperature for up to 1 week.

BISCOFF CHOCOLATE COOKIES

MAKES *about 10 large cookies*
TOTAL TIME: *30 minutes*

- 10 teaspoons Biscoff cookie butter
- ¾ cup turbinado sugar
- 8 tablespoons (1 stick/4 ounces) unsalted vegan butter
- 3 tablespoons plain unsweetened vegan milk
- 1 teaspoon vanilla extract
- 1 cup all-purpose flour
- 2 tablespoons cornstarch
- ½ teaspoon baking soda
- ⅓ cup semisweet chocolate chips (about 2 ounces)
- Ice cream or milk, for serving

Preheat the oven to 350°F. Line a baking sheet with parchment paper.

Recipes Continue

Using a teaspoon measure and your hands, roll the cookie butter into little balls. Place the balls on the prepared baking sheet and freeze while you make the dough.

In a large bowl, using a hand mixer, cream together the sugar, butter, milk, and vanilla until completely smooth, about 4 minutes. (Alternatively, you could do this in a stand mixer fitted with the paddle.)

In a medium bowl, whisk together the flour, cornstarch, and baking soda. Add the flour mixture to the sugar-butter mixture and beat on medium speed until well combined and smooth. Fold in the chocolate chips with a silicone spatula or wooden spoon.

Use a tablespoon measure to scoop a portion of the dough. Flatten it a bit, then place a ball of cookie butter on the dough, followed by another tablespoon of cookie dough. Wrap the dough around the cookie butter and use your hands to roll it into a larger ball. Place it on the baking sheet and repeat with the remaining dough and cookie butter balls.

Arrange the dough balls evenly on the baking sheet about 1 inch apart. Bake until golden brown, 12 to 13 minutes.

Serve warm with ice cream or milk.

Store the leftovers in a sealed container at room temperature for up to 1 week.

OATMEAL RAISIN COOKIES

MAKES *8 to 12 large cookies*
TOTAL TIME: *35 minutes*

2 sticks (8 ounces) cold unsalted vegan butter, diced

1 packed cup light brown sugar

1 flax egg (1 tablespoon flaxmeal mixed with 3 tablespoons water)

2 cups all-purpose or gluten-free flour

1 cup rolled oats

1 cup raisins

½ cup walnuts

1 teaspoon ground cinnamon

¾ teaspoon baking soda

½ teaspoon baking powder

½ teaspoon sea salt

In a large bowl, using a hand mixer, beat together the butter and sugar until light and fluffy, about 4 minutes. (Alternatively, you could use a stand mixer fitted with the paddle, or a fork will also work!) Add the flax egg and beat again until combined.

Using a silicone spatula or wooden spoon, stir in the flour, oats, raisins, walnuts, cinnamon, baking soda, baking powder, and salt until combined. Chill the dough in the refrigerator for 10 to 15 minutes.

Preheat the oven to 400°F. Line two baking sheets with parchment paper.

Divide the dough into 8 to 12 portions and roll the dough into balls with your hands. Arrange the dough balls on the prepared baking sheets with at least 2 inches between them. Lightly press on each dough ball to flatten slightly.

Bake until the tops are golden brown, 10 to 12 minutes. Transfer the cookies to a cooling rack and let them rest for at least 10 to 15 minutes before eating.

Store any leftovers in a sealed container at room temperature for up to 1 week.

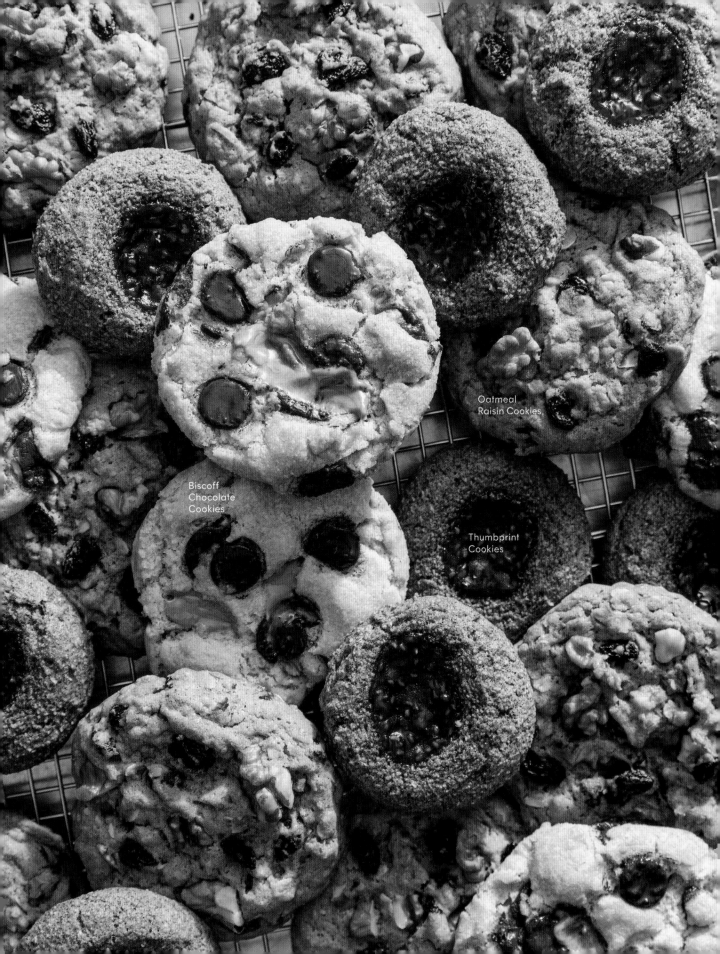

Oatmeal
Raisin Cookies

Biscoff
Chocolate
Cookies

Thumbprint
Cookies

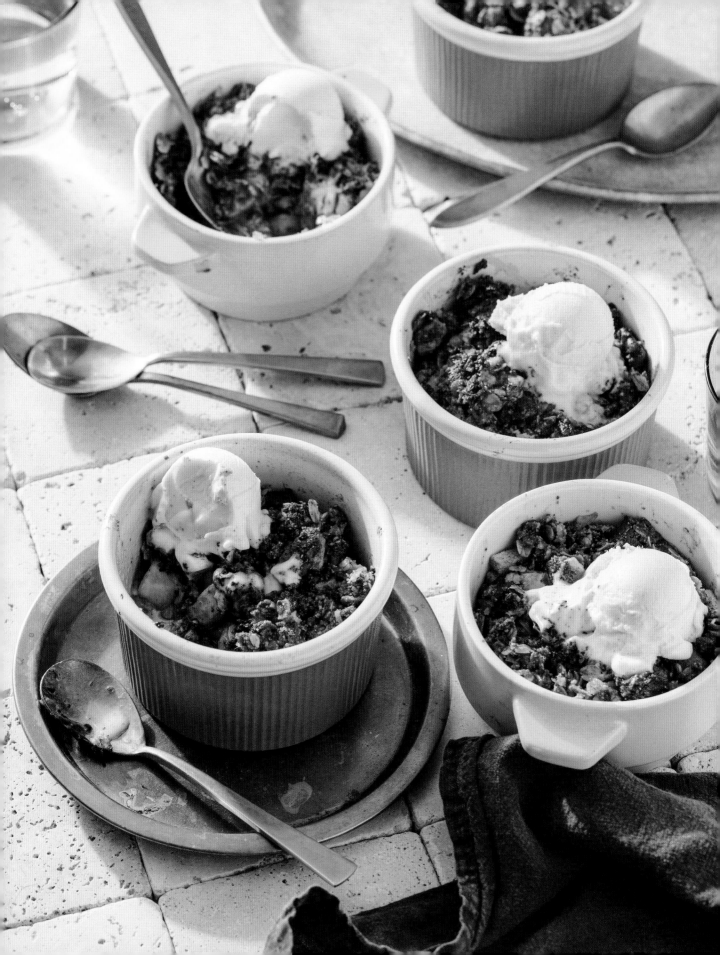

DIDI'S PEAR AND CHOCOLATE CRUMBLE

Didi is the queen of crumbles, and actually the queen of making really yummy, quick desserts in general, especially on the nights my family spontaneously comes together to have dinner. There are some people (cough cough . . . my husband . . .) who believe that once you add a fruit to a dessert, it can no longer be classified as such. But while I respect everyone's opinions about what they find satisfying and delicious . . . I can't help but feel like I can maybe prove this wrong? And if there were ever a recipe to make a believer of the doubters, it would be this one. The pears submit into pudding-like, caramelized richness while they bake, which is the perfect contrast for a crunchy, chocolatey crumble topping and basically begs for a big scoop of ice cream. And if that *still* doesn't do anything for you, then there's always Chocolate Mud Pie (page 273).

SERVES *4 to 6*
TOTAL TIME: *1 hour 5 minutes*

- 5 pears (such as Bosc, Bartlett, or Anjou), peeled, cored, and cut into ¼-inch dice
- ⅓ cup maple syrup
- 2 tablespoons cornstarch
- 2 tablespoons fresh lemon juice
- 1½ teaspoons ground cinnamon
- ½ teaspoon ground ginger
- 1 cup old-fashioned oats
- ½ cup almond flour
- ½ cup walnuts or pecans
- ½ cup chopped dark chocolate (2.8 ounces)
- ⅓ cup coconut sugar
- 3 tablespoons unsalted vegan butter
- 3 tablespoons plain vegan yogurt
- ¼ teaspoon sea salt
- Vegan vanilla ice cream, store-bought custard, or Sweet Cashew Cream (page 263), for serving (optional)

Preheat the oven to 350°F.

In a large bowl, gently toss together the pears, maple syrup, cornstarch, lemon juice, cinnamon, and ginger. Set aside.

In another large bowl, combine the oats, almond flour, nuts, chocolate, sugar, butter, yogurt, and salt. Use your hands to rub the butter into the mixture until the texture is sandy. Don't worry if you have some unmixed bits.

Dividing evenly, fill four 8-ounce or six 5-ounce ramekins (or a 1½- to 2-quart baking dish) with the pear filling. Dollop spoonfuls of the chocolate-oat topping on top, distributing it evenly.

Bake until golden brown and bubbling on top, 30 to 35 minutes for the ramekins or 45 to 50 minutes for the larger dish. Let the crumble rest for a good 10 minutes before serving.

Serve warm. If desired, top with ice cream, custard, or sweet cream.

Leftovers can be stored in a sealed container in the refrigerator for up to 3 days.

BAKLAVA CHEESECAKE

Need I even say anything more to convince you that you will fall in love with this creamy, dreamy dessert? I shan't, as no words will do it justice. Except maybe to tell you that this makes for an extremely memorable treat. And it's so easy: just a flaky phyllo base topped with a crushed buttery cookie layer, followed by a baklava topping, then finished off with a cheesecake filling. That's it. Nothing else to add. Okay, *maybe* a drizzle of cashew cream . . .

SERVES *8*

TOTAL TIME: *1 hour 30 minutes, plus soaking and setting time*

PHYLLO AND COOKIE CRUST

- Softened vegan butter for the pan
- 7 ounces graham crackers, vanilla cookies, or another crunchy cookie
- 2 tablespoons unsalted vegan butter, melted
- 10 sheets phyllo (see Notes)

NUT CRUMBLE

- 2 cups walnuts
- ½ cup pistachios
- Grated zest of 1 orange
- 1 teaspoon ground cinnamon
- ½ cup agave nectar or vegan honey

CHEESECAKE FILLING

- 1 cup cashews, soaked for 30 minutes and drained
- ¾ cup coconut cream (see Notes)
- 6 ounces plain vegan cream cheese
- ¼ cup maple syrup or agave nectar
- ¼ cup fresh lemon juice (about 2 lemons)
- 1 tablespoon cornstarch

FOR SERVING

- Sweet Cashew Cream (page 263), made loose enough to drizzle, for serving

MAKE THE PHYLLO AND COOKIE CRUST: Preheat the oven to 350°F. Lightly butter the bottom and sides of an 8-inch springform pan.

In a food processor, combine the cookies and melted butter and pulse until the mixture looks like wet sand.

Working quickly so the phyllo doesn't dry out, layer the phyllo sheets all along the sides and bottom of the pan, covering the whole pan. Press the cookie crumb mixture on top of the phyllo. Set aside while you make the nut crumble.

MAKE THE NUT CRUMBLE: In a food processor, combine the walnuts, pistachio, orange zest, and cinnamon and pulse until roughly ground. Add the agave and pulse again to combine.

Dollop about half of the nut mixture over the crust and set the remainder aside until serving time.

MAKE THE CHEESECAKE FILLING: In a high-powered blender, combine the cashews, coconut cream, cream cheese, maple syrup, lemon juice, and cornstarch and blend until completely smooth. Taste and adjust the flavors as you like, adding more lemon juice for tang or maple syrup for sweetness.

Pour the filling over the nut mixture. Give the pan a good tap on the counter to remove any air bubbles. Bake until the edges of the cheesecake start browning and come away from the sides, 45 minutes to 1 hour. The center should still be a little jiggly but not wet.

Let the cheesecake cool for about 15 minutes at room temperature. Cover and transfer the cake to the fridge for at least 5 hours, but ideally overnight.

Dollop the top of the cheesecake with the reserved nut crumble. Slice and serve with a drizzle of cream.

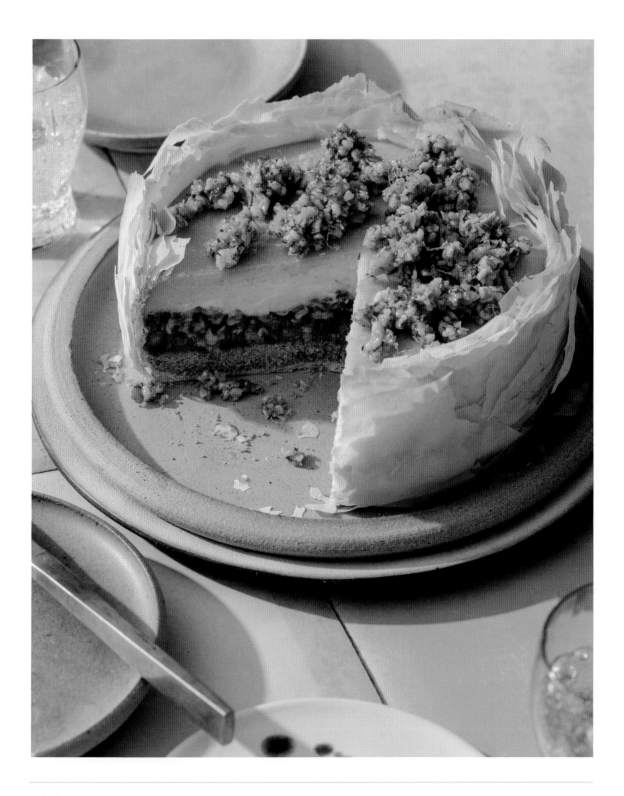

NOTE   You could also make this cheesecake without the phyllo layer. You would just start by pressing the cookie layer into the pan without buttering it first. You can either buy a can of coconut cream or you can refrigerate coconut milk for 30 minutes and skim off the thick cream at the top. Thai coconut milk is perfect for this as it tends to be creamier.

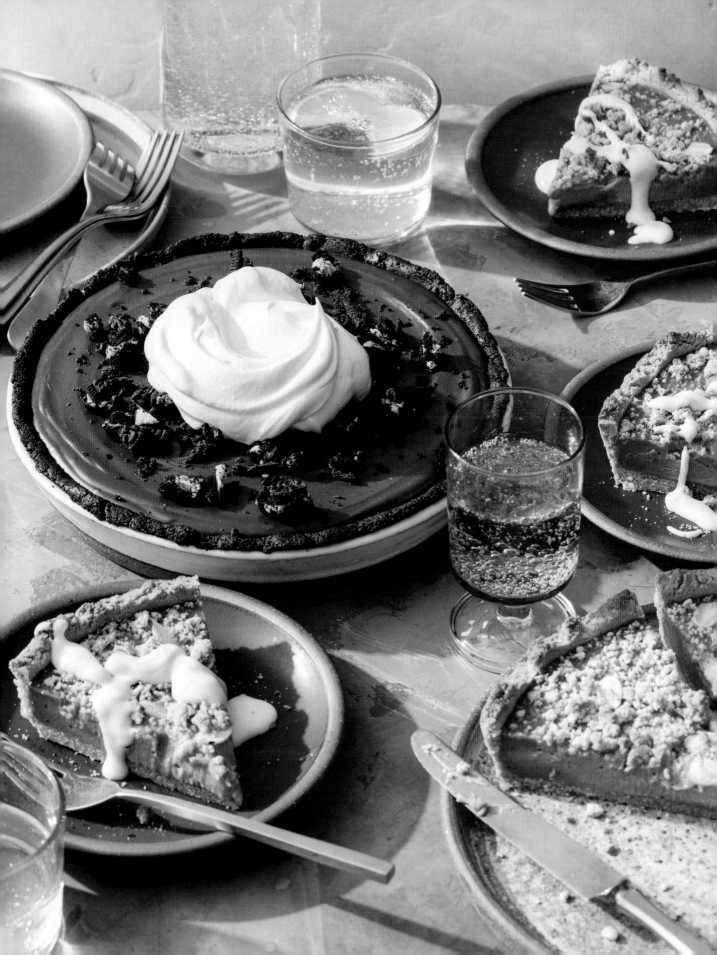

CHOCOLATE MUD PIE

I see you, chocolate lovers. Don't worry—I wouldn't dream of writing a dessert chapter without giving you the creamiest, silkiest, cheekiest chocolate dessert you could possibly imagine. This beauty has a rich chocolate cookie base plus mousse-y chocolate filling that gets its luxurious texture from silken tofu.

SERVES *6 to 8*
TOTAL TIME: *20 minutes*

CRUST

- 11 ounces crisp chocolate cookies of choice, homemade or store-bought, such as Simple Mills Dark Chocolate cookies or Oreos
- 4 tablespoons (2 ounces) unsalted vegan butter or coconut oil, melted (omit if using Oreos)

FILLING

- 12 ounces semisweet chocolate
- 16 ounces silken tofu
- 1 cup canned coconut cream
- ½ cup unsweetened cashew butter (optional)
- ¼ cup maple syrup
- Sweet Cashew Cream (page 263), for serving

MAKE THE CRUST: In a food processor, pulse the cookies until they're sandy in texture. Add the melted butter and pulse until finely crumbled. (It will look a bit like soil.) Measure out a few tablespoons to use for decorating the pie and set aside.

Transfer the remaining crumb mixture to an 8-inch pie plate and use your hand to press the mixture into the bottom and up the sides of the dish. Transfer the crust to the refrigerator to chill while you make the filling.

MAKE THE FILLING: Add 2 inches of water to a medium saucepan and bring to a simmer over high heat. Set a heatproof bowl over the pan, making sure it is not touching the water. Add the chocolate to the bowl and allow it to melt completely, stirring occasionally, about 5 minutes. Carefully remove the bowl from the pan (oven mitts recommended here and watch the steam!), set aside, and remove the pan from the heat.

In a high-powered blender, combine the tofu, coconut cream, cashew butter (if using), and maple syrup. With the blender running, add the melted chocolate and continue blending until the mixture is super smooth and creamy.

Pour the chocolate mixture into the chilled crust and sprinkle the reserved cookie mixture on top. Chill the pie for at least 1 hour, or ideally overnight, until firmly set.

Serve chilled with a generous amount of the sweet cashew or coconut cashew cream.

PECAN UPSIDE DOWN CAKE

The minute I feel the tiniest bit of chill in the air, I know I'm going to need a few things STAT: snuggly socks, cozy sweaters, and a whole lotta baked treats. I came up with this recipe when daydreaming about how everyone needs a gooey, caramelly, moist, fluffy pecan pie they can enjoy come holiday time. Consider this my heartfelt gift to you!

SERVES *6 to 8*

TOTAL TIME: *45 minutes*

PECAN TOPPING

- 1 cup pecans
- 4 tablespoons unsalted vegan butter
- ½ packed cup light brown sugar

CAKE

- 1½ cups all-purpose flour, sifted
- ½ packed cup light brown sugar
- 1 teaspoon baking powder
- ½ teaspoon baking soda
- 1 cup plain unsweetened oat milk
- 8 tablespoons (1 stick/4 ounces) unsalted vegan butter, melted
- 1 tablespoon apple cider vinegar
- ½ teaspoon vanilla extract

FOR SERVING

- Sweet Cashew Cream (optional; page 263), for serving

Preheat the oven to 350°F. Line an 8-inch square baking dish with parchment paper.

MAKE THE PECAN TOPPING: Spread the pecans over the bottom of the prepared baking dish. In a medium saucepan, melt the butter over low heat. Add the brown sugar and cook, stirring, until the mixture is syrupy, 2 to 4 minutes. Drizzle the syrup over the pecans and give everything a toss to coat well. Set aside.

MAKE THE CAKE: In a large bowl, whisk together the flour, brown sugar, baking powder, and baking soda. In a medium bowl, whisk together the oat milk, melted butter, vinegar, and vanilla until smooth. Add the milk mixture to the flour mixture and gently whisk until smooth. Pour the batter over the pecan layer in the baking dish.

Bake until the cake is fragrant and a cake tester or knife comes out clean, about 30 minutes.

Let the cake cool in the baking dish for a few minutes. Place a plate over the baking dish and, using a kitchen towel or oven mitts to protect your hands, grab the baking dish and plate and flip to invert the cake.

Carefully peel off and discard the parchment paper. If some pecans come off, simply stick them back on.

Serve hot or at room temperature. If desired, serve cream on the side.

Leftovers can be stored in an airtight container for up to 3 days.

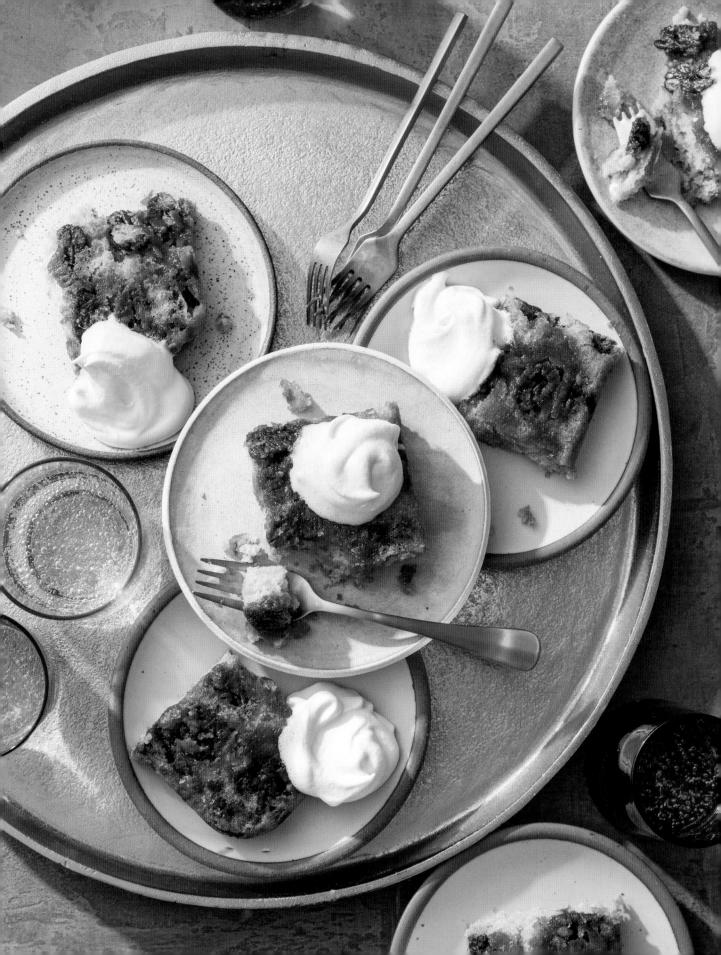

UMM ALI

Behold your new favorite dessert: an Egyptian bread pudding scented with cinnamon and studded with raisins, walnuts, pistachios, and coconut. And to make it even more luxurious, I've swapped day-old bread out for buttery, flaky vegan croissants (which you can handily buy from the store and pop into the oven before you assemble everything). It's the kind of dish that you want to dive into headfirst, and I'm not going to be the one to stop you.

SERVES 6
TOTAL TIME: *35 minutes*

6 plain vegan croissants

3 cups plain unsweetened oat milk

½ cup unsweetened oat or vegan cream

¼ packed cup light brown sugar, plus more for sprinkling

1 teaspoon ground cinnamon

1 cup vegan whipping cream

½ cup unsweetened shredded coconut

¼ cup raisins

¼ cup walnuts, toasted in a dry pan until fragrant

¼ cup pistachios, toasted in a dry pan until fragrant

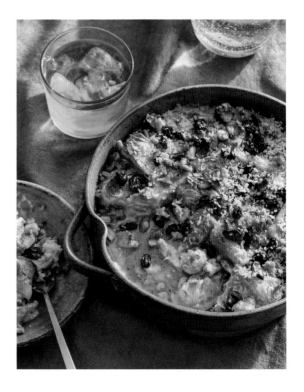

Bake the croissants according to the package directions.

Cut the croissants into 1½-inch pieces and arrange them in a broilerproof 9 × 11-inch baking dish. Set aside.

In a medium saucepan, combine the milk, cream, brown sugar, and cinnamon. Cook over medium heat, stirring, until warmed through and the sugar has dissolved, about 5 minutes. Remove the pan from the heat and set aside.

Preheat the broiler on high.

In a medium bowl, using a whisk or hand mixer (or in a stand mixer fitted with the whisk), whip the cream until medium peaks form. Set aside.

Sprinkle the coconut, raisins, and both nuts over the croissant pieces. Pour the sweet milk mixture evenly over the croissants. Spoon the whipped cream over everything and smooth the top. Sprinkle the top generously with brown sugar.

Slide the dish under the broiler until the sugar has melted and caramelized, about 5 minutes. Be sure to check frequently to ensure that the sugar doesn't burn. Serve immediately.

Leftovers can be stored in a sealed container in the refrigerator for up to 3 days.

TRIPLE-CHOCOLATE BROWNIE BLACK FOREST CELEBRATION CAKE

I love all my sister's baking, but this recipe of hers is the one to beat. Black forest may just be my dream cake, with its mixture of juicy sweet cherries and rich dark chocolate plus an indulgent ganache that gets drizzled over the top. (It also just so happens to be gluten- and refined sugar–free, though you'd never guess from the look or taste of it.) To serve it is to celebrate, no matter how ordinary the occasion. And while it can be a labor of love to assemble, just remember my sister's words: *This cake is all about joy over perfection.*

MAKES *one 8-inch triple-layer cake*
TOTAL TIME: *2 hours 45 minutes*

BROWNIE CAKE

Olive oil cooking spray or avocado oil

10 Medjool dates, pitted

¼ cup maple syrup

2 tablespoons plain unsweetened vegan milk

1 tablespoon unsalted vegan butter, melted

1 teaspoon vanilla extract

1 tablespoon ground chia seeds

½ cup sorghum flour

¼ cup plus 1 tablespoon raw cacao powder

¼ cup coconut sugar

1 tablespoon carob powder (or an extra tablespoon cacao powder)

1 teaspoon maca root powder

½ teaspoon baking soda

Pinch of sea salt

¼ cup finely chopped dark chocolate (about 1½ ounces)

WHIPPED CREAM

2 cups cold coconut whipping cream

½ teaspoon cornstarch

1 teaspoon plain unsweetened vegan milk

3 tablespoons maple syrup

1 teaspoon vanilla extract

Pinch of sea salt

DARK CHERRY COMPOTE

3 cups frozen pitted black cherries, thawed

2 tablespoons maple syrup

1 tablespoon chia seeds

CHOCOLATE GANACHE

1 cup raw cacao powder or cocoa powder

¾ cup maple syrup

¾ cup plain unsweetened oat milk

1 tablespoon unsweetened cashew butter (optional)

1 teaspoon vanilla extract

ASSEMBLY

Dark chocolate shavings, for garnish

MAKE THE CAKE: Preheat the oven to 350°F. Mist an 8-inch cake pan with cooking spray (see Note).

In a high-powered blender, combine the dates and ½ cup water and blend until smooth.

Transfer the date puree to a large bowl and whisk in the maple syrup, milk, melted butter, and vanilla. Stir in the chia seeds and let sit for 10 minutes to let the batter thicken.

In another large bowl, whisk together the sorghum flour, cacao powder, sugar, carob powder, maca powder, baking soda, and salt. Add the dry mixture to the date-chia mixture and mix well to combine. Fold in the chopped chocolate. Pour the cake batter into the prepared pan.

Bake until the cake feels fairly firm when you press lightly on the top or a cake tester or toothpick inserted in the center comes out clean, about 20 minutes. Let the cake cool in the pan for at least 15 minutes. Gently invert the cake onto a cooling rack to cool completely. The cake will firm up as it cools.

Recipe Continues

Repeat the process (see Note), making two more batches of batter and baking two more layers for a total of three.

MAKE THE WHIPPED CREAM: In a stand mixer fitted with the whisk (or in a large bowl with a hand mixer or whisk), whip the coconut cream to soft, fluffy peaks.

In a medium bowl, whisk together the cornstarch and milk until smooth. Whisk in the maple syrup, vanilla, and salt to combine. Add the mixture to the cream and whip to medium-firm peaks. Cover the bowl and refrigerate the whipped cream until you're ready to assemble the cake.

MAKE THE DARK CHERRY COMPOTE: In a medium saucepan, combine the cherries, maple syrup, ¼ cup water, and the chia seeds. Stir and bring the mixture to a simmer over medium heat. Cook, stirring occasionally, until the cherries have softened and the liquid is slightly thickened, 10 to 12 minutes.

Remove the pan from the heat and let the compote cool completely—it will thicken as it cools. Transfer to a sealed container and refrigerate until you're ready to assemble the cake.

MAKE THE CHOCOLATE GANACHE: In a medium saucepan, whisk together the cacao powder, maple syrup, oat milk, cashew butter (if using), and vanilla. Bring the mixture to a simmer over medium-low heat and cook, whisking occasionally, until thickened, 3 to 5 minutes. Remove the pan from the heat.

Transfer the ganache to a jar and let cool completely at room temperature, then refrigerate until you're ready to assemble the cake.

ASSEMBLE THE CAKE: Place a cake layer on a cake board or plate and top with 3 large dollops of the ganache. Spread the ganache outward from the center of the cake, bringing it all the way to the edge.

Top the ganache with 3 large dollops of whipped cream. Spread it outward from the center of the cake, leaving a ¼-inch border around the outside edge.

Add a thin layer of compote on top of the whipped cream, again leaving a ¼-inch border around the outside edge.

Repeat with the remaining cake layers so you end up with 3 layers of cake finished with ganache, whipped cream, and cherry compote on top. Garnish the cake with any leftover ganache and some dark chocolate shavings.

Leftovers can be stored in a sealed container in the refrigerator for up to 5 days.

NOTE   The cake batter is enough for just one 8-inch cake, so to make a triple layer cake, you will need to repeat the process three times. I know this seems a little fussy, but it ensures that you don't need to purchase more cake pans than you already have, as well as that the cake will turn out perfectly every time. To help the cake-building process go more quickly, you could make the compote and ganache ahead of time and store them in the refrigerator for up to 2 days.

VARIATION   *Brownie Black Forest Sundae:* For a fun twist, make all the components, then break up the cake pieces and layer on the ganache, whipped cream, and compote. Top with your favorite ice cream and dive in.

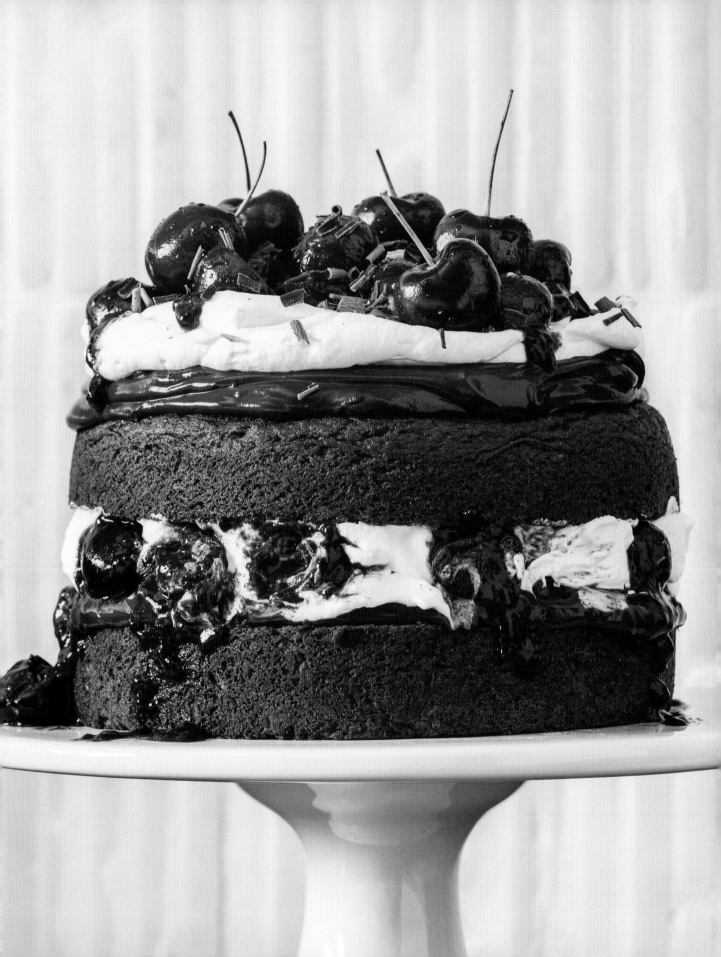

Appendix: SPICE UP YOUR LIFE

Spice/Herb	Health Benefits	Taste	Contraindications	Best Way to Use
Ajwain	• Alleviates gas, bloating, and indigestion • Stimulates appetite • Helps regulate cholesterol and blood pressure	Slightly bitter, herbal taste with notes of oregano, celery seed, and a hint of anise.		Can be used as whole seeds or ground.
Asafoetida	• Aids digestion • Relieves gas and bloating • Fights viral infection • Nourishes nervous tissue • Improves circulation • Supports ovulation	Similar to onions or leeks with a more floral character. Very strong and pungent smell in its raw form.	Avoid using large quantities during pregnancy or breastfeeding as it stimulates the uterus.	Cook in fat before enjoying. Use in small amounts owing to pungency.
Basil	• Reduces mucus, phlegm, and congestion • Helps release toxins through sweat	A balance between sweet and savory, with hints of mint, anise, and pepper.		Best added near the end of cooking or sprinkled on top of a finished dish to maintain its flavor. But if added during cooking, you will still get a lingering subtle taste.
Bay leaf	• Clears sinuses • Moves fluid in the body • Regulates blood sugar • Removes toxins from intestines • Soothes IBS • Reduces stress hormones in the body	Subtle hints of black pepper and pine.		Can be used fresh or dried.
Black pepper	• Stimulates the production of digestive juice • Stokes the appetite • Improves circulation • Antibacterial • Antioxidant • Feeds the skin • Aids weight loss and fertility in men • Prevents premature aging	A complex flavor with piney, woody, citrusy notes.	Avoid large amounts if you get acid reflux or too much heat in the body.	Can be infused into dishes whole or used ground.
Caraway	• Alleviates acid reflux, menstrual cramps, and heartburn	Nutty, bittersweet flavor with hint of citrus and anise.		Can be used as whole seeds or ground.

Spice/Herb	Health Benefits	Taste	Contraindications	Best Way to Use
Cardamom	• Relieves nausea and morning sickness • Relaxes muscle tissue • Breaks up mucus • Opens pores for detoxification and cleansing • Cleanses the lymphatic system • Opens the airways to aid breathing	Herbal warmth, like a fragrant cross between eucalyptus, mint, and pepper—more citrusy than fennel and sweeter than cumin.		Whole pods can be used to infuse milks, teas, or dishes. Seeds can be ground.
Cinnamon	• Improves circulation in the lungs • Supports joint health • Elevates mood • Loosens lung mucus • Soothes the throat	Sweet and woody flavor with a slight citrusy note and a punch of spice.		Can be used ground or infused into dishes or drinks in whole form.
Cloves	• Supports dental hygiene, circulation, and metabolism • Alleviates toothache, gas, bloating, and nausea • Antibacterial	Intensely aromatic with a subtly sweet, warm flavor and a hint of astringency.		Can be used whole or ground.
Coriander/cilantro	• Calms the immune system • Cools the body (especially the liver) • Removes heavy metals from the body • Helps the body flush out toxins • Encourages movement of fluid in the body	Cilantro leaves are refreshing, tart, and citrusy. Coriander seeds are the plant's dried fruit. Its flavor is earthy, tart, and sweet, with a floral aroma that releases when toasted.	To some, cilantro tastes like soap. Crushing the leaves releases enzymes that break down aldehydes and destroys the "soapy" or "buggy" taste that some people experience.	Coriander seeds can be used whole or ground. Toasting or sautéing in fat helps release their aroma. Heat diminishes the flavor of fresh cilantro quickly; it is best used as a raw garnish.
Cumin	• Aids digestion • Stimulates blood flow to digestive organs • Purifies the blood • Flushes out toxins • Supports metabolism	Rich and hearty, slightly peppery, earthy, and warm, with an edge of citrus.		Cook in fat before using. Roast the seeds in a dry pan to release the oils before grinding.

Spice/Herb	Health Benefits	Taste	Contraindications	Best Way to Use
Curry leaves	• Antioxidant, antimicrobial, and anticarcinogenic • Encourages hair growth • Prevents premature graying • Protects the liver from oxidative damage • Regulates blood glucose levels	Flavor similar to basil, Thai lime leaves, and lemongrass.		Can be used fresh or dried.
Dill	• Blood and liver cleanser • Diuretic • Reduces gas • Increases milk production in lactating mothers	Like a gentler version of caraway.		Can be used fresh or dried.
Fennel	• Stimulates appetite • Primes digestion • Increases flow of milk in lactating mothers • Freshens the breath	Anise-like with a warm, sweet aroma.	Avoid in large quantities and in tea during pregnancy.	Can be enjoyed whole or ground. Chew the seeds before or after meals, add as a powder to meals or drinks.
Fenugreek	• Supports lactation, healthy bowel movements, stable blood glucose, and hair growth	Tangy and bitter but imparts a sweet, slightly nutty, maple syrup-like flavor when cooked.	Avoid in large quantities during pregnancy.	Can be used as whole seeds or ground.
Ginger	• Whets the appetite • Stokes the digestive fire • Improves assimilation and transportation of nutrients in the body • Clears microcirculatory channels • Alleviates motion or air sickness • Supports joint health	Earthy, peppery, and sweet with a pungent and spicy aroma.	Ginger increases heat in the body, so large quantities can cause heartburn.	Can be enjoyed fresh or dried and ground.
Kalonji/Nigella	• Reduces inflammation • Strengthens hair and fingernails • Balances blood sugar • Supports liver function • Supports kidney function	Slightly bitter with some of the pungency of onion. Strong aroma and a flavor profile that has notes of onion, oregano, and black pepper.	Large quantities can decrease blood pressure and blood glucose levels.	Cook in fat before using. Roast the seeds in a dry pan to release the oils before grinding.

Spice/Herb	Health Benefits	Taste	Contraindications	Best Way to Use
Mustard seeds	• Improves circulation • Breaks up mucus • Clears sinuses	Spicy, pungent, slightly bitter, sharp.	Avoid in large quantities if you get acid reflux or too much heat in your body. Avoid large quantities during pregnancy.	
Nutmeg	• Natural sedative, anti-inflammatory • Relieves insomnia, sore throats, bloating, and abdominal pain • Boosts immunity and blood circulation	Warm, nutty, slightly sweet.		Use in its whole form to grate into savory dishes, desserts, or drinks. Buy preground (less potent).
Oregano	• Antibacterial and anti-inflammatory • Boosts immunity and digestion	Earthy, "green" flavor with hints of mint and hay.		Can be used fresh or dried.
Paprika	• Antioxidant • Relieves gas • Boosts immunity • Prevents premature wrinkles • Increases circulation • Brings healthy color to skin	Domestic paprika is mild and sweet. Spanish paprikas can be smoky.		Found in powdered form and can be used to season dishes.
Saffron	• Helps with mood regulation, blood glucose stabilization, and inflammation • Reduces fevers • Cleanses the skin	Sweet, floral, and earthy.		
Star anise	• Supports digestion, lactation, and reproductive health • Alleviates gas, bloating, and mucus • Anti-inflammatory	Licorice-like, slightly sweet flavor.		Used as whole pods.
Turmeric	• Supports liver function • Stimulates digestion • Boosts immunity • Antiseptic • Antiviral • Purifies the blood • Protects against allergies • Improves skin luminosity	Overwhelmingly earthy and bitter, almost musky, with a bit of peppery spice.		Combine with black pepper for optimal digestion. Ideally cook in fat before eating.

Index